Volume 1

Practical Manual & Logbook in Community Medicine

(Based on Latest CBME)

(Includes Family Adoption Programme)

Revised and Updated

Authors

Dr. Priya Arora
Professor, Community Medicine
Army College of Medical Sciences
New Delhi

Dr. Pooja Goyal
Professor & Head, Community Medicine
ESIC Medical College and Hospital
Faridabad, Haryana

Dr. Shveta Lukhmana
Associate Professor, Community Medicine
VMMC and Safdarjung Hospital
New Delhi

Dr. Abhishek Singh
Associate Professor, Community Medicine
SHKM Government Medical College
Mewat, Haryana

Foreword By

- Col. (Dr) Puja Dudeja
- Dr. Abhishek V. Raut
- Dr. Prasanna Mithra P.
- Dr. Avijit Roy

Peepee Publishers and Distributors Private Limited®

Practical Manual & Logbook in Community Medicine (Based on Latest CBME)

Published by
Pawaninder P. Vij and Anupam Vij

Peepee Publishers and Distributors (P) Ltd.
Head Office: 160, Shakti Vihar, Pitam Pura, Delhi-110 034 (India)

Correspondence Address:
7/31, First Floor, Ansari Road, Daryaganj
New Delhi-110 002 (India)
Ph: 41512412, 9811156083
e-mail: peepee160@yahoo.co.in
e-mail: peepee160@gmail.com
www.peepeepub.com
join us on facebook.com/pp.publishers

LM-03

First Edition: 2022

Revised and Updated: 2025

ISBN: 978-81-9651-878-3

Foreword

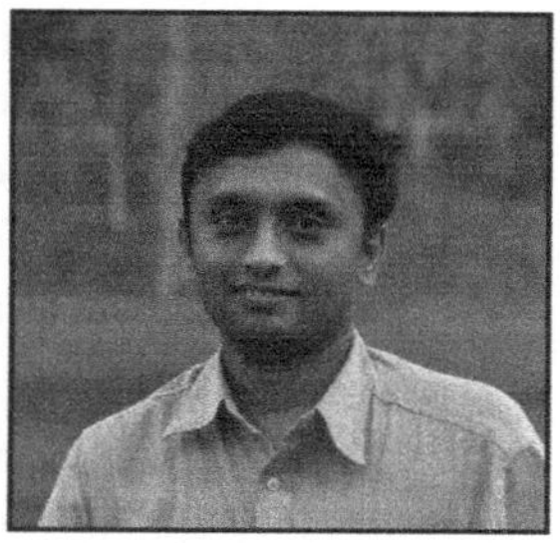

It is indeed a pleasure to pen down the foreword for this Practical Manual and Logbook in Community Medicine. This book has been written in alignment with the newer Competency Based Medical Education (CBME) guidelines for the subject of Community Medicine. It is heartening to see that the book is striving to catalyze *'contextual'* learning through linkage with the field practice area. The cross-cutting competencies that the students will be able to build in topics like epidemiology, biostatistics, dietary and nutritional assessment should serve them good as future professionals irrespective of the discipline of their post-graduation. The example-based approach for clinic-social cases that the book has adopted should facilitate in-depth learning of students. The specimen case scenarios for case-based learning may act as a stimulus for some of the learners to innovate and try these active learning methods. The book has made a conscious attempt to try and touch base on delineated topics and competencies for Community Medicine including exposure field visits, self-directed learning, AETCOM modules among others.

Considering the comprehensive nature of the book and the deliberate effort that has gone into making it practical and competency oriented, I am sure that this book will pave the way for the students to learn the nuances in the discipline of Community Medicine in an *experiential* and *authentic* manner.

I congratulate the authors for coming out with something like this and with them all the very best for this and their future endeavors!!!

Abhishek V. Raut
MD, DNB
Professor, Department of Community Medicine
Mahatma Gandhi Institute of Medical Sciences, Sevagram

Foreword

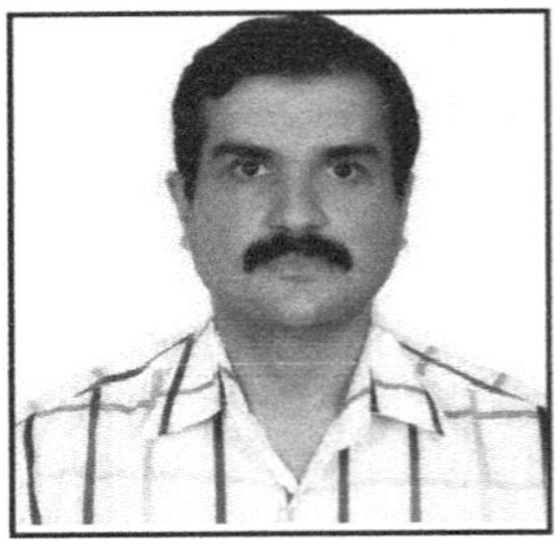

It gives me immense pleasure to pen down the foreword for this **Practical Manual and Logbook in Community Medicine**, which has been prepared keeping in mind the existing CBME guidelines and requirements. I have no doubt while I mention that this manual will prove to be a milestone in practical teaching of Community Medicine. Currently the requirements and guidelines of CBME are challenging for both the teacher and the medical student. To add on, the Covid-19 pandemic has paved the way for an enhanced level of challenges for community health professionals. Also, a medical graduate is expected to possess reasonable expertise in practical aspects related to Community Medicine; irrespective of the future journey into specialties.

Hence, considering all these points, this unique manual will definitely act as an aid to practical learning by medical students, streamline the ongoing teaching-learning process, while helping in suitable documentation of all the works done. In addition, the authors have taken the brunt of efforts in dividing the entire practical teaching into suitable, relevant topics and arrange the exercises according to competencies. This work also brings out the contrast with already available manuals in the market. I wish the authors all the very best for this endeavor and let this work come out with flying colors !!

Dr. Prasanna Mithra P.
MBBS, MD, DNB, FAGE
Associate Professor of Community Medicine
Kasturba Medical College, Mangalore
(Manipal Academy of Higher Education, Manipal)
Lighthouse Hill Road, Mangalore - 575001

Foreword

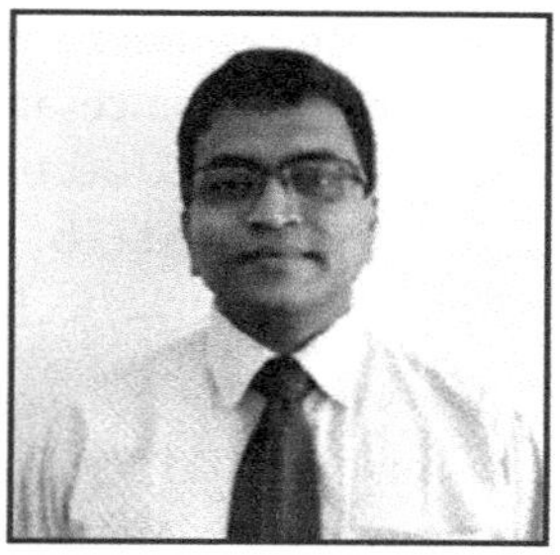

From the time of appearance of human beings we are trying our best for a healthy life-style for which we are trying to take control over the diseases and promote a healthy behavior which after a long struggle gave rise to the concept of health and that too was achieved by the integrated approach to health care through Community Medicine. Sanitary awakening lead to the birth of the concept of public health and started dated back in 1869 in India with the first Municipal Act passed on 1884 in Bengal.

The Community Medicine field is mainly concerned with the study of health and disease in the population of a defined community or group. Its main goal is to identify the health problems and needs of defined community diagnosis and to plan implement and evaluate the extent of which health measures effectively met this need.

The Community Medicine needs a practical approach and also involves record keeping along with better understanding of health seeking behavior of the people. The CBME based Practical Manual and Logbook in Community Medicine written by the authors is an exemplary example of CBME to serve the purpose of teaching Community Medicine. The authors have taken utmost care in delivering the clear concept of CBME and the Community Medicine as a subject and learning through practical approach.

If we want to achieve Health for All Community Medicine will definitely be the key factor during this era. Best wishes for the authors.

Dr. Avijit Roy
MD, MHA
Deputy Director (Health)
(Public Health Specialist Gr-I, CHS)
Andaman and Nicobar Administration
Office of the Deputy Director (Health)
Directorate of Health Services

Preface

In 2019, "Regulations on Graduate Medical Education (Amendment)" released by National Medical Commission came into existence and is applicable to the MBBS course from academic year 2019-20 onwards. Competency Based Medical Education (New Curriculum) mandates medical education to be learner centric, patient centric and outcome oriented. The epicenter of learning has shifted from cognitive approach to inclusive learning that focuses on psychomotor, affective and communication domains as well.

As per the new curriculum, transformation in the methodology of teaching has also been recommended, wherein only 30% of teaching hours should comprise lectures and rest should be interactive learning including small group discussions, self directed learning, case based learning and other interactive teaching learning methods. Structured guidelines for attitude, ethics and communication have been developed that need to be included in the teaching curriculum.

Implementation of competency based undergraduate curriculum for the Indian medical graduate is a big challenge. To attain a competency, there must be a perfect alignment between learning objectives, teaching learning methods and assessment. This can be achieved by a meticulous upkeep of logs of skill-based training and documentation of students' performance through structured periodic (formative and summative) assessment.

Authors of the book felt the necessity of having a comprehensive, all-inclusive competency based manual in Community Medicine, that would not only provide in-depth conceptual and hands-on learning for the students but also facilitate the instructors in teaching, assessment and record keeping of the students' progress. Through this manual we have attempted to integrate newer concepts like pre-clinical exposure for first year, Case based and Self Directed Learning, AETCOM and Pandemic Management Module, alongside concise logbook and in-built assessment of all the competencies making it an all-inclusive single repository for skill-based training. In order to facilitate seamless implementation of practical training at undergraduate level, the book can be adapted by various institutions in accordance with their respective teaching schedules.

Developing such an extensive resource has not been easy and we extend a heartfelt gratitude to all those who have helped in this journey, especially the seniors, colleagues, families and friends who have supported in this endeavor. A special thanks to our publishers M/s Peepee Publishers and Distributors (P) Ltd.

Constructive criticism and suggestions for improvement are always welcome.

Dr. Priya Arora
Dr. Pooja Goyal
Dr. Shveta Lukhmana
Dr. Abhishek Singh

Contents

Volume 1

Section I: Pre-Clinical Exercise

Section II: Family Adoption Programme

Volume 2

Section IV: Epidemiology and Biostatistics

Section V: Visits to Institutions of Public Health Importance

Section VI: Spots

Volume 3

Section VII: Self Directed Learning (SDL)

Section VIII: Logbook

TIME DISTRIBUTION OF MBBS PROGRAMME AND EXAMINATION SCHEDULE

Academic calendar for admission batch 2024-2025												
	JAN	FEB	MAR	APR	MAY	JUN	JUL	AUG	SEP	OCT	NOV	DEC
Adm year										1 14 Oct	2	3
Phase 1 exam	4	5	6	7	8	9	10	11	12 Phase 1 exam, result	13 Phase 2 starts	14	15
Phase 2 exam	16	17	18	19	20	21	22	23	24 Phase 2 exam, result	25 Phase 3 part 1 starts	26	27
Phase 3 part 1 exam	28	29	30	31	32	33	34	35	36 Phase 3 Part 1 exam, result	37 Phase 3 part 2 starts	38	39
	40	41	42	43	44	45	46	47	48	49	50	51
Phase 3 part 1 exam	52	53	54 Proposed NExT step1	1 CRMI	2	3	4	5	6	7	8	9
Internship	10	11	12 Proposed NExT step2									

Legends:

CRMI-Compulsory rotating medical internship.

PROFESSIONAL-WISE TEACHING HOURS IN COMMUNITY MEDICINE

Professional	Lectures (hours)	Small Group Teaching / Tutorials / Integrated learning / Practical (hours)	Self directed learning (hours)	FAP	Total
First Prof	20	20	–	24	40+24
Second Prof	25	–	10	24	35+24
Third Prof (Part 1)	50	80	20	36	150+36

PANDEMIC MANAGEMENT MODULE

A. Learning Modules for Professional Year II

- Number of modules: 2
- Number of hours: 12

B. Learning Modules for Professional Year III Part I

- Number of modules: 3
- Number of hours: 18s

CLINICAL POSTINGS IN COMMUNITY MEDICINE

Period of training in weeks			Total weeks
II MBBS	III MBBS Part I	III MBBS Part II	
4	4	-	8

AETCOM

Paper I: Module 3.2: Case studies in bioethics—Disclosure of medical errors.

Paper II: Module 3.5: Case studies in bioethics—Fiduciary duty.

COMMUNITY MEDICINE ASSESSMENT

ASSESSMENT SCHEDULE AS PER NMC GUIDELINES

Phase	Minimum Number of Internal Assessment Tests (Summative Assessment)	Minimum Number of Clinical End of Posting Test (Theory and Practical)
I	1	-
II	2	1
III	2*	1

*One of these should be Prelim / Preuniversity Exam

UNIVERSITY EXAM–At the End of Phase III (Part 1)

Written Theory Total Marks – 200 (2 Papers)

Practicals / Orals/ Clinicals – 100 Marks

For passing, mandatory to get 40% marks separately in theory and practical; and total 50% for theory plus practical.

(Practical = practical / clinical + viva)

(Theory = theory papers only)

INTERNAL ASSESSMENT

50% combined in theory and practical (not less than 40% in each) for eligibility for appearing for University Examinations).

Internal assessment marks are not to be added to the marks of the University examination and should be shown separately in the grade card.

LIST OF CERTIFIABLE COMPETENCIES

Number	**COMPETENCY** **The student should be able to**	Domain K/S/A/C	Level K/KH/ SH/P	Core Y/N	Suggested Teaching learning methods	Suggested Assessment method	Number required to certify P
CM 2.1	Describe the steps and perform clinico socio-cultural and demographic assessment of the individual, family and community	S	SH	Y	LGT,SGT, DOAP FAP Clinical posting	Written/ Viva voce/ Skill assessment	5
CM 2.2	Describe the socio-cultural factors, family (types), its role in health and disease & demonstrate in a simulated environment the correct assessment of socio-economic status	S	SH	Y	LGT,SGT, DOAP FAP Clinical posting	Written/ Viva voce/ Skill assessment	5
CM 4.4	Conduct a health education session for community awareness in a simulated environment/FAP/ clinical posting	S	SH	Y	SGT, DOAP, FAP, Clinical posting	Written/ Viva voce/ Skill assessment /OSCE	1
CM 5.9	Perform nutritional assessment of individual, family and community using appropriate method and plan a diet for health promotion based on the assessment	S	SH	Y	LGT, SGT	Written/ Viva voce/ OSCE	5
CM 5.10	Recommend a dietary plan for a person with DM/ HTN/ Obesity in a simulated environment/FAP/ Clinical posting	S	SH	Y	LGT, SGT	Written/ Viva voce/ OSCE	5
CM 5.11	Plan a diet for an adult which meets the protein (macro nutrients) requirements as per latest RDA-NIN guidelines for vegetarian/ ovo-vegetarian/non-vegetarian	S	SH	Y	LGT, SGT	Written/ Viva voce/ OSCE	5
CM 5.12	Demonstrate different types of breastfeeding holds, latching, manual expression of breast milk using a baby model and breast model.	S	SH	Y	LGT, SGT	Written/ Viva voce/ OSCE	5
CM 5.13	Counsel a mother about complementary feeding for different age groups of the child covering the 8 dietary diversity food groups, quantity, frequency, consistency of the food.	S	SH	Y	LGT, SGT	Written/ Viva voce/ OSCE	5
CM 6.6	Perform descriptive statistics of a given data-set and interpret	S	SH	Y	LGT, SGT	Written/ Viva voce/ OSCE	5
CM 7.4	Define, calculate and interpret morbidity and mortality indicators based on given set of data	S	SH	Y	SGT,DOAP	Written/ Viva voce/ OSCE	5

Section I

Pre-Clinical Exercise

Section I: Pre-Clinical Exercise

	Topic	Competency	Signature of Supervisor with Date	Grade
1.	Concept of Health and Disease	CM 1.2 – Define health; describe the concept of holistic health including concept of spiritual health and the relativeness and determinants of health. CM 1.3 – Describe the characteristics of agent, host and environmental factors in health and disease and the multifactorial etiology of disease. CM 1.4 – Describe and discuss the natural history of disease. CM 1.5 – Describe the application of interventions at various levels of prevention CM 1.7 – Enumerate and describe health indicators. CM 17.3 – Describe primary health care, its components and principles.		
2.	Health Education	CM 1.6 – Describe and discuss the concepts, the principles of health promotion and education, IEC and Behavioral change communication (BCC). CM 4.1 – Describe various methods of health education with their advantages and limitations CM 4.2 – Describe the methods of organizing health promotion and education and counselling activities at individual, family and community settings		
3.	Air Pollution	CM 3.1 – Describe the health hazards of air, water, radiation and noise pollution. CM 3.2 – Describe concepts of safe and wholesome water, sanitary sources of water, water purification processes, water quality standards, concepts of water conservation and rainwater harvesting CM 3.3 – Describe the etiology and basis of water borne diseases/ jaundice, Hepatitis/ diarrheal diseases PA 12.1 – Enumerate and describe the pathogenesis of disorders caused by air pollution, tobacco and alcohol.		

4.	Demography	CM 1.8 – Describe the demographic profile of India and discuss its impact on health. CM 9.1 – Define and describe the principles of demography, demographic cycle, vital statistics. CM 9.4 – Enumerate and describe the consequences of population explosion and population dynamics of India. CM 9.7 – Enumerate the sources of vital statistics including census, SRS, NFHS, NSSO etc.		
5.	Vectors of Public Health Importance	CM 3.6 – Describe the role of vectors in the causation of diseases. Also discuss national vector borne disease control program. CM 3.7 – Identify and describe the identifying features and life cycles of vectors of Public health importance and their control measures		
6.	Biomedical Waste Management	CM 14.1 – Define and classify hospital waste. CM 14.2 – Describe various methods of treatment of hospital waste. CM 14.3 – Describe laws related to hospital waste management.		
7.	Nutrition and Health	CM 5.1 – Describe the common sources of various nutrient and special nutritional requirements according to age, sex, activity, physiological conditions. CM 5.3 – Define and describe common nutrition related health disorders (including macro-PEM, micro-iron, Zn, iodine, Vitamin A), their control and management.		
Hints and Answers to Exercises				

Objective of the Pre-Clinical Exercises

The overall objective is to impart requisite knowledge to the medical student about factors related to health care delivery, health promotion and disease prevention. This knowledge shall empower the student to acquire skills to demonstrate the same in the subsequent semesters.

The specific learning objectives are: At the end of Phase 1, student should be able to:

1. Discuss in detail determinants of health and disease.
2. Enlist indicators of health and disease.
3. Describe methods and principles of health education.
4. Enlist barriers in communication process and steps to overcome the same.
5. Describe role of physical and biological environment on health.
6. Discuss the public health importance of demography.
7. Enumerate the steps to segregate, transport and dispose biomedical waste.
8. Describe the role of nutrients in disease causation.

CHAPTER 1

Concept of Health and Disease

Date: ___________

Specific learning objectives: At the end of the session, Phase III (Part-1) student should be able to:

1. Define Health.
2. Enumerate determinants and indicators of health and disease.
3. Discuss in detail the concept of natural history of disease.
4. Enlist levels of prevention and modes of intervention.

Suggested reading before the session: Lecture notes on "Concept of Health and Disease", Health care delivery system in India, epidemiology of communicable diseases.

1. As defined by WHO, 'Health' is a ____________________

____

____

2. Match the following:

Concept of health	Definition
Ecological concept	Health is absence of disease
Holistic concept	Health is dynamic equilibrium between man and his environment
Biomedical concept	Health is also influenced by social, psychological, cultural, economic, political factors
Psychosocial concept	Health is a multi-dimensional process involving health and well-being of a person in the context of his environment

3. ____________ **concept has its basis in 'germ theory of disease'.**

4. Holistic concept = ____________ **+** ____________ **+** ____________ **concept.**

5. Enumerate components of well-being of an individual.

____

6. **Standard of living includes:**
   (a) Income and occupation
   (b) Standards of housing and sanitation
   (c) Nutrition and health
   (d) Educational, recreational and other services
   (e) All of the above

7. **Enlist components of level of living.**

____

____

____

____

____

8. **Define Quality of life.**

____

____

____

____

9. **Physical quality of life comprises of three indicators namely:-**
   (a) ____
   (b) ____
   (c) ____

10. **Enlist components of Human Development Index.**
   (a) ____
   (b) ____
   (c) ____

11. **What are the different levels of health care?**
   (a) ____
   (b) ____
   (c) ____

12. **Define Primary health care.**

____

____

____

____

13. **Give examples for principles of Primary health care.**

Principle of primary health care	Examples
Equitable distribution	
Community participation	
Inter-sectoral coordination	
Appropriate technology	

14. **Natural history of disease comprises of ______________________ and ______________________ phase.**

15. **What does the inverted triangle represent?**

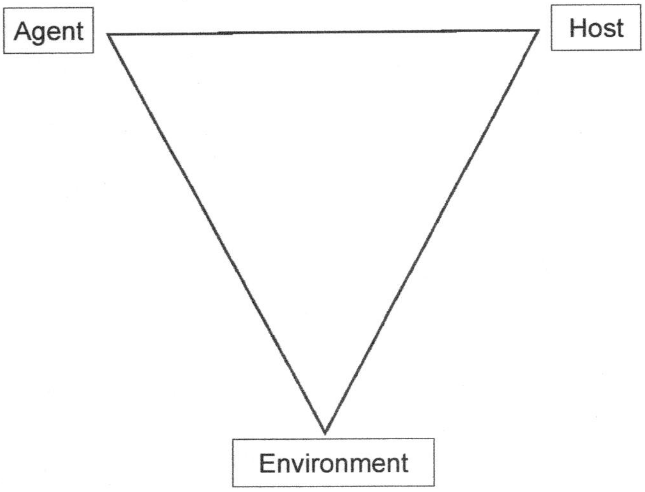

____

____

____

____

____

16. **Define**

(a) Agent: ______________________________________

(b) Host: ______________________________________

(c) Environment: ____

(d) Time: ____

17. Web of causation model of disease causation was given by ____________________ .

18. Web of causation considers all the ____________________ factors and their complex ____________________ with each other.

19. 'In a multifactorial causation, predisposing factors do not have equal weight'. Interpret the statement.

20. Draw an illustrative diagram for web of causation for malnutrition/ tuberculosis/ depression.

21. Draw an epidemiological triad of measles/poliomyelitis/cholera/dengue/rabies and clearly outline all the components.

22. Match the following:

Factors	Items to be matched
Virus, rickettsia, fungi, bacteria	Physical environment
Anaemia, goitre, obesity	Mechanical agent
Heat, cold, humidity, radiation	Psychosocial environment
Ketone, bilirubin, uric acid, urea	Physical agent
Crushing, tearing, sprains, dislocations	Nutrient agent
Alcohol, poverty, social isolation	Biological agent
Overcrowding, poor ventilation, air pollution	Chemical agent
Customs, beliefs, attitudes	Social agent

23. Match the following:

Ability of infectious agent to invade and multiply in a host	Pathogenicity
Ability to introduce clinically apparent illness	Virulence
Proportion of clinical cases resulting in a severe clinical manifestation	Infectivity

24. **Draw sickness spectrum of Leprosy.**

25. **Draw a diagram depicting iceberg phenomenon of disease in context of COVID-19. Clearly outline/ label all its components.**

26. For each of the following scenarios, select the most appropriate answer from the following list of options:

i. Chicken pox
ii. Small pox
iii. Measles
iv. Polio
v. Yaws
vi. Guineaworm

(a) Transmission of an acute infectious disease, characterized by sudden onset of fever, headache, backache, accompanied by development of a maculopapular rash (on third day) with centrifugal distribution eventually resulting in scarring, has been terminated as the infectious agent has been exterminated.

(b) A chronic, contagious, non-veneral disease which was transmitted by direct contact with secretions from infected lesions and characterized by a primary lesion on exposed body parts such as legs, arms, buttocks or face followed by a generalized eruption and a late stage of destructive lesions of skin and bone which may develop, subside and relapse at irregular intervals. Transmission of this disease has been interrupted.

27. For each of the following statements, select the most appropriate answer from the following list of options:

i. Primordial prevention
ii. Primary prevention
iii. Secondary prevention
iv. Tertiary prevention
v. Health promotion
vi. Specific protection
vii. Early diagnosis and treatment
viii. Disability limitation
ix. Rehabilitation
x. Prevention of emergence of risk factors

(a) Action taken prior to onset of disease, which removes the possibility that a disease will ever occur.

____

(b) Action which halts the progress of a disease at its incipient stage and prevents complication.

____

(c) All measures available to reduce or limit impairments and disabilities, minimize suffering caused by existing departures from good health and to promote patient's adjustment to irremediable conditions.

____

(d) Fortification of salt, oil and wheat flour in mid-day meal distributed to primary school children.

____

(e) Use of goggles by workers involved in cutting and welding at glass furnace.

____

(f) Administration of oral polio vaccine to protect against poliomyelitis disease.

____

(g) Opportunistic screening among individuals aged more than 30 years for identification of diabetes mellitus and hypertension so as to identify patients and initiate timely treatment among the same.

____

(h) Providing knee ankle foot orthosis for walking among children with permanent muscle weakness after poliomyelitis.

____

(i) Managing disabilities by reconstructive surgeries including tendon transfer for hands, feet and eyelids among leprosy patients. _______________

(j) Providing specialised protective footwear to leprosy patients for anaesthetic feet.

____

(k) Stringent legislative measures to ban tobacco production. _______________

(l) Breast self-examination to pick up breast lump. _______________

28. Impairment refers to any loss or abnormality of _______________, _______________ or _______________ structure or function.

29. Disability refers to any _______________ or _______________ to perform an activity in the manner or within the range considered _______________ for a human being.

30. Handicap is a disadvantage for a given individual resulting from an _______________ or a _______________, that _______________ the fulfilment of a role that is normal for that individual.

31. Match the following:

A driver lost his left foot in a road traffic accident	Handicap
A driver cannot drive because he lost his left foot in RTA	Impairment
A driver lost his job because he cannot drive due to limb amputation after RTA	Disability

32. Pick the odd one out. Substantiate your choice with explanation.

(a) Primary prevention, specific protection, primordial prevention, tertiary prevention.

____

(b) Agent, host, environment, time, prevention.

(c) Disability limitation, early diagnosis, overcrowding, health promotion.

(d) Bacteria, protozoa, metazoan, heat.

(e) Crushing, tearing, sprain, ketones.

(f) Age, gender, education, occupation, income, physical exercise.

(g) Overcrowding, Kucha house, cross-ventilation, natural light, open drains.

(h) Yaws, guineworm, neonatal tetanus, polio, small pox.

33. Draw a schematic diagram for natural history of disease for Measles:

Supervisor's Signature

CHAPTER 2

Health Education

Date: ___________

Specific learning objectives: At the end of the session, Phase III (Part-1) student should be able to:

1. Define health education, IEC and BCC.
2. Discuss principles of health education.
3. Discuss in detail communication process and its barriers.
4. Enumerate methods of health education.

Suggested reading before the session: Lecture notes of "Health Education".

1. Enumerate components of communication process.

____

____

2. Which if the following is correct?

(a) Sender → receiver → message → channel → feedback → sender

(b) Sender → message → channel → receiver → feedback → sender

(c) Sender → channel → message → receiver → feedback → sender

(d) Sender → receiver → channel → message → feedback → receiver

3. Indicate true or false in the following statements.

In a communication process-

(a) Sender should only be aware of the message he intends to give. (True/ False)

(b) Receiver may be a single person or a group of people. (True/ False)

(c) Message need not be culturally appropriate. (True/ False)

(d) Message should be based on felt needs. (True/ False)

(e) Message should be specific. (True/ False)

(f) Message may or may not be in line with the objective. (True/ False)

(g) Feedback is the most important component of any communication process. (True/ False)

4. Enumerate few channels of communication.

____

____

5. Match the following

Learning components	**Domains of learning**
Cognitive	Emotions
Psychomotor	Knowledge
Affective	Skill

6. For each of the following statements, select the most appropriate answer from the following list of options:-

Didactic method of communication

Dialectic method of communication

Verbal communication

Non-verbal communication

Interpersonal communication

(a) Flow of communication is one way from sender/source to audience. Learning is usually authoritative with little or no participation and feedback from audience.

(b) Flow of communication is two-way where sender/ source is a facilitator. Learning is democratic and audience is an equal stakeholder, where they participate and give feedback.

(c) Flow of communication is through facial expressions including smile, raised eye brows, widened eyes, raised upper lip, mouth open, staring, silence, not making eye contact, yawning, looking at the watch while communicating, taking notes.

7. Define Information, Education and Communication (IEC) and Behaviour change and communication (BCC).

____

____

____

____

____

____

____

____

8. Define health education.

9. Justify the statement, "Health education alone is insufficient to achieve optimum health".

10. Match the following:

Principle of health education	Items to be matched
Credibility	If I hear, I forget; if I see, I remember; If I do, I know. e.g., making people demonstrate handwashing after a demonstration of the same.
Participation	Language/ jargons used to communicate with patients/ community should be easily understood. e.g., cut down on intake of papad, chutney, pickle, namkeen, extra salt in curd or salad instead of saying reduce the amount of salt in diet
Comprehension	Health educator won't be very successful in explaining the hazards of smoking if he/ she is a smoker himself
Reinforcement	It helps to know if the recipient has understood the message in the same way as was intended by the sender. e.g., Rogi Kalyan Samiti
Learning by doing	The people have a right and duty to participate individually and collectively in the planning and implementation of their health care. e.g., VHSNC
Setting an example	A message is repeated in different ways at different times using different methods of communication. e.g., spreading awareness for pulse polio immunization day through advertisements on television, radio, newspaper, announcements through autorickshaw/rickshaw, interpersonal communication through ASHA and ANM's in their respective areas.
Feedback	It is the degree to which the message to be communicated is perceived as trustworthy by the receiver.

11. Enumerate different approach(s) in health communication.

12. Enlist few barriers in a communication process with examples.

13. Enumerate models of behaviour change.

14. Match the following:

Method in health communication	Items to be matched
Lecture	It is an instructional process that substitutes real patient encounters with artificial models, live actors, or virtual reality patients
Tutorial	A series of prepared talks given by few experts on many aspects of a topic under a chair person
Seminar	It is a form of simulation that focusses attention on the interaction of people with one another
Case study	An orderly and logical conversation on an assigned topic by 4 or more experts with moderator in front of audience
Bedside teaching	A small group of learners are guided by a facilitator to help clear doubts, improve understanding and enhance knowledge
Simulation	A method of group work, active involvement of participants and problem solving with the help of colleagues and professional peers under guidance from experts who act as resource persons
Role play	A formal event where researchers/ academicians present their work in speeches, workshop or posters
Symposium	It consists of group of persons engaged in advanced study of a subject who meet under the general direction of an expert staff member
Panel discussion	Any teaching done in the presence of the patient, regardless of the setting
Workshop	An intensive description and analysis of a single individual (unit)
Conference	A way of presentation of facts with organized thoughts and ideas by a qualified person

15. All of the following are true for lecture except:

(a) Learning in a lecture is passive.
(b) Does not cater to individual pace of learning.
(c) Communication is a two-way process.
(d) Teacher's time consumed per learner is very less.

16. Which of the following is true for tutorial?

(a) Communication is a one-way process.
(b) Helps to discover and correct mistakes in learning.
(c) Effective way of transmitting information to a large audience.
(d) Ineffective in problem solving.

17. A case study:

(a) Provides detailed insight into a particular case.
(b) Provides opportunity to study rare disorders.
(c) Has potential for hypothesis generation.
(d) All of the above are true for case study.

18. Bedside teaching:

(a) Does not help in skill development.
(b) Includes teaching done in a conference room in presence of a patient.
(c) Does not integrate knowledge and skill.
(d) Does not lack confidentiality.

19. Learning includes ability to rewind, rehearse and practice without negative patient outcomes in

(a) Tutorial (b) Workshop
(c) Simulation (d) Bedside teaching

20. Which of the following are examples of learning through simulation?

(a) Resusci-Ani (b) Harvey
(c) Role play (d) All of the above

21. In a symposium:

(a) Comprehensive coverage of subject is possible.
(b) Role of audience is passive.
(c) Little opportunity for discussion between speakers.
(d) Gives a fair analysis of several sides of a controversial issue.

i. a and c are correct. ii. a, b, c, d is correct.
iii. b and c are correct. iv. a, b, d is correct.

22. Which of the following is true for conference?

(a) Conference can be either general or themed.
(b) Allows exchange of ideas among scholars.
(c) Allows networking among scholars.
(d) Cannot be organised at international level.

i. a and c are correct. ii. a, b, c, d is correct.
iii. b and c are correct. iv. a, b, c is correct.

Supervisor's Signature

CHAPTER 3

Air Pollution

Date: ___________

Specific learning objectives: At the end of the session, Phase III (Part-1) student should be able to:

1. Discuss the relevance of environment and its impact on health.
2. Enlist major air pollutants and sources of air pollution.
3. Enumerate steps in prevention and control of air and water pollution.

Suggested reading before the session: Lecture notes of Environment and Health, guidelines on air quality management, national air quality monitoring program (NAMP). (can be accessed from website of Central Pollution Control Board)

In order to understand the relevance of learning concepts related to environment and health for an Indian Medical Graduate, let's review the historical perspective.

A. **Fog in Meuse Valley 1930**: The area of Liege on the River Meuse, was one of the most heavily industrialised areas of continental Europe, with steelworks, zinc smelters, glass manufacturers and fertiliser and explosive plants established since the industrial revolution. Between Dec 1 and Dec 5, 1930, a thick fog covered a large part of Belgium. From Dec 3 onwards, hundreds of people in the villages situated in the narrow portion of the Meuse Valley between the towns of Huy and Liege started to have severe respiratory signs and symptoms. More than 60 people died in the entire country and almost 6000 people became ill with respiratory disease. The weather was characterised by anticyclonic conditions with high atmospheric pressures and a very feeble (1-3 km/h) easterly wind that blew from the city of Liege into the narrow valley, which had 90-120 m hills on each side. These conditions produced a persistent fog with a temperature of 1-2 deg C. However, a temperature inversion of about 70-80 m above ground, i.e., just above the tallest chimneys in the valley- prevented the fumes from rising. This atmospheric ceiling forced emitted gases and impurities to accumulate in the corridor formed by the valley between Liege and Huy. Investigators established, for the first time, the roles of temperature inversion and fog in air pollution. It was further concluded that sulphur dioxide produced due to coal burning by industry and private households coupled with fog that resulted in H_2SO_4 production resulted in such high morbidity and mortality.

B. IN **1940'S Los Angeles**, California became one of the first cities in the US to experience severe air pollution problems then called "gas attacks". L.A.'s location in a basin like area ringed by mountains makes it susceptible to accumulation of auto exhaust and emissions from local petroleum refineries.

C. A similar air pollution occurred in **Donora, Pennsylvania in 1948**. Donora is located in the inside of a sharp horse shoe valley in the Monongahela River. The area along the riverbank was occupied by a large steel mill, a sulfuric acid plant, and a large zinc production plant. During October 1948, a heavy fog settled over the area surrounding Donora because of temperature inversion. This prolonged stable atmospheric condition permitted the accumulation of air pollutants emitted from plants along the riverbank. Nearly 42% of the population got affected with varying severity of upper respiratory tract symptoms and 20 persons died.

D. In **1969**, sulphur dioxide pollution emitted by industries near Gary, Indiana and East Chicago became potent acid rain that burnt lawns, ate away the tree leaves and caused birds to lose their feathers. The episodes demonstrated that severe air pollution can cause death and serious morbidity effects in those human/ animal populations that are exposed to it, and that PM and SO_2 are among the air pollutants that can contribute to the induction of such health effects.

1. **Environmental health requires services of health and non-health personnel like__________, __________, __________, __________, __________and__________ to name a few.**

2. **Match the following:**

Water related diseases	Items to be matched
Typhoid	Water based disease
Scabies	Water related disease
Malaria	Water borne disease
Guinea worm	Water washed disease

3. **According to Global burden of Disease estimates, the diseases (globally) that can be attributed to air pollution are __________, __________, __________, __________, __________, __________, __________**

4. **Define 'chlorine demand' of water.**

5. **Air pollution is the __________ leading risk factor for premature death globally, accounting for nearly __________ of all deaths worldwide.**

6. **Define ash, rubbish and garbage.**

7. **Who are most vulnerable to air pollution?** __________

8. **Enumerate features of 'Safe and wholesome water'.**

9. **Which of the following are indicators of faecal contamination of water?**
   (a) Coliforms
   (b) Coliforms, Fecal streptococci
   (c) Coliforms, fecal streptococci and clostridium perfringens
   (d) None of the above

10. Enlist sources of air pollution:

(a) ____________________

(b) ____________________

(c) ____________________

(d) ____________________

(e) ____________________

(f) ____________________

(g) ____________________

(h) ____________________

11. ____________________ is used to calculate the amount of bleaching powder required for disinfection.

12. Stock solution is made in ____________________ cup in horrocks apparatus.

13. In horrocks apparatus, addition of starch iodide solution to white cups results in development of ______________ color which indicates presence of ____________________.

14. Which of the following is a primary pollutant?

(a) SO_3 (b) H_2SO_4

(c) O_3 (d) SO_2

15. Which disease is associated with use of step well?

____

16. Septic tank is a ____________________ tank which holds ____________________ from individual dwellings or small groups of houses but it does not have access to ____________________.

17. Which of the following is a secondary pollutant?

(a) CO (b) H_2SO_4

(c) NO_2 (d) SO_2

18. Enumerate methods of waste disposal.

____

____

____

____

19. What is National air Quality Index?

____

____

____

____

20. How many categories are there in AQI?

(a) Five (b) Six

(c) Seven (d) Eight

21. Draw an illustrative diagram to depict the transmission of faecal borne diseases.

22. Which of the following is correct with respect to AQI categories?

(a) Good, satisfactory, moderately polluted, poor, severe.

(b) Good, satisfactory, moderately polluted, poor, very poor, severe.

(c) Good, satisfactory, moderately polluted, poor, very poor, severe, very severe.

(d) Good, satisfactory, moderately polluted, poor, very poor, severe, very severe, extremely severe.

23. Sand bed gets covered with a slimy growth known as 'Schmutzdecke' in ______________ filter.

24. Biochemical oxygen demand is the amount of ______________ absorbed by a sample of sewage during a specified period of______________, at a specified temperature of ______________ for ______________destruction.

25. **Answer the following as Yes/No.**

Name of pollutant	Use for calculation of AQI (Yes/No)
PM_{10}	
$PM_{2.5}$	
NO_2	
O_3	
CO	
SO_2	
NH_3	
Pb	

26. **Match the following:**

AQI score	AQI category
0-50	Moderate
51-100	Very poor
101-200	Good
201-300	Severe
301-400	Satisfactory
401-500	Poor

27. **Venturi-meter measures loss of head in a ______________________ filter.**

28. **______________________ was introduced by Rockfeller Foundation in 1930's to address the menace of ______________________ infestation.**

29. **Free residual chlorine of ______________ provides a margin of safety against subsequent microbial contamination.**

30. **Indicate the health impact against each AQI category.**

AQI category	Health impact
Good	
Satisfactory	
Moderate	
Poor	
Very poor	
Severe	

31. **Filter cleaning is done by ______________________ in a slow sand filter and by ______________________ in rapid sand filter.**

32. **What are the major pollutants from the following sources?**

Source of air pollution	Major pollutant
Vehicular/ Transport	
Industrial process	
Agriculture	
Power	
Waste treatment and biomass burning	
Residential	
Construction and demolition waste	

33. **CPCB has categorised the polluting industries into 17 types, out of which seven have been marked as 'critical' industries that include____.**

34. **Water seal in a latrine refers to____**

35. **Before the water is led into sedimentation tank of rapid sand filter, it is treated with ________________, followed by rapid mixing in ____________________ followed by slow and gentle stirring in ____.**

36. **Classify air pollutants (with examples):**

(a) Based on source of origin

i. ____

ii. ____

(b) Based on method of origin

i. ____

ii. ____

(c) Based on chemical composition

i. ____

ii. ____

(d) Based on state of matter

i. ____

ii. ____

37. **In multiple tube method used for estimation of most probable numbers of coliform organisms, positive test is indicated by ______________________, which gets collected in the inverted ______________________ tube.**

38. **In India, air quality (including air pollution) is being monitored by __________________ which is a statutory body under Ministry of ________________________________.**

39. What is the health impact of air pollution?

(a) Due to short term exposure:

____

____

____

____

(b) Due to long term exposure:

____

____

____

____

40. Which of the following methods can be used for treatment of hardness?

(a) Boiling

(b) Addition of sodium carbonate

(c) Permutit process

(d) Base exchange process

i. Both a and b ii. a, b and c

iii. a, b, c, and d iv. a, c and d

41. Point at which chlorine demand of water is met is termed as ______________________________

____

42. Outline steps for prevention and control of air pollution with suitable examples.

43. Differentiate between sewage and sullage.

44. Indicate true/false for the following statements.

(a) Orthotolidine test can assess only free chlorine. (True/ False)

(b) Breakpoint chlorination refers to appearance of free residual chlorine. (True/ False)

(c) Contact period of one hour is essential to kill bacteria and viruses. (True/ False)

(d) Chlorine acts best as a disinfectant when the pH of water is around 8.5. (True/ False)

(e) A disinfectant should not be amenable to detection. (True/ False)

(f) Washing of filter is more tedious in rapid sand filter as compared to slow sand filter. (True/ False)

(g) Boiling as a method of disinfection alters taste of water. (True/ False)

(h) Chlorine tablets used for disinfection of water are available at anganwadi. (True/ False)

(i) Horrocks apparatus has 7 cups, 7 stirring rods and 2 droppers. (True/ False)

(j) Multiple tube method is used for presumptive coliform test. (True/ False)

Supervisor's Signature

CHAPTER 4

Demography

Date: __________

Specific learning objectives: At the end of the session, Phase III (Part-1) student should be able to:

1. Discuss public health importance of Demography.
2. Enlist demographic characteristics of India.
3. Enumerate fertility related statistics.

Suggested reading before the session: Lecture notes of Demography, Census 2011 report, NFHS-5 factsheets, SRS bulletin (May 2020), Special bulletin on Maternal mortality in India 2016-2018 (SRS), SRS Statistical report 2018, Annual report on vital statistics of India based on CRS-2019.

1. **The total population of India as per Census 2011 is __________ .**
2. **Total population of India has increased from __________ in 1901 to __________ in 2011.**
3. **The total population of India is almost equal to the combined population of ______, ______, ______, ______, ______ and ______ put together.**
4. **India accounts for ______,and ______ of world's surface area but supports and sustains ______% of the world's population.**
5. **Enumerate names of States and Union Territories in India.**

6. **Demography is** ______________________________

____

7. **Demography takes into account three observable human phenomenon namely** __________, __________, __________ **and** __________.

8. **Demography deals with five processes namely** __________, __________, __________, __________ **and** __________.

9. **Demographic cycle depicts** ______________________________

____

10. **Demographic cycle has** ______________________________ **stages.**

11. **Match the following:**

Stage of demographic cycle	Items to be matched
Late expanding	High birth rate and high death rate
Low stationary	Death rate starts to decline and birth rate remains unchanged
Declining	Death rate continues to decline and birth rate starts to fall
High stationary	Low birth rate and low death rate
Early expanding	Birth rate is lower than death rate

12. **Number of administrative units in Census 2011 were** __________ **States,** __________ **Districts,** __________ **sub-districts,** __________ **Towns,** __________ **villages.**

13. **With the exception for 1911-1921, 2001-2011 has been the first decade which has added** __________ **population compared to previous decade.**

14. **The percentage decadal growth rate has** __________ **from** __________ **in 1991-2001 to** __________ **in 2001-2011.**

15. **Match the following:**

State	Items to be matched
Uttar Pradesh	Least populous UT
Maharashtra	Least populous state
Bihar	Fourth most populous state
West Bengal	Most populous State
Sikkim	Third most populous state
Lakshadweep	Second most populous state

16. **Population of Uttar Pradesh is more than the population of** __________ **(Country).**

17. **Which age group is included to calculate Child Sex Ratio?**

(a) 1-6 years (b) 0-5 years

(c) 0-6 years (d) 0- 6 months

18. In how many years is the official enumeration of population carried out for census.

(a) 1 year
(b) 5 years
(c) 10 years
(d) 2 years

19. Which of the following is an important social indicator to measure the extent of equality between males and females in a society at a given time?

(a) Age composition
(b) Literacy Rate
(c) Sex ratio
(d) Death Rate

20. Birth rate is the number of live births per thousand persons in:

(a) 10 years
(b) 5 years
(c) 2 years
(d) 1 year.

21. What year is considered a great demographic divide in India?

(a) 1911
(b) 1921
(c) 1931
(d) 1751

22. Birth rate of India (2018) is ____________.

23. Birth rate in rural areas has declined from ____________ in 2009 to ____________ in 2018, while in urban areas it has declined from ____________ in 2009 to ____________ in 2018.

24. Death rate of India is____________.

25. Death rate in rural areas has declined from ____________in 2009 to ____________ in 2018, while in urban areas it has declined from ____________in 2009 to ____________ in 2018.

26. Infant mortality rate of India was ____________ in 2009 which has reduced to ____________ in 2018.

27. Infant mortality rate for rural and urban areas is ____________ and ____________ respectively.

28. Match the following:

State	Birth rate
Delhi	26.2
Uttar Pradesh	13.9
Bihar	14.7
Rajasthan	15.6
Kerala	24
Maharashtra	25.6

29. Maternal mortality ratio of India is____________.

30. Births and deaths are to be reported within ____________days of occurrence of event.

31. Birth and death certificate are issued at a price of ____________ if reported within 21 days of occurrence of event.

32. Birth and deaths can be reported:

(a) After 21 days but within 30 days
(b) After 30 days but within one year
(c) After one year
(d) All of the above

33. Birth can be registered ______________________ (with/ without) the name of the child.

34. Mid-year population is defined as ______________________

____

____

35. Proportion of males and females in India as per Census 2011 are ________ % and ________ %.

36. Sex ratio of India, as per Census 2011 is ______________________ .

37. Match the following:

State	Sex Ratio
Delhi	916
Uttar Pradesh	866
Bihar	1084
Rajasthan	877
Kerala	908
Haryana	618
Daman and Diu	926

38. Proportion of children in the age group 0-6 years is ______________________ %.

39. Child sex ratio of India in the age group 0-6 years is ______________________ .

40. Literate is a person ______________________

____

____

41. As per census 2011, literates comprise ______________________% of total population aged seven and above and illiterates comprise ______________________% of total population.

42. According to Census 2011, literacy rate for males and females are ____________ and ____________ respectively.

43. State and UT with highest literacy rate in India are ______________________ and ____________ respectively.

44. State with lowest literacy rate in India is ______________________ .

45. Population density of India has increased to ______________ persons per square kilometre in 2011 from ______________ persons per square kilometre in 2001.

46. Match the following:

State/ Union Territory	Population density per square km
NCT of Delhi	11,297
India	382
Chandigarh	9252
Bihar	1102
Maharashtra	365
Andaman and Nicobar Islands	46

47. Please indicate true/ false for the following statements:

(a) There has been a decline in number of illiterates from census 2001 to Census 2011. (True/False)

(b) Formal education is important for a person to be classified as literate. (True/False)

(c) Out of the total literates added during 2001-2011, females outnumber males. (True/False)

(d) Male-female gap in literacy rate has reduced from the year 2001 to year 2011. (True/False)

48. What is fertility? Enlist factors affecting fertility.

____

____

____

49. Enumerate fertility related statistics.

____

____

____

____

____

____

____

50. Define General fertility rate.

____

____

____

____

____

51. What is the current GFR for India? Please indicate the rural-urban difference for the same.

____

____

____

____

____

52. GFR for India has declined from ________________ in 2006-08 to ________________ in 2016-18.

53. **What is age specific fertility rate?**

54. **Comment on Age-specific fertility rate in India.**

55. **What do you understand by Total fertility rate?**

56. **What is the current TFR of India?**

57. **What do you understand by Gross reproduction rate?**

58. **What is the current GRR of India?**

59. **Please indicate life expectancy at birth for the period 2014-2018 the following:**

i. India: ____________________

ii. Rural India: ____________________

iii. Urban India: ____________________

iv. Males: ____________________

v. Females: ____________________

Supervisor's Signature

Chapter 5

Vectors of Public Health Importance

Date:____________

Specific learning objectives: At the end of the session, Phase III (Part-1) student should be able to:

1. Enlist vectors of public health importance and their identifying features.
2. Discuss in detail life cycle of these vectors.
3. Enumerate disease(s) transmitted by vectors of public health importance.
4. Enlist prevention and control measures for vectors of public health importance.

Suggested reading before the session: Lecture notes of "Medical Entomology" and insecticides, guidelines on integrated vector management (IVM).

1. Enlist vectors of public health importance.

____

____

2. Name some common species of the following genus:

(a) Anopheles: ____________________

(b) Aedes: ____________________

(c) Culex: ____________________

(d) Musca: ____________________

(e) Phlebotomus: ____________________

(f) Pediculus: ____________________

(g) Xenopsylla: ____________________

(h) Guineaworm: ____________________

3. Identify the vector:

(a) ____________________ lays her eggs singly, and eggs are boat shaped and possess lateral floats.

(b) Larvae of ____________________ floats horizontally in water, and does not have a siphon tube.

(c) ____________________ lays her eggs in small clusters/ rafts and eggs do not possess lateral floats.

(d) ____________________ lays her eggs singly, eggs are cigar shaped and do not possess lateral floats.

(e) ____________________ lays her eggs in star shaped clusters attached to the under surface of leaves of pistia plant.

(f) Larvae of ____________________ are suspended in water with their heads downwards, and have a siphon tube on the 8th abdominal segment.

(g) At rest ____________________ sits at an angle of 45 deg to the surface.

(h) ____________________ is also known as Tiger mosquito because it has ____________________.

(i) The period between blood meal and oviposition is termed as ____________________.

(j) ____________________ has lanceolate shaped wings, wherein the second longitudinal vein branches twice and has hairy antennae, abdomen and wings.

(k) ____________________ has dorso-ventrally flattened body, three pair of legs, pair of 5-jointed antennae.

(l) ____________________ has bilaterally compressed body, three pairs of legs, no wings.

(m) Rocky mountain spotted fever is caused by bite of ____________________ which has ____________________ legs and dorsal surface is covered with ____________________.

(n) Q fever is caused by ____________________ which has ____________________ legs and ____________________ have chitinous covering.

(o) ____________________ has a pear shaped body, forked tail and five pair of legs.

4. Match the following:

Vector (at different stage of development)	Identifying feature
Egg of Aedes	Lay horizontally without a siphon tube
Eggs of anopheles	Suspended in water with siphon tube on 8th abdominal segment
Eggs of Mansonia	Tiger mosquito
Sand fly	Cigar/Boat shaped
Eggs of Culex	Dorso-ventrally flattened body
Larvae of Anopheles	At rest, sits at an angle of 45 degrees/ Spotted wings
Larvae of Aedes, Culex, Mansonia	Have lateral floats
Adult Anopheles	Hairy antennae
Adult Aedes	Eggs laid in clusters/rafts
Louse	Star shaped clusters

5. **Please indicate vector for the following potential breeding sites.**

Breeding place	Vector
Decaying vegetables and fruits (including peels)	
Broken tyre	
Dirty polluted water	
Garbage	
Dirty water puddles	
Open drains	
Cesspool	
Clean slow-moving water	
Overhead tank	
Dead and decaying organic matter	
Human excreta	
Manure of animals	
Freshwater collection	
Septic tank (if open and leaking)	
Flower pot	
Desert cooler	
Artificial collection of water	
Salt water collection	

6. **Anopheles transmits** ____________________.

7. **Which if the following diseases are transmitted by Culex**
   (a) Bancroftian filariasis, Japanese encephalitis
   (b) Bancroftian filariasis, Japanese encephalitis, West nile fever
   (c) Bancroftian filariasis, Japanese encephalitis, West nile fever, Viral arthritis
   (d) Bancroftian filariasis, West nile fever, Viral arthritis

8. **Which of the following is true for Aedes?**
   (a) Aedes transmits Dengue, DHF, Chikungunya and filaria
   (b) Aedes transmits Dengue, DHF, Chikungunya, rift valley fever, filaria and yellow fever
   (c) Aedes transmits Dengue, DHF, rift valley fever and yellow fever
   (d) Aedes transmits Dengue, DHF and Chikungunya.

9. **Name some diseases transmitted by house fly.**

____

____

10. **Sand fly transmits** ____________________ **and** ____________________

11. Louse transmits

(a) Epidemic typhus
(b) Relapsing fever
(c) Trench fever
(d) Dermatitis

i. a, b, c are correct
ii. a, c are correct
iii. a, b, c, d are correct
iv. a, c, d are correct

12. Bubonic plague, endemic typhus and chiggerosis are transmitted by ____________________.

13. Enlist few diseases transmitted by Ticks.

____

____

14. Scabies is transmitted by ____________________________.

15. Match the following:

Vector	Flight range
Anopheles	Hops up to 4 inches
Aedes	3-12 km
Culex	Mostly hop within 50 metres
Sand fly	11 km
Rat flea	Less than 100 m

16. Indicate true or false for the following statements.

(a) Pupa is a feeding stage. (True/False)

(b) Pupa is a resting stage. (True/False)

(c) Pupa swims rapidly into the water when disturbed. (True/False)

(d) Male mosquitoes never bite. (True/False)

(e) Chemical agents used under NVBDCP have only larvicidal action. (True/False)

(f) Temephos and insect growth regulators are used as chemical larvicide. (True/False)

(g) Temephos is used as a larvicide in a dosage of 10 ppm. (True/False)

(h) Insecticidal residual spray is one of the most cost-effective measure for control of malaria and Kala azar in India. (True/False)

(i) DDT and malathion are used for insecticidal residual spray in India. (True/False)

17. What is Aedes aegypti index?

____

____

____

18. What is a blocked flea?

____

____

____

19. A woman comes to your OPD with two children, with complaints of itching in between fingers, over wrist, extensor aspect of elbow which gets worse at night. She reported that both her children have been having similar complaints for the past few days. On examining the affected sites, follicular lesions were seen. What is your provisional diagnosis?

____

____

____

____

20. What is integrated vector management?

____

____

____

21. Enlist tools of vector control.

(a) ______________________________

(b) ______________________________

(c) ______________________________

(d) ______________________________

22. All of the following are environmental measures of vector control except:

(a) Improved water supply
(b) Mosquito proofing of overhead tanks
(c) Insecticide treated nets
(d) Solid waste disposal

23. Which of the following is an environmental management method of vector control?

(a) Repellents
(b) Protective clothing
(c) Temephos
(d) Inspection of tyre depots

24. Mosquito proofing of overhead tank is ______________________________ method of vector control.

(a) Environmental management method
(b) Source reduction method
(c) Biological method
(d) Chemical method

25. Environmental methods to control Aedes aegypti are:

(a) Source reduction, insecticide-treated nets, modification of man-made breeding sites and repellents

(b) Source reduction, solid waste management, modification of man-made breeding sites and improved housing design

(c) Temephos, solid waste management, Bacillus sphaericus and improved housing design

(d) Source reduction, solid waste management, modification of man-made breeding sites and improved housing design

26. All of the following is a personal protective measure of vector control except

(a) Protective clothing (b) Repellents, mats, coils, aerosols

(c) Larvivorus fish (d) Insecticide treated nets

27. Biological agents used under the program are against the ________________ stage of mosquito.

28. Name the biological agents used under NVBDCP for vector control.

(a) ________________________

(b) ________________________

29. What are the characteristics of NICD cooler?

Supervisor's Signature

Chapter 6

Biomedical Waste Management

Date:____________

Specific learning objectives: At the end of the session, Phase III (Part-1) student should be able to:

1. Define Biomedical waste.
2. Discuss the public health importance of biomedical waste.
3. Categorize biomedical waste into colour coded categories.
4. Enumerate steps involved in segregation, transport and disposal of biomedical waste.

Suggested reading before the session: Lecture notes of "Biomedical waste management" and visit to CSSD, guidelines on biomedical waste (management and handling) rules 2016.

1. Define Biomedical waste.

____

____

____

____

2. Biomedical waste comprises of ________________% total waste generated from the health care facility.

3. There are________________________ categories of biomedical waste.

4. Enlist the categories used to segregate biomedical waste

____

____

____

____

____

5. What type of waste is segregated in each of the colour coded bags enlisted above?

____

____

____

____

____

____

____

6. Biomedical waste management and handling rules do not apply to ______________________ waste.

7. Define Biomedical waste treatment and disposal facility.

____

____

____

8. Enumerate the steps involved in bio-medical waste management.

____

____

____

____

9. Biomedical waste should be segregated at ______________________ of waste.

10. What do you understand by point of generation of biomedical waste?

____

____

____

____

11. Biomedical waste should be segregated in ______________________ bags/ bins/ containers.

12. Please indicate true or false for the following statements.

(a) Interim storage of bio-medical waste should be done in respective departments. (True/False)

(b) General waste should be stored in central waste collection room meant for bio medical waste. (True/False)

(c) Biomedical waste can be transported from site of generation to central waste collection centre in patient trolleys. (True/False)

(d) Non-chlorinated plastic bags should be used for collection and segregation of bio medical waste. (True/False)

(e) Yellow waste including human and animal anatomical and soiled waste are permitted for deep burial only in rural or remote areas where there is no access to common biomedical waste treatment facility. (True/False)

13. Discuss in detail the type of waste segregated in yellow bag.

(a) ______________________________

____

(b) ______________________________

____

(c) ______________________________

____

(d) ______________________________

____

(e) ______________________________

____

(f) ______________________________

____

(g) ______________________________

____

(h) ______________________________

____

14. Please indicate the type of bag/bin/ container used for storage and method of ultimate disposal.

Type of biomedical waste	Type of bin used for storage and ultimate disposal
(a) Human anatomical waste	
(b) Animal anatomical waste	
(c) Soiled waste	
(d) Expired or discarded medicines	
(e) Chemical solid waste	
(f) Chemical liquid waste	
(g) Discarded linen, mattresses, beddings contaminated with blood or body fluid	
(h) Microbiology, biotechnology and other clinical laboratory waste	

15. Which of the following biomedical waste can be sent to incinerator?

(a) Biomedical waste segregated in yellow bag

(b) Biomedical waste segregated in red bag

(c) Biomedical waste segregated in white translucent container

(d) Biomedical waste segregated in puncture proof container with blue coloured marking

i. All of the above can be incinerated

ii. a and b can be incinerated

iii. a, c and d can be incinerated

iv. Only a can be incinerated

16. If a hospital is in a rural or remote area with no access to CBWTF, how should the biomedical waste segregated in yellow bag be disposed?

(a) Incineration

(b) Plasma pyrolysis

(c) Deep burial pits

(d) All of the above

17. An attempt should be made to return the following to the manufacturer:

(a) Expired antibiotic

(b) Expired chemotherapeutic agents along with vial

(c) Expired vaccines

(d) Both a and b

18. Which of the following biomedical waste should be pre-treated with autoclave/ microwave/ hydroclave before final disposal?

(a) Culture plates, vaccines, waste blood bags

(b) Biomedical waste segregated in red bag

(c) Biomedical waste segregated in white translucent container

(d) Biomedical waste segregated in puncture proof container with blue coloured marking

i. Only a

ii. a, b, c and d

iii. a, c and d

iv. a, b and c

19. Biomedical waste bags and sharp containers should be filled to ________________ capacity after which they should be sealed for collection.

20. All the bags/containers/ bins used for collection and storage of bio-medical waste, must be labelled with symbol of ______________________________ or ______________________________ whichever is applicable.

21. As per biomedical waste management and handling rules, 2016, ________________health care facility shall establish on-site treatment and disposal facility for BMW, if a CBWTF is available within ________________ km of health care facility.

22. **As In charge of health care facility, how will you ensure occupational safety of the staff involved in handling biomedical waste?**

23. **Give some examples of general waste generated in a health care setting.**

Supervisor's Signature

CHAPTER 7

Nutrition and Health

Date:______________

Specific learning objectives: At the end of the session, Phase III (Part-1) student should be able to:

1. Classify foods.
2. Enlist sources of macronutrients.
3. Discuss the role of fatty acids in disease causation.
4. Enumerate diseases caused by deficiency or excess of various macro and micronutrients.

Suggested reading before the session: Lecture notes of Nutrition, Report of expert group, ICMR, on nutrient requirements for Indians (2020), guidelines on nutrition, lifestyle and immunity, ICMR.

1. How do you classify foods?

(a) By origin

____

(b) By chemical composition

____

(c) By predominant function

____

(d) By nutritive value

____

2. What are proximate principles?

____

____

3. Enlist essential and non-essential amino acids.

____

____

4. 'Biologically complete' protein is one which contains:

____

____

____

5. Enlist sources of protein.

____

____

6. What do you mean by supplementary action of proteins?

____

____

____

7. How do you classify fatty acids?

____

____

8. What is Vanaspati? What is the current recommendation for use of vanaspati?

____

____

____

9. Trans fatty acids are ______________________________

____

10. Nutritionally significant unsaturated fatty acids (MUFA and PUFA) have double bonds in ______________ configuration.

11. Humans ______________ (can/cannot) synthesize parent PUFA's namely linoleic acid and alpha-linolenic acid.

12. Linoleic acid and alpha-linolenic acid are metabolized into.

____

____

13. Recommended dietary ratio for LA:ALA is ______________

14. Give some examples of visible fat consumed in Indian diet.

____

____

15. Give some examples of dietary fats rich in Saturated fatty acids (SFA's).

____

____

16. **Main source of trans fatty acids (TFA) in Indian diet is** ____________________

____

17. **Dietary oils rich in Linoleic acid and alpha linolenic acid are:**

____

____

18. **Dietary oils with high linoleic acid content are** ____________________

____

____

19. **Classify the following into good sources of linoleic acid and both linoleic and alpha-linolenic acid:- Cereals, millets, pulses, green leafy vegetables, fenugreek, soyabean flax seed, mustard seed.**

____

____

____

____

20. **Egg is a rich source of** ____________________ **fatty acid.**

21. **How can cooking oils be combined to ensure adequate consumption of LA and ALA?**

____

____

____

____

____

____

22. **Indicate true or false against each of the following:**

(a) Replacing SFA's with PUFA/ MUFA increases LDL cholesterol. (True/False)

(b) Replacing SFA's with PUFA/ MUFA decreases the total/HDL cholesterol ratio. (True/False)

(c) Replacing carbohydrate with MUFA decreases HDL cholesterol concentrations. (True/False)

(d) LA and ALA are indispensable since they cannot be synthesised by humans. (True/False)

(e) 20-30% of energy should come from dietary fats to ensure adequate consumption of essential fatty acids and fat-soluble vitamins for adults. (True/False)

(f) To ensure appropriate balance of fatty acids in cereal-based diets, it is necessary to increase the ALA intake and reduce the quantity of LA obtained from cooking oil. (True/False)

(g) Carbohydrates from whole grains, legumes, vegetables and whole fruits are associated with reduced risk of type-2 diabetes mellitus and cardiovascular disease. (True/False)

23. Enumerate major dietary sources of carbohydrate.

____

____

____

24. In Indian diet, ______________ of energy should be from carbohydrates, ______________ from proteins, and ______________ from fats.

25. What is the difference between glycaemic index and glycaemic load?

____

____

____

26. What are the important determinants of post prandial glucose response?

____

____

27. What is the public health importance of parboiling?

____

____

____

____

28. Dietary fibre is defined as ______________________________

____

____

29. What is the significance of dietary fibre in diet?

____

____

30. Name some foods with high dietary fibre content.

____

____

31. Indicate relevant nutrient responsible for the following deficiency diseases:

Deficiency disease	Nutrient
Rickets	
Scurvy	
Angular stomatitis	
Peripheral neuritis	
Anaemia	
Bitot spots	
Pellagra	
Conjunctival xerosis	
Anaemia	
Beriberi	
Osteomalacia	
Night blindness	
Dental caries	
Genu valgum	

Supervisor's Signature

Hints and Answers to Exercises

CHAPTER 1

1. State of complete physical, mental and social well-being and not merely an absence of disease or infirmity. It further includes the ability to lead a 'socially and economically productive life'.
2. Match the following concepts of health with respective definition.

Concept of health	Definition
Biomedical concept	Health is absence of disease
Ecological concept	Health is dynamic equilibrium between man and his environment
Psychosocial concept	Health is also influenced by social, psychological, cultural, economic, political factors
Holistic concept	Health is a multi-dimensional process involving health and well-being of a person in the context of his environment

3. Biomedical concept.
4. Biomedical; ecological; psychosocial concept.
5. (Objective components)Standard of living, level of living and quality of life (subjective component).
6. e. All of the above.
7. Level of living includes nine components: health, food consumption, education, occupation and working conditions, housing, social security, clothing, recreation and leisure and human rights.
8. As defined by WHO, QOL is a composite measure of physical, mental and social well being as perceived by each individual or by group of individuals, i.e. happiness, satisfaction and gratification as it is experienced in such life concerns as health, marriage, family work, financial situation, educational opportunities, self-esteem, creativity, belongingness and trust in other.
9. Infant mortality, life expectancy at age 1 and literacy.
10. Longevity (life expectancy at birth), knowledge (mean and expected years of schooling), income (GNI per capita/ PPP US$).
11. Primary level e.g. Subcentre, PHC. Secondary level e.g. community health centre (CHC), tertiary level e.g. regional/ central level institutions including medical colleges.
12. Primary health care refers to essential health care based on practical, scientifically sound and socially acceptable methods and technology made universally accessible to individuals and families in the community through their full participation and at a cost that the community and the country can afford to maintain at every stage of their development in the spirit of self-determination.
13.

Principle of primary health care	Examples
Equitable distribution	Poor distribution of health care services in remote, tribal, rural areas
Community participation	Village health nutrition and sanitation committee, Jan sunways, lok manch, rogi kalyan samiti
Inter-sectoral coordination	NACP with NHAI and Ministry of petroleum for social marketing of condoms
Appropriate technology	ORS, MCTS, GIS for spatial mapping in NUHM, auto-disabled syringes, hub cutter, vaccines, laproscopic technology for MTP, No-scalpel vasectomy

14. **Pre-pathogenesis; pathogenesis phase**
15. **Represents interaction and interdependence of A, H and E and time.**
16.
    (a) Cause of disease
    (b) Organism that harbours the disease
    (c) Surroundings external to agent and host that facilitate transmission
    (d) Incubation period/ life expectancy of the host and/ or pathogen/ duration of illness
17. **MacMohan and Pugh**
18. **Predisposing; interrelationships.**
19. **Removal or elimination of only one link may be sufficient to control disease provided that link is sufficiently important in the pathogenic process.**
20. **Diagram to be drawn**
21. **Epidemiological triad to be drawn**
22. **Match the following:**

Virus, rickettsiae, fungi, bacteria	Biological agent
Anaemia, goitre, obesity	Nutrient agent
Heat, cold, humidity, radiation	Physical agent
Ketone, bilirubin, uric acid, urea	Chemical agent
Crushing, tearing, sprains, dislocations	Mechanical agent
Alcohol, poverty, social isolation	Social agent
Overcrowding, poor ventilation, air pollution	Physical environment
Customs, beliefs, attitudes	Psychosocial environment

23. **Match the following:**

Ability of infectious agent to invade and multiply in a host	Infectivity
Ability to introduce clinically apparent illness	Pathogenicity
Proportion of clinical cases resulting in a severe clinical manifestation	virulence

24. **Tuberculoid, borderline tuberculoid, borderline (BB), borderline lepromatous and lepromatous (LL)**
25. **Diagram to be drawn**
26. (a) Small pox, (b) Yaws
27. **Most appropriate answer**
    (a) Primary prevention
    (b) Early diagnosis and treatment
    (c) Tertiary prevention
    (d) Health promotion; primary prevention
    (e) Specific protection
    (f) Specific protection

(g) Early diagnosis and treatment

(h) Rehabilitation

(i) Disability limitation

(j) Rehabilitation

(k) Primordial prevention

(l) Early diagnosis

28. Psychological, physiological, anatomical

29. Restriction, lack of ability, normal

30. Impairment, disability, limits

31. Match the following:

A driver lost his left foot in a road traffic accident	Impairment
A driver cannot drive because he lost his left foot in RTA	Disability
A driver lost his job because he cannot drive due to limb amputation after RTA	Handicap

32. Pick the odd one out. Substantiate your choice with explanation.

(a) Specific protection; rest are all levels of prevention

(b) Prevention; rest are part of epidemiological triad

(c) Overcrowding; rest are interventions at different levels of prevention

(d) Heat; rest are all biological agents

(e) Ketones; rest are mechanical agents

(f) Physical exercise; rest are all socio-demogrpahic host factors

(g) Open drains; rest are all components of physical environment

(h) Small pox; rest have only been eliminated.

33. Diagram to be drawn

CHAPTER 2

1. Sender, receiver, message, channel, feedback

2. Sender → message →channel →receiver→feedback→sender

3. Indicate true or false in the following: - In a communication process

(a) False; he should also know about his objectives, audience, channels of communication and his limitations at all levels

(b) True

(c) False

(d) True

(e) True

(f) False

(g) True

4. Interpersonal communication, print media, electronic media, traditional or folk media, melas/ festivals, trialogue approach, workshop/ seminar, health camps etc.

5. **Match the following:**

Learning components	Domains of learning
Cognitive	Knowledge
Psychomotor	Skill
Affective	emotions

6. **Most appropriate answer:**
   (a) Didactic method of communication
   (b) Dialectic method of communication
   (c) Non-verbal communication

7. **IEC is a public health approach aiming at changing or reinforcing health related behaviours in a target audience, concerning a specific problem and within a pre-defined period of time, through communication methods and principles.**

   BCC is a process of working with individuals, communities and societies to develop communication strategies to promote positive behaviours which are appropriate to their settings; and provide a supportive environment which will enable people to initiate and sustain positive behaviours.

8. **Health education is the process by which individuals and groups of people learn to behave in a manner conducive to the promotion, maintenance or restoration of health (John M. Last). The dynamic definition of health education given after Alma-Ata declaration is 'a process aimed at encouraging people to want to be healthy, to know how to stay healthy, to do what they can individually and collectively to maintain health, and to seek help when needed.**

9. **Community must have access to proven preventive measures. They must have access to health and health related information so as to identify problems/ risk factors at the earliest and be able to set their own targets and priorities so as to modify the risk factor. Community must have access to solutions to health-related problems, in terms of diagnostic and treatment modalities and rehabilitative measures, if need arises.**

10. **Match the following:**

Principle of health education	Items to be matched
Credibility	It is the degree to which the message to be communicated is perceived as trustworthy by the receiver.
Participation	The people have a right and duty to participate individually and collectively in the planning and implementation of their health care, e.g., VHSNC
Comprehension	Language/ jargons used to communicate with patients/ community should be easily understood, e.g., Cut down on intake of papad, chutney, namkeen, extra salt in curd or salad instead of saying reduce the amount of salt in diet
Reinforcement	A message is repeated in different ways at different times using different methods of communication, e.g., Spreading awareness for pulse polio immunization day through advertisements on television, radio, newspaper, announcements through autorickshaw/ rickshaw, interpersonal communication through ASHA and ANM's in their respective areas.
Learning by doing	If I hear, I forget; if I see, I remember; If I do, I know, e.g., Making people demonstrate handwashing after a demonstration of the same.
Setting an example	Health educator won't be very successful in explaining the hazards of smoking if he is a smoker himself
Feedback	It helps to know if the recipient has understood the message in the same way as was intended by the sender, e.g., Rogi Kalyan Samiti

11. Individual approach, group approach, mass approach

12. Barriers can be classified at the level of

1. Sender (Physiological barriers: difficulty in hearing, poor speech or hand writing; Psychological barrier: emotional disturbance, stressed, tired; Cultural barrier: customs, beliefs, values, perceptions; Socio-demographic barrier: age, gender, marital status)
2. Receiver (Physiological barriers: impaired hearing and/or eyesight, poor comprehension; Psychological barrier: emotional disturbance, stressed, anxious; Cultural barrier: customs, beliefs, values, perceptions; Socio- demographic barrier: age, gender, marital status, education status)
3. Message (Components of message: difficult language, too much information, complex message, technical jargon, inappropriate weak content, ambiguity)
4. Channel
5. Environment (noise, poor ventilation; overcrowding, lack of privacy etc.)

13. Transtheoretical model, health belief model, theory of reasoned action, diffusion of innovation theory

14. Match the following:

Method in health communication	Items to be matched
Lecture	A way of presentation of facts with organized thoughts and ideas by a qualified person
Tutorial	A small group of learners are guided by a facilitator to help clear doubts, improve understanding and enhance knowledge
Seminar	It consists of group of persons engaged in advanced study of a subject who meet under the general direction of an expert staff member
Case study	An intensive description and analysis of a single individual (unit)
Bedside teaching	Any teaching done in the presence of the patient, regardless of the setting
Simulation	It is an instructional process that substitutes real patient encounters with artificial models, live actors, or virtual reality patients
Role play	It is a form of simulation that focusses attention on the interaction of people with one another
Symposium	A series of prepared talks given by few experts on many aspects of a topic under a chair person
Panel discussion	An orderly and logical conversation on an assigned topic by 4 or more experts with moderator in front of audience
Workshop	A method of group work, active involvement of participants and problem solving with the help of colleagues and professional peers under guidance from experts who act as resource persons
Conference	A formal event where researchers/ academicians present their work in speeches, workshop or posters

15. Communication is a two-way process

16. Helps to discover and correct mistakes in learning

17. All of the above is true for case study

18. Includes teaching done in a conference room in presence of a patient

19. Simulation

20. All of the above

21. a, b, c, d is correct

22. a, b, c is correct

CHAPTER 3

1. Doctor, epidemiologist, public health engineer, town planner, sociologist, economist, health inspector.

2.

Water related diseases	Items to be matched
Typhoid	Water borne disease
Scabies	Water washed disease
Malaria	Water related disease
Guinea worm	Water based disease

3. 40% of COPD deaths, 20% of diabetes deaths, 20% of ischemic heart disease deaths, 19% of lung cancer deaths, 26% of stroke deaths, 30% of lower respiratory infection deaths, 20% of neonatal deaths.
4. Chlorine demand is the difference between the amount of chlorine added to the water, and the amount of residual chlorine remaining at the end of a specific period of contact (usually 60 minutes), at a given temperature and pH of water.
5. 4th, 12%
6. Ash refers to residue from fire used for cooking and heating

   Rubbish includes paper, clothing, bits of wood, metal, glass, dust and dirt etc.

   Garbage is the waste matter arising from preparation, cooking and consumption of food (e.g., waste food, vegetable peelings, organic matter etc.)
7. Children, pregnant women, elderly, people with heart and lung diseases.
8. Free from pathogenic agents, free from harmful chemical substances, pleasant to taste (Free from color and odour) and usable for domestic purposes.
9. Coliforms, fecal streptococci, clostridium perfringens
10. Sources of pollution
    (a) Road and soil dust and its re-suspension
    (b) Vehicular emission
    (c) Domestic fuel burning
    (d) Open waste burning; burning of dry leaves/ garbage
    (e) Construction and demolition activities
    (f) Industrial pollution emission
    (g) Trans state movement of pollutants especially due to burning of crop residue in neighbouring states
    (h) Industrial sources/ thermal power stations
11. Horrocks apparatus
12. Black
13. Blue color, free residual chlorine
14. SO_2
15. Guineaworm
16. Water-tight masonry tank; household sewage; public sewerage system
17. H_2SO_4
18. Dumping, controlled tipping/ sanitary landfill, incineration, composting, manure pits, burial.

19. It is a tool for effective communication of air quality status to people in terms which are easy to understand. It transforms complex air quality data of various pollutants into a single number (index value), nomenclature and colour. Each of the NAQI category is decided based on ambient concentration values of air pollutants and their likely health impacts.
20. Six
21. Draw diagram
22. Good, satisfactory, moderately polluted, poor, very poor, severe.
23. Slow sand filter
24. Oxygen; 5 days; 20 degrees C; aerobic
25. Yes for all
26. Match the following:

AQI score	AQI category
0-50	Good
51-100	Satisfactory
101-200	Moderate
201-300	Poor
301-400	Very poor
401-500	Severe

27. Slow sand filter

28. Bore hole latrine; Hookworm
29. 0.5 mg/l
30. Please indicate the health impact against each AQI category

AQI category	Health impact
Good	Minimal impact
Satisfactory	Minor breathing discomfort to sensitive people
Moderate	Breathing discomfort to people with respiratory problems, asthma and heart diseases
Poor	Breathing discomfort to most people on prolonged exposure
Very poor	Respiratory illness on prolonged exposure
Severe	Affects healthy people and seriously impacts those with existing diseases

31. Scraping off the top portion of the sand bed; backwashing
32. What are the major pollutants from the following sources?

Source of air pollution	Major pollutants
Vehicular/ Transport	CO, NOX, NMVOC's (trace: CH4, CO2, Sox, total suspended particles)
Industrial process	SPM, SOX, NOX, CO2
Agriculture	NH3, N2O, CH4, nitrogen excretions from animal manure
Power	SO2, TSP, PM10
Waste treatment and biomass burning	PM10, PM2.5, CH4, NH3
Residential	Fossil fuel burning, kerosene, wood, crop residue, cow dung cakes
Construction and demolition waste	Greenhouse gas

33. Steel, sugar, paper, cement, fertiliser, copper and aluminium

34. Small depth of water that seals off the night soil from flies. This water is contained in a bent pipe called the trap

35. Chemical coagulant alum, mixing chamber, flocculation chamber

36. Air pollutants (with examples):

(a) Based on source of origin

i. Natural air pollutants emitted from natural sources such as volcanic activity, dust, sea-salt, forest fires, lightening etc.

ii. Anthropogenic air pollutants: emissions from stationary point sources (industry), mobile sources (vehicular emission, marine vessel, airplane), waste disposal landfill, etc

(b) Based on method of origin

i. Primary: emitted directly from any emission source in atmosphere e.g., sulphur dioxide, SO2, CO, lead, ammonia etc.

ii. Secondary: formed by reactions between primary pollutants and normal atmospheric constituents, e.g., ozone, smog etc.

(c) Based on chemical composition

i. Organic: hydrocarbons, aldehydes, ketones, amines, alcohols etc.

ii. Inorganic: carbon compounds (carbonates), nitrogen compounds (NOx, and NH3), sulphur compounds (H2S, SO2, SO2, H2SO4), halogen compounds (HF, HCL etc.), fly ash, silica etc.

(d) Based on state of matter

i. Gaseous: pollutants in the form of gas, SO2, NOx, O3, CO

ii. Particulate air pollutant: microscopic solid or liquid matter suspended in the earths atmosphere, e.g., total suspended particulate matter (TSPM), PM10 (less than 10 micron m in diameter-coarse particles), PM 2.5 (less than 2.5 micron m in diameter- fine particles), PM1.0 (less than 1 micron m in diameter-ultra-fine particles)

37. Production of gas, Durrhams tube

38. Central pollution control board, Environment, forest and climate Change, GoI

39. Health impact of air pollution

(a) Short term exposure: exposure over a few hours or few days: contribute to ear, nose and throat irritation, which usually disappears as air pollution levels decline. It may further cause or aggravate lower respiratory and chronic conditions such as allergies, asthma, chronic obstructive pulmonary disease, and bronchitis. People who have a pre-existing heart condition, it can lead to arrythmias, heart attacks and even premature death.

(b) Long term exposure: increases chances of developing or even dying from a chronic heart disease, respiratory disease, lung infections, lung cancer, diabetes etc. It can have neurological effects in childhood and adolescence, neurodegenerative diseases in adulthood and poorer birth outcomes in terms of low birth weight or per-term labour.

40. a, b, c and d

41. Break point chlorination

42. According to WHO, following steps should be taken for prevention and control of air pollution: containment, replacement, dilution, legislation.

Let's discuss this w.r.t. Delhi and try to place the abovementioned measures in line with AQI

AQI category	Broad procedure	Steps to be taken by the concerned agency
Severe + or Emergency*	Legislation	Stop entry of trucks in to city
		Stop construction activities
		Introduce odd-even scheme
Severe	Legislation	Close brick kilns, power plants, stone crushers
	Replacement	Generation of power from existing natural gas plant instead of coal-based power plant
		Intensify public transport services
	Dilution	Increase frequency of mechanized cleaning of road and sprinkling water on roads
Very poor	Legislation	Stop use of diesel generator sets
		Stop use of coal/ firewood in hotels/restaurants
	Replacement	Increase bus and metro service
Moderate	Legislation	Enforce pollution control in thermal power plant
		Stop plying of visibly polluting vehicles
		Enforce rules for dust control in construction sites
		Regulate truck entry and movement in city
		Enforce ban on firecrackers
	Dilution	Periodic mechanized sweeping on roads and water sprinkling on unpaved roads

(*) A new category Severe + or Emergency category has been added from January 2017

43. **Waste water from community containing solid and liquid excreta is sewage. Sullage is waste water from community that does not contain human excreta.**

44. **True/false**
    (a) False, OT test can assess both free and combined chlorine; OTA can determine free and combined chlorine separately.
    (b) True, the point at which the residual chlorine appears and when all the combined chlorine has been completely destroyed is termed as breakpoint
    (c) True
    (d) False, best around pH of 7 because of predominance of HOCl, at pH of 8.5, HOCl gets ionized to OCl-]
    (e) False; should be amenable to detection by practical, rapid and simple analytical techniques.
    (f) False; easier in rapid sand filter
    (g) True
    (h) True
    (i) True
    (j) True

CHAPTER 4

1. **121,019,3422**
2. **238.4 million to 1210.19 million**

3. USA, Indonesia, Brazil, Pakistan, Bangladesh and Japan.
4. 2.4%, 135.79 million sq. km; 17.5%
5. States: Andhra Pradesh, Arunachal Pradesh, Assam, Bihar, Chhatisgarh, Goa, Gujarat, Haryana, Himachal Pradesh, Jharkhand, Karnataka, Kerala, MP, Maharashtra, Manipur, Meghalaya, Mizoram, Nagaland, Odisha, Punjab, Rajasthan, Sikkim, Tamil Nadu, Telangana, Tripura, Uttarakhand, UP, West Bengal.
   UT: A and N Islands, Chandigarh, D and N Haveli, Daman and Diu, NCT of Delhi, Lakshadweep, Puducherry, Jammu and Kashmir and Ladakh.
6. Demography is the scientific study of human population, its size, composition and distribution
7. Changes in population; composition of population, distribution of population in space
8. Fertility, mortality, marriage, migration and social mobility
9. Changes in population growth rates over time. It describes and analyses the transition from a stable population with high mortality and high fertility to a stable population with low mortality and low fertility
10. Five
11. Match the following:

Stage of demographic cycle	Items to be matched
High stationary	High birth rate and high death rate
Early expanding	Death rate starts to decline and birth rate remains unchanged
Late expanding	Death rate continues to decline and birth rate starts to fall
Low stationary	Low birth rate and low death rate
Declining	Birth rate is lower than death rate

12. 35, 640, 5924, 7936, 6.41 lakh
13. Lesser
14. Declined; 21.54; 17.64
15. Match the following:

State	Items to be matched
Uttar Pradesh	Most populous State
Maharashtra	Second most populous state
Bihar	Third most populous state
West Bengal	Fourth most populous state
Sikkim	Least populous state
Lakshadweep	Least populous UT

16. Brazil
17. 0-6 years
18. 10 years
19. Sex ratio
20. 1 year
21. 1921

22. 20
23. Rural: 24.1, 21.6; Urban: 18.3, 16.7
24. 6.2
25. Rural: 7.8, 6.7; Urban: 5.8, 5.1
26. 50, 32
27. 36, 23
28. Match the following

State	Birth rate
Delhi	14.7
Uttar Pradesh	25.6
Bihar	26.2
Rajasthan	24
Kerala	13.9
Maharashtra	15.6

29. 113
30. 21
31. Rs. 0/-; free of charge
32. All of the above
33. Without
34. Mid-year population is defined as population at the mid-point of the year, i.e. 1st July of the year provided by population projections based on 2011). (Ref: Source: Population Projections for India and States 2011–2036, Report of the Technical Group on Population Projections constituted by National Commission on Population, July. 2020)
35. 51.54%; 48.46%
36. 940
37. Match the following:

State	Sex Ratio
Delhi	866
Uttar Pradesh	908
Bihar	916
Rajasthan	926
Kerala	1084
Haryana	877
Daman and Diu	618

38. 914
39. 13.1%; 158.8 million
40. Aged seven years and above, who can both read and write with understanding in any language. A person who can read but cannot write is not literate. To be classified as literate, it is not necessary to have received any formal education or acquired any minimum educational standard.

41. 74%; 26%
42. 82.14%; 65.46%
43. Kerala, 93.91%; Lakshadweep, 92.28%
44. Bihar, 63.82%
45. 382; 325
46. Match the following:

State/Union Territory	Population density per square km
NCT of Delhi	11, 297
India	382
Chandigarh	9252
Bihar	1102
Maharashtra	365
Andaman and Nicobar Islands	46

47. True/false for the following statements:
    (a) True
    (b) False; not necessary
    (c) True
    (d) True
48. Fertility refers to number of children borne by a woman. A woman's reproductive period ranges from 15 to 49 years which implies that a woman can give birth during this period. Fertility depends on a host of factors some of which are age at marriage, duration of marriage, level of literacy, economic status, spacing between children, use of contraceptives, caste, religion, nutrition etc.
49. Birth rate, General fertility rate (GFR), General marital fertility rate (GMFR), Age-specific fertility rate (ASFR), Age-specific marital fertility rate (ASFMR), Total fertility rate (TFR), Total marital fertility rate (TFMR), Gross reproduction rate (GRR), Net reproduction rate (NRR)
50. GFR is the number of live births per thousand women in the reproductive age group of 15-49 years
51. According to SRS statistical report 2018, current GFR is 70.4 per thousand women, rural: 77.4, urban: 56.7
52. 90.3 to 72.4
53. ASFR is the number of live births to 1000 women in a year in a specified age group
54. ASFR increases and reached peak in the age group 25-29 years and shows a steep decline thereafter.

Age group	Total	Rural	Urban
15-19	12.2	13.5	8.4
20-24	122.9	135.9	91.5
25-29	146.4	160.1	119.1
30-34	94.7	101.3	81.7
35-39	36.9	40.7	30.2
40-44	12.7	14.8	9.1
45-49	4.4	5.5	2.4

55. TFR represents average number of children expected to be born per woman during her entire span of reproductive period assuming that the age specific fertility rates, to which she is exposed to, continue to be the same and that there is no mortality. It is the cumulative value of the age specific fertility rates at the end of the child bearing ages.

56. According to SRS statistical report 2018, TFR for India is 2.2 per woman and varies from 2.4 in rural areas to 1.7 in urban areas.

57. GRR measures average number of female children a woman is expected to give birth during her entire span of reproductive period assuming that the age specific fertility rates, to which she is exposed to, continue to be the same and that there is no mortality.

58. According to SRS statistical report 2018, GRR for India is 1.0 per woman and varies from 1.1 in rural areas to 0.8 in urban areas.

59. Life expectancy at birth for the period 2014-2018:

(a) 69.4 years
(b) 68 years
(c) 72.6 years
(d) 68.2 years
(e) 70.7 years

CHAPTER 5

1. **Vectors of public health importance.**
   (a) Anopheles, Aedes, Culex, House fly, Sand fly, Head louse, body louse, rat flea
   (b) Hard tick, soft tick, Itch mite, Cyclops
2. **Common species of the following genus:**
   (a) Anopheles Culicifacies, Stephensi, fluviatilis, sundaicus, philippinensis, minimus
   (b) Aedes aegypti, albopictus
   (c) Culex fatigans, vishnui, tritaeniorhyncus
   (d) Musca domestica, nebulo, sorbens
   (e) Phlebotomus Argentipes, papatasii
   (f) Pediculus capitis
   (g) Cheopis, astia, braziliensis
   (h) Diphyllobothrium karvei
3. **Identify the vector:**
   (a) Anopheles
   (b) Anopheles
   (c) Culex
   (d) Aedes
   (e) Mansonia
   (f) Culex, Aedes, Mansonia
   (g) Adult Anopheles
   (h) Adult Aedes, white stripes on black coloured body
   (i) Gonotrophic cycle
   (j) Sandfly
   (k) Louse
   (l) Rat flea
   (m) Hard tick, four pair of legs, scutum
   (n) Soft tick, four pair of legs, does not
   (o) Cyclops

4. **Match the following:**

Vector (at different stage of development)	Identifying feature
Egg of Aedes	Cigar shaped/Boat shaped
Eggs of anopheles	Have lateral floats
Eggs of Mansonia	Star shaped clusters
Eggs of Culex	Eggs laid in clusters/rafts
Larvae of Anopheles	Lay horizontally without a siphon tube
Larvae of Aedes, Culex, Mansonia	Suspended in water with siphon tube on 8th abdominal segment
Adult Anopheles	At rest, sits at an angle of 45 degrees/Spotted wings
Adult Aedes	Tiger mosquito
Sand fly	Hairy antennae
Louse	Dorso-ventrally flattened body

5. **Please indicate vector for the following potential breeding sites:**

Breeding place	Vector
Decaying vegetables and fruits (including peels)	Housefly
Broken tyre	Aedes
Dirty polluted water	Culex
Garbage	Housefly
Dirty water puddles	Culex
Open drains	Culex
Cesspool	Culex
Clean slow-moving water	Anopheles
Overhead tank	Aedes
Dead and decaying organic matter	Housefly
Human excreta	Housefly
Manure of animals	Housefly
Freshwater collection	Anopheles
Septic tank (if open and leaking)	Culex
Flower pot	Aedes
Desert cooler	Aedes
Artificial collection of water	Aedes
Salt water collection	Anopheles

6. **Malaria, filaria (not in India)**
7. **Bancroftian filariasis, Japanese encephalitis, West nile fever, Viral arthritis**
8. **Aedes transmits Dengue, DHF, Chikungunya, rift valley fever, filaria and yellow fever**
9. **Typhoid, Cholera, Amoebiases, conjunctivitis**
10. **Kala azar and oriental sore**
11. **a, b, c, d are correct**
12. **Rat flea.**

13. **Hard tick transmits tick typhus, viral encephalitis, viral hemorrhagic fever (KFD), tularemia, tick paralysis, human babesiosis. Soft tick transmits Q fever, relapsing fever, KFD**
14. **Itch mite.**
15. **Match the following:**

Vector	Flight range
Anopheles	3-12 km
Aedes	Less than 100 m
Culex	11 km
Sand fly	Mostly hop within 50 metres
Rat fles	Hops up to 4 inches

16. **Please indicate true or false for the following statements.**
    (a) False
    (b) True
    (c) True
    (d) True
    (e) False, both adulticide and larvicide
    (f) True
    (g) False; 1ppm
    (h) True
    (i) Truee
17. **Aedes aegypti index is the ratio which is expressed as percentage of houses in a limited well-defined area on the premises of which actual breeding is found and the total number of houses examined in that area. It should be less than 1% in endemic areas to ensure control of yellow fever**
18. **Fleas which ingest plague bacilli become blocked due to multiplication of bacilli in their stomach. Such fleas are called as 'blocked fleas'. Blockage of the food passage renders the flea unable to obtain anymore blood feeds. Because of hunger, flea begins to bite more ferociously and makes frantic efforts to suck blood. Each time it bites, instead of sucking blood, it injects plague bacilli into the wound. Blocked fleas play a huge role in spread of plague**
19. **Scabies**
20. **IVM is a rational decision-making process to optimize the use of resources for vector control. It includes implementation of all feasible strategies safely with or without insecticides to manage vector population in such a way so that disease transmission is kept under check. It also includes management of insecticide resistance.**
21. **Tools of vector control.**
    (a) Source reduction and environmental management
    (b) Personal protection
    (c) Biological
    (d) Chemical: larvicide, adulticide
22. **Insecticide treated nets**
23. **Inspection of tyre depots**
24. **Source reduction method**
25. **Source reduction, solid waste management, modification of man-made breeding sites and improved housing design**
26. **Larvivorus fish**
27. **Larval**

28. **Biological agents used under NVBDCP for vector control.**
    (a) Larvivorus fish: gambusia affinis, poecilia reticulata
    (b) Bacillus thuringenesis, H-14 and Bacillus sphaericus
29. **Water tank of the NICD cooler is completely covered to prevent the entry of mosquitoes in the water tank for breeding. Weekly cleaning of tank is not required. Since there's no breeding, no need of chemical larvicide.**

CHAPTER 6

1. **Biomedical Waste refers to any waste that is generated during the diagnosis, treatment or immunization of human beings or animals or research activities pertaining thereto or in the production or testing of biological or in health camps.**
2. **10-15%**
3. **Four**
4. **Yellow, red, white and blue**
5.

Category	Type of waste
Yellow	(a) Human anatomical waste (b) Animal anatomical waste (c) Soiled waste (d) Expired or discarded medicines (e) Chemical solid waste (f) Chemical liquid waste (g) Discarded linen, mattresses, beddings contaminated with blood or body fluid (h) Microbiology, biotechnology and other clinical laboratory waste
Red	Contaminated recyclable waste
White	Waste sharps including metals
Blue	Glassware and metallic body implants

6. **Radioactive waste, wastes covered under municipal solid waste rules, lead acid batteries, hazardous chemicals waste, e-waste, hazardous micro-organism**
7. **Bio-medical waste treatment and disposal facility refers to any facility wherein treatment, disposal of biomedical waste or processes incidental to such treatment and disposal is carried out, and includes common bio-medical waste treatment facilities**
8. **Segregation, collection, pre-treatment, transportation within the health care facility, storage, treatment and disposal**
9. **Point of generation**
10. **Point of generation of bio-medical waste refers to location where wastes are initially generated while providing treatment to the patient. It is under the control of treating doctor or nurse.**
11. **Color coded bags/bins/container**
12. **True or false:**
    (a) False; it should be stored in central waste collection rooms
    (b) False; it should not be stored there, should be stored separately
    (c) False; it should be transported in closed trolleys designated for the purpose of bio medical waste collection only
    (d) True
    (e) True
13. **Type of waste segregated in yellow bag.**
    (a) Human anatomical waste: Human tissue, amputated limb, products of conception, placenta, extracted tooth

(b) Animal anatomical waste: Animal viscera, animal carcasses

(c) Soiled waste: Dressing soiled with blood/ pus, soiled plaster cast, used and soiled caps, shoe-cover, mask and disposable gowns, used diapers and sanitary pads.

(d) Expired or discarded medicines: Expired antibiotic, Expired chemotherapeutic agents along with vial.

(e) Chemical solid waste: Chemical used in production of biological, discarded containers of chemicals and disinfectants etc.

(f) Chemical liquid waste: Discarded formalin, discarded povidone iodine, aspirate from ascitic and pleural tap

(g) Discarded linen, mattresses, beddings contaminated with blood or body fluid: Discarded mattress, bedsheet, bedding, mask, reusable gown

(h) Microbiology, biotechnology and other clinical laboratory waste: Used culture plates from microbiology lab, Cell culture plates used for vaccine production, vaccines, waste blood bags, vacutainers, vials with blood samples

14. Please indicate the type of bag/bin/ container used for storage and method of ultimate disposal.

Type of biomedical waste	Type of bin used for storage and ultimate disposal
(i) Human anatomical waste	Yellow bag; stored in yellow bin and handed over to CBWTF
(j) Animal anatomical waste	Yellow bag; stored in yellow bin and handed over to CBWTF
(k) Soiled waste	Yellow bag; stored in yellow bin and handed over to CBWTF
(l) Expired or discarded medicines	Yellow bag; stored in yellow bin and handed over to CBWTF
(m) Chemical solid waste	Yellow bag/ container (for liquid) and handed over to CBWTF
(n) Chemical liquid waste	Liquid waste collected through a separate collection system for pre-treatment (through neutralization/ precipitation followed by disinfection) before mixing with rest of waste water for further treatment
(o) Discarded linen, mattresses, beddings contaminated with blood or body fluid	Disinfect with non-chlorinated chemical and hand over to CBWTF for incineration
(p) Microbiology, biotechnology and other clinical laboratory waste	Yellow bag; pre-treatment by autoclave/ microwave/ hydroclave and hand over to CBWTF

15. Only a can be incinerated

16. All of the above

17. Both A and B

18. A, B, C and D

19. No more than three quarters full.

20. Biohazard, cytotoxic hazard.

21. No; within 75 km

22.

1. Provide adequate personal protective equipment (PPE) to the staff handling bio medical waste including, heavy duty gloves, gum boots or safety shoes, face mask, head cap, splash proof gowns or aprons, disposal gloves.
2. Conducting health check-up of all employees at the time of induction followed by regular health check-up once every year.
3. Immunization of this staff against hepatitis B and tetanus toxoid.

23. Newspaper, paper, cardboard boxes, plastic water bottles, aluminium cans of soft drinks, packaging materials, food containers after emptying residual food, food waste from leftover food from hospital kitchen, construction and demolition waste.

CHAPTER 7

1. **Foods can be classified as:**
   (a) Foods of animal origin and plant origin
   (b) Protein, carbohydrate, fats, protein, minerals
   (c) Energy giving foods, body building foods and protective foods
   (d) Cereals and millets, pulses, vegetables, nuts and oilseeds, fruits, animal foods, fats and oils, sugar and jaggery, condiments and spices, miscellaneous foods
2. **Proteins, fats and carbohydrates because they form main bulk of food.**
3. **Essential amino acids: leucine, isoleucine, lysine, methionine, phenylalanine, threonine, valine, tryptophan and histidine. Non-essential amino acids: arginine, asparaginic acid, serine, glutamic acid, proline and glycine.**
4. **All the essential amino acids in amounts corresponding to human needs.**
5. **Milk, meat, eggs, fish, cereals, pulses, nuts, soyabean etc.**
6. **When two or more vegetarian foods are eaten their proteins supplement one another and provide a protein comparable to animal protein w.r.t. essential amino acids. e.g. cereals are deficient in lysine and threonine and pulses are deficient in methionine, when they are eaten together as a mixed diet, deficiency of essential amino acid in one item is compensated by that in other.**
7. **Saturated fatty acids, monounsaturated fatty acids (MUFA), polyunsaturated fatty acids (PUFA)**
8. **Vanaspati is prepared by hydrogenation of vegetable oils. During hydrogenation, liquid oils become solid because mono- and poly unsaturated fatty acids are converted to saturated fatty acids and trans fatty acids. Saturated fatty acids and trans fatty acids increase the risk of heart disease. Vanaspati is used as a substitute for ghee in cooking and preparation of bakery products, sweets and snack foods. Therefore, consumption of these foods should be limited.**
9. **Unsaturated fatty acids (MUFA and PUFA) containing one or more double bonds in trans configuration.**
10. **Cis configuration.**
11. **Cannot synthesize.**
12. **Arachidonic acid, eicosapentaenoic acid (EPA), docosapentaenoic acid (DPA), docosahexaenoic acid (DHA).**
13. **5:1 to 10:1.**
14. **Vegetable oil, vanaspati, ghee.**
15. **Butter, ghee, coconut oil, palm kernel oil.**
16. **Vanaspati.**
17. **Soyabean oil, canola oil, mustard oil, flax seed oil.**
18. **cotton seed oil, corn oil, safflower oil, sunflower oil.**
19. **LA (cereals, millets), ALA (green leafy vegetables, fenugreek, soyabean flax seed, mustard seed).**
20. **LA, ALA and DHA.**
21.
    1. Ground nut or Sesame or rice bran + Mustard.
    2. Ground nut or Sesame or rice bran + Canola
    3. Ground nut or Sesame or rice bran + Soyabean
    4. Palmolein + Soyabean
    5. Safflower or Sunflower + Palmolein + Mustard
22. **Indicate true or false against each of the following:**
   (a) False; decreases
   (b) True
   (c) False; increases
   (d) True
   (e) True
   (f) True
   (g) True

23. **Sugars, cereals, millets, roots and tubers, pulses and legumes and limited extent from vegetables, fruits and dairy.**
24. **55-60%, 10-15%, 20-30%.**
25. **Glycaemic index of a food is the blood glucose response after consuming a carbohydrate containing food relative to a carbohydrate containing reference food (usually 50 gm available carbohydrate). Glycaemic load considers glycaemic index and total amount of available carbohydrate present in the food consumed.**
26. **Glycaemic index, glycaemic load, portion size of food consumed, type of carbohydrate component, amount of protein and fat, nutrient interactions, type of food processing etc.**
27. **Parboiling is a method to preserve the nutritive quality of rice. This process comprises of following steps-**

Steps of parboiling	Nutritional significance
Soaking the unhusked rice in hot water at 65-70 deg. C for 3-4 hours	Swells the grain
Drain the water and steam the soaked paddy in the same container for 5-10 minutes	Vitamins and minerals present in outer aleurone layer of the rice grain are driven into the endosperm
Dried	Germ gets attached more firmly to the grain and it hardens the grain
Home pounded or milled	Nutrients are not removed due to above steps

28. **Dietary fibre is endogenous edible component present in plant materials or analogous carbohydrates which are resistant to digestion by the enzymes secreted in small intestine.**
29. **Insoluble dietary fibre promote laxation, speed up intestinal transit time, add bulk to stool, thereby preventing constipation, hemorrhoids and diverticulitis. Soluble dietary fibre delays gastric emptying and intestinal transit time, reduce blood cholesterol levels. It reduces the risk of hyperlipedemia, hypercholesterolemia and hyperglycemia.**
30. **Whole wheat, ragi, bajra, Bengal gram, soya bean, tamarind leaves, drumstick leaves, drumstick, sapota, carrot, fenugreek seeds, mustard seeds, almond, dried oyster mushroom.**
31. **Please indicate relevant nutrient responsible for the following deficiency diseases.**

Deficiency disease	Nutrient
Rickets	Vitamin D
Scurvy	Vitamin C
Angular stomatitis	Riboflavin
Peripheral neuritis	Pyridoxine
Anaemia	Folate
Bitot spots	Vitamin A
Pellagra	Niacin
Conjunctival xerosis	Vitamin A
Anaemia	Vitamin B12
Beriberi	Thiamine
Osteomalacia	Vitamin D
Night blindness	Vitamin A
Dental caries	Deficiency of fluorine
Genu valgum	Excess of fluorine

Section II

Family Adoption Programme

Section II: Family Adoption Programme

	Topic	Competency	Signature of Supervisor with Date	Grade
.	**Record of Family Adoption Programme Visits**	FAP		
	An Overview of Field Practice Area	-		
		FAMILY NUMBER 1		
1.	Identification and Demographic Data	CM 1.9- Demonstrate the role of effective communication skills in health in a simulated environment CM 2.1- Describe the steps and perform clinico socio-cultural and demographic assessment of the individual, family and community		
2.	Socio-Economic Data	CM 1.9, CM 2.2- Describe the socio-cultural factors, family (types), its role in health and disease and demonstrate in a simulated environment the correct assessment of socio-economic status		
3.	Environmental Data	CM 1.9, CM 3.5- Describe the standards of housing and the effect of housing on health, IM 25.13- Counsel the patient and family on prevention of various infections due to environmental issues		
4.	Socio-Cultural Environment	CM 1.9, CM 2.2, CM 2.3- Describe and demonstrate in a simulated environment the assessment of barriers to good health and health seeking behavior CM 10.3 Describe local customs and practices during pregnancy, childbirth, lactation and child feeding practices		

5.	Dietary Assessment	CM 1.9, CM 5.2- Describe and demonstrate the correct method of performing a nutritional assessment of individuals, families and the community by using the appropriate method CM 5.4- Plan and recommend a suitable diet for the individuals and families based on local availability of foods and economic status, etc in a simulated environment PE 9.4- Elicit, Document and present an appropriate nutritional history and perform a dietary recall PE 9.5 Calculate the age-related calorie requirement in health and disease PE 9.7 Plan an appropriate diet in health and disease		
6.	Immunization	CM 1.9, CM 1.10- Demonstrate the important aspects of the doctor patient relationship in a simulated environment, CM 10.5 Describe Universal Immunization Program; Integrated Management of Neonatal and Childhood Illness (IMNCI) and other existing Programs.		
7.	Health Records of Vulnerable Groups A. ANC/ B. PNC C. Under-Five Child D. Adolescent Health Record (10-19 years) E. Eligible Couple Health Record F. Geriatric Health Record (60 years and above)	CM 1.9, CM 1.10, CM 10.3 PE 18.3 - Conduct Antenatal examination of women independently and apply at-risk approach in antenatal care PE 18.6 - Perform Postnatal assessment of newborn and mother, provide advice on breast feeding, weaning and on family planning OG 19.2- Counsel in a simulated environment, contraception and puerperal sterilization PE 8.4- Elicit history on the Complementary Feeding habits, PE 8.5- Counsel and educate mothers on the best practices in Complimentary feeding, PE 9.6 Assess and classify the nutrition status of infants, children and adolescents and recognize deviations CM 12.2- Describe health problems of aged population CM 12.3- Describe the prevention of health problems of aged population		
8.	Summary, Conclusion and Recommendations	-		

FAMILY NUMBER 2				
1.	Identification and Demographic Data	CM 1.9- Demonstrate the role of effective communication skills in health in a simulated environment CM 2.1- Describe the steps and perform clinico socio-cultural and demographic assessment of the individual, family and community		
2.	Socio-Economic Data	CM 1.9, CM 2.2- Describe the socio-cultural factors, family (types), its role in health and disease and demonstrate in a simulated environment the correct assessment of socio-economic status		
3.	Environmental Data	CM 1.9, CM 3.5- Describe the standards of housing and the effect of housing on health, IM 25.13- Counsel the patient and family on prevention of various infections due to environmental issues		
4.	Socio-Cultural Environment	CM 1.9, CM 2.2, CM 2.3- Describe and demonstrate in a simulated environment the assessment of barriers to good health and health seeking behavior CM 10.3 Describe local customs and practices during pregnancy, childbirth, lactation and child feeding practices		
5.	Dietary Assessment	CM 1.9, CM 5.2- Describe and demonstrate the correct method of performing a nutritional assessment of individuals, families and the community by using the appropriate method CM 5.4- Plan and recommend a suitable diet for the individuals and families based on local availability of foods and economic status, etc in a simulated environment PE 9.4- Elicit, Document and present an appropriate nutritional history and perform a dietary recall PE 9.5 Calculate the age-related calorie requirement in health and disease PE 9.7 Plan an appropriate diet in health and disease		
6.	Immunization	CM 1.9, CM 1.10- Demonstrate the important aspects of the doctor patient relationship in a simulated environment, CM 10.5 Describe Universal Immunization Program; Integrated Management of Neonatal and Childhood Illness (IMNCI) and other existing Programs.		

7.	Health Records of Vulnerable Groups A. ANC/ B. PNC C. Under-Five Child D. Adolescent Health Record (10-19 years) E. Eligible Couple Health Record F. Geriatric Health Record (60 years and above)	CM 1.9, CM 1.10, CM 10.3 PE 18.3 - Conduct Antenatal examination of women independently and apply at-risk approach in antenatal care PE 18.6 - Perform Postnatal assessment of newborn and mother, provide advice on breast feeding, weaning and on family planning OG 19.2- Counsel in a simulated environment, contraception and puerperal sterilization PE 8.4- Elicit history on the Complementary Feeding habits, PE 8.5- Counsel and educate mothers on the best practices in Complimentary feeding, PE 9.6 Assess and classify the nutrition status of infants, children and adolescents and recognize deviations CM 12.2- Describe health problems of aged population CM 12.3- Describe the prevention of health problems of aged population		
8.	Summary, Conclusion and Recommendations	-		
FAMILY NUMBER 3				
1.	Identification and Demographic Data	CM 1.9- Demonstrate the role of effective communication skills in health in a simulated environment CM 2.1- Describe the steps and perform clinico socio-cultural and demographic assessment of the individual, family and community		
2.	Socio-Economic Data	CM 1.9, CM 2.2- Describe the socio-cultural factors, family (types), its role in health and disease and demonstrate in a simulated environment the correct assessment of socio-economic status		
3.	Environmental Data	CM 1.9, CM 3.5- Describe the standards of housing and the effect of housing on health, IM 25.13- Counsel the patient and family on prevention of various infections due to environmental issues		
4.	Socio-Cultural Environment	CM 1.9, CM 2.2, CM 2.3- Describe and demonstrate in a simulated environment the assessment of barriers to good health and health seeking behavior CM 10.3 Describe local customs and practices during pregnancy, childbirth, lactation and child feeding practices		

5.	Dietary Assessment	CM 1.9, CM 5.2- Describe and demonstrate the correct method of performing a nutritional assessment of individuals, families and the community by using the appropriate method CM 5.4- Plan and recommend a suitable diet for the individuals and families based on local availability of foods and economic status, etc in a simulated environment PE 9.4- Elicit, Document and present an appropriate nutritional history and perform a dietary recall PE 9.5 Calculate the age-related calorie requirement in health and disease PE 9.7 Plan an appropriate diet in health and disease		
6.	Immunization	CM 1.9, CM 1.10- Demonstrate the important aspects of the doctor patient relationship in a simulated environment CM 10.5 Describe Universal Immunization Program; Integrated Management of Neonatal and Childhood Illness (IMNCI) and other existing Programs		
7.	Health Records of Vulnerable Groups A. ANC/ B. PNC C. Under-Five Child D. Adolescent Health Record (10-19 years) E. Eligible Couple Health Record F. Geriatric Health Record (60 years and above)	CM 1.9, CM 1.10, CM 10.3 PE 18.3 - Conduct Antenatal examination of women independently and apply at-risk approach in antenatal care PE 18.6 - Perform Postnatal assessment of newborn and mother, provide advice on breast feeding, weaning and on family planning OG 19.2- Counsel in a simulated environment, contraception and puerperal sterilization PE 8.4- Elicit history on the Complementary Feeding habits, PE 8.5- Counsel and educate mothers on the best practices in Complimentary feeding, PE 9.6 Assess and classify the nutrition status of infants, children and adolescents and recognize deviations CM 12.2- Describe health problems of aged population CM 12.3- Describe the prevention of health problems of aged population		
8.	Summary, Conclusion and Recommendations	-		
9.	Community Diagnosis	CM 17.2- Describe community diagnosis		
Annexure (1 to 7) ***Viva Voce***				

Record of Family Adoption Programme Visits

CURRICULUM FOR FAMILY ADOPTION PROGRAMME (FAP)

The National Medical Commission (NMC) envisages the FAP as an opportunity for the Institute(s) to discharge its social responsibility and as a critical platform to facilitate *Authentic learning* of the under-graduate students to sensitize them with the real-life challenges of working for the Universal health coverage (UHC). The FAP will present an opportunity for the students to experience the health inequities and understand the social factors contributing to it.

The FAP is expected to complement the other Competency-Based Medical Education (CBME) reforms e.g., posting of interns in the public health facilities under the Compulsory Rotating Medical Internship (CRMI) and the District Residency Program (DRP) for producing socially-responsive competent Indian Medical Graduates who would contribute for the cause of reducing inequities in health and society in the future. Institute(s) should leverage collaboration and partnership with the community and the public health care delivery system for effective implementation of the FAP so as to serve the larger purpose of the CBME reforms in the country.

TARGETS TO BE ACHIEVED BY STUDENTS

Phase 1:

1. Rapport building and connect with the families
2. Learning communication skills and inspire trust building amongst families
3. Understand the dynamics of community set-up of that region
4. Mobilize families for participation in Screening programs
5. Undertake detailed family study and prepare the family diagnosis to identify diseases/ ill-health/ malnutrition of allotted families/ risk factors / scope for health promotion
6. Formulate objectives to be achieved for each family

Phase 2:

1. Continue active involvement to become the first doctor /reference point of the family by continued active interaction
2. Ensure follow-up of members from adopted families for vaccination, growth monitoring and promotion, menstrual hygiene, IFA prophylaxis, health lifestyle adoption, nutrition, vector control measures, compliance to medications etc.
3. Work collaboratively with adopted families to achieve the formulated objectives
4. Inform families about ongoing government sponsored health related programs
5. Ensure appropriate referral of family members considering their choice for additional or annual screening at higher health facilities.

Phase 3:

1. Work collaboratively with adopted families to achieve the formulated objectives
2. Observation of services delivered at the community level during Village Health Nutrition Days (VHND), Community-Based Events (CBEs), Health and Wellness Centres (HWC) camps under the different national health program
3. Build understanding regarding work of frontline workers (ANM, ASHA/USHA, AWW, MPW) through interaction
4. Build understanding around intersectoral action for health through Local self-governing bodies, NGOs, SHGs etc for health promotion
5. Undertake short term action projects for improving health in the adopted families or community
6. Analysis of their own involvement and impact on improving the health conditions in the adopted families

Final visit to have last round of active interaction with families - prepare a report to be submitted to department addressing:

1. Improvement in overall health of the family
2. Immunization
3. Sanitation
4. De-addiction
5. Whether healthy lifestyles like reading good books. Sports/yoga activities have been inculcated in the house-holds
6. Improvement in anaemia, tuberculosis control
7. Health awareness
8. Any other issues
9. Role of the student in supporting family during illness / medical emergency
10. Social responsibility in the form of environment protection programme in form of plantation drive (medicinal plants/trees) cleanliness and sanitation drive with the initiative of the medical student

Phase wise competencies to be achieved through the FAP

Professional year and topics for visit	Competency	Objectives	Suggested T-L methods	Suggested assessment methods	Teaching hours
First year Visit 1– Rapport building with the Families and Orientation Socio-demographic and socio-economic profile Visit 2– Environmental health Drinking Water supply, Sanitation and Vector control Visit 3– Individual health profile including Anthropome try Visit 4– Addictions Tobacco, Alcohol, Screen addiction and other addictions	Collect demographic profile of allotted families, take history and conduct clinical examination of all family members	By the end of this visit, students should be able to compile the basic demographic profile of allocated family members and formulate objectives for each family	Family survey, Screening camps Field visit clinics	Community case presentation, OSPE, Observation, FAP logbook Multi-source feedback Reflections Case studies	Total 24 hours [A minimum of 4 visits of full day of around 6 hours] OR [If 3 hours visit then 8 visits to be conducted]
	Mobilize the adopted family members for participation in screening camps and coordinate treatment of adopted family under overall guidance of mentor	By the end of this visit, students should be able to report the basic health profile and treatment history of allocated family members	Screening camps Field visit clinics PLA techniques (sorting, ranking etc.)	Community case presentation OSPE, Observation, FAP logbook Multi-source feedback Reflection case studies	
	Maintain communication and follow-up of remedial measures	By the end of this visit, students should be able to provide details of communication maintained with family members for follow-up of treatment and suggested remedial neasures	Family survey, Screening camps Field visit clinics Reporting of follow-up visits	Community case presentation. OSPE, FAP logbook based verification of competency, Multi-source feedback Reflections	
	Take part in health promotion, environment protection and sustenance activities	By the end of this visit, students should be able to report the activities undertaken for health promotion, environment protection and sustenance like tree plantation, herbal plantation activities conducted in the community	Participation in and process documentation of activities (NSS activities) along with reporting of case studies	Community case presentation. OSPE, Observation, FAP logbook Multi-source feedback Reflections Case studies	

Second year Visit 5– Healthy Lifestyle Dietary assessment, Physical activity and Exercise Visit 6– Micronutrient deficiencies- Nutritional anemia, Iodine deficiency disorders Care of under-5 children Visit 7– Feeding, vaccination, HBYC Maternal health Visit 8– Care of Pregnant and Lactating mothers	Take history and conduct clinical examination of all family members	By the end of this visit, students should be able to compile the updated medical history of family members through family follow-up	Family survey, Field visit clinics Referral and follow-up	Community case presentation. OSPE, Observation, FAP logbook Multi-source feedback Reflections Case studies	Total 24 hours [A minimum of 4 visits of full day of around 6 hours] OR [If 3 hours visit then 8 visits to be conducted]
	Facilitate checkup and/or referral of adopted family under overall guidance of mentor	By the end of this visit, students should be able to report the details of clinical examination and investigations like HB %, blood group urine routine and blood sugar or any other investigation along with treatment history. compliance to treatment, of allocated family members	Field visit clinics Referral Field visit clinics Reporting of follow-up visits	Community case presentation. OSPE, FAP logbook Case studies Multi-source feedback	
	Maintain communication and follow-up of remedial measures	By the end of this visit, students should be able to provide details of communication maintained with family members including information about National programs provided.. Students should also be able to follow up on treatment and suggested remedial measures under the guidance of a mentor. Documentation of referral in logbook	Family survey. Screening camps Field visit clinics Reporting of follow-up visits	Community case presentation. OSPE, FAP logbook based verification of competency, Multi-source feedback Reflections	

Third year Visit 9– Communicable diseases - Tuberculosis, Influenza and others Visit 10– Non-communicable diseases - HTN, DM and others Visit 11– Adolescent health / School health Menstrual hygiene, Life skills Visit 12– Healthy ageing Health care of the Elderly Visit 13– Mental health Healthy coping strategies and Resilience Visit 14– Well-being of the Families Final visit and Report submission	Take history and conduct clinical examination of all family members and facilitate health check-up if required	By the end of this visit, students should be able to maintain follow-up with the families and update the medical history of family members	Family survey, Field visit clinics Referral and follow-up	Community case presentation. OSPE, Observation, FAP logbook Multi-source feedback Reflections Case studies	Total 36 hours [A minimum of 6 visits of full day of around 6 hours] OR [If 3 hours visit then 12 visits to be conducted]
	Maintain communication and follow-up of remedial measures	By the end of this visit, students should be able to provide details of communication maintained with family members and collaborative efforts undertaken with family members for improving their health.	Family survey, Field visit clinics Referral and tracking Reporting of follow up visits.	Community case presentation. OSPE, Observation, FAP logbook based verification of competency, Multi-source feedback Reflections	
	Counsel the family members of allotted families and analyze the health trajectory of adopted family under overall guidance of mentor	By the end of this visit, students should able to analyze and report the findings of short term action projects and its effect on health trajectory at individual Family and community level	Participation in and process documentation of activities (NSS activities) along with reporting of photographic evidences, Small group discussion (report of the health trajectory of adopted family)	Community case presentation. OSPE, Logbook based verification of competency. Observation Viva-voce Multi-source feedback Reflections	
	Work as a member of Health Team and facilitate intersectoral action for health	By the end of this visit, students should able to report the role of various frontline functionaries' delivery primary health care and Local self-governing bodies, NGOs, SHGs etc. for health promotion	Observation and reporting of events Exposure visits Interaction with frontline functionaries	Logbook based verification of competency, Observation Viva-voce Multi-source feedback Reflections	

FIRST PROFESSIONAL YEAR

Visit number:

Date of Visit:

Objective of Visit:

Activities conducted and Problems Identified:

Family 1:

Family 2:

Family 3:

Action taken for the problems:

Family 1:

Family 2:

Family 3:

Student's Reflection for the Visit:

Supervisor's Grading and Signature with Date:

FIRST PROFESSIONAL YEAR

Visit number:

Date of Visit:

Objective of Visit:

Activities conducted and Problems Identified:

Family 1:

Family 2:

Family 3:

Action taken for the problems:

Family 1:

Family 2:

Family 3:

Student's Reflection for the Visit:

Supervisor's Grading and Signature with Date:

FIRST PROFESSIONAL YEAR

Visit number:

Date of Visit:

Objective of Visit:

Activities conducted and Problems Identified:

Family 1:

Family 2:

Family 3:

Action taken for the problems:

Family 1:

Family 2:

Family 3:

Student's Reflection for the Visit:

Supervisor's Grading and Signature with Date:

FIRST PROFESSIONAL YEAR

Visit number :

Date of Visit :

Objective of Visit:

Activities conducted and Problems Identified:

Family 1:

Family 2:

Family 3:

Action taken for the problems:

Family 1:

Family 2:

Family 3:

Student's Reflection for the Visit:

Supervisor's Grading and Signature with Date:

FIRST PROFESSIONAL YEAR

Visit number:

Date of Visit:

Objective of Visit:

Activities conducted and Problems Identified:

Family 1:

Family 2:

Family 3:

Action taken for the problems:

Family 1:

Family 2:

Family 3:

Student's Reflection for the Visit:

Supervisor's Grading and Signature with Date:

FIRST PROFESSIONAL YEAR

Visit number:

Date of Visit:

Objective of Visit:

Activities conducted and Problems Identified:

Family 1:

Family 2:

Family 3:

Action taken for the problems:

Family 1:

Family 2:

Family 3:

Student's Reflection for the Visit:

Supervisor's Grading and Signature with Date:

FIRST PROFESSIONAL YEAR

Visit number:

Date of Visit:

Objective of Visit:

Activities conducted and Problems Identified:

Family 1:

Family 2:

Family 3:

Action taken for the problems:

Family 1:

Family 2:

Family 3:

Student's Reflection for the Visit:

Supervisor's Grading and Signature with Date:

FIRST PROFESSIONAL YEAR

Visit number:

Date of Visit:

Objective of Visit:

Activities conducted and Problems Identified:

Family 1:

Family 2:

Family 3:

Action taken for the problems:

Family 1:

Family 2:

Family 3:

Student's Reflection for the Visit:

Supervisor's Grading and Signature with Date:

FIRST PROFESSIONAL YEAR

Visit number:

Date of Visit:

Objective of Visit:

Activities conducted and Problems Identified:

Family 1:

Family 2:

Family 3:

Action taken for the problems:

Family 1:

Family 2:

Family 3:

Student's Reflection for the Visit:

Supervisor's Grading and Signature with Date:

FIRST PROFESSIONAL YEAR

Visit number:

Date of Visit:

Objective of Visit:

Activities conducted and Problems Identified:

Family 1:

Family 2:

Family 3:

Action taken for the problems:

Family 1:

Family 2:

Family 3:

Student's Reflection for the Visit:

Supervisor's Grading and Signature with Date:

SECOND PROFESSIONAL YEAR

Visit number:

Date of Visit:

Objective of Visit:

Activities conducted and Problems Identified:

Family 1:

Family 2:

Family 3:

Action taken for the problems:

Family 1:

Family 2:

Family 3:

Student's Reflection for the Visit:

Supervisor's Grading and Signature with Date:

SECOND PROFESSIONAL YEAR

Visit number:

Date of Visit:

Objective of Visit:

Activities conducted and Problems Identified:

Family 1:

Family 2:

Family 3:

Action taken for the problems:

Family 1:

Family 2:

Family 3:

Student's Reflection for the Visit:

Supervisor's Grading and Signature with Date:

SECOND PROFESSIONAL YEAR

Visit number:

Date of Visit:

Objective of Visit:

Activities conducted and Problems Identified:

Family 1:

Family 2:

Family 3:

Action taken for the problems:

Family 1:

Family 2:

Family 3:

Student's Reflection for the Visit:

Supervisor's Grading and Signature with Date:

SECOND PROFESSIONAL YEAR

Visit number:

Date of Visit:

Objective of Visit:

Activities conducted and Problems Identified:

Family 1:

Family 2:

Family 3:

Action taken for the problems:

Family 1:

Family 2:

Family 3:

Student's Reflection for the Visit:

Supervisor's Grading and Signature with Date:

SECOND PROFESSIONAL YEAR

Visit number:

Date of Visit:

Objective of Visit:

Activities conducted and Problems Identified:

Family 1:

Family 2:

Family 3:

Action taken for the problems:

Family 1:

Family 2:

Family 3:

Student's Reflection for the Visit:

Supervisor's Grading and Signature with Date:

SECOND PROFESSIONAL YEAR

Visit number:

Date of Visit:

Objective of Visit:

Activities conducted and Problems Identified:

Family 1:

Family 2:

Family 3:

Action taken for the problems:

Family 1:

Family 2:

Family 3:

Student's Reflection for the Visit:

Supervisor's Grading and Signature with Date:

SECOND PROFESSIONAL YEAR

Visit number:

Date of Visit:

Objective of Visit:

Activities conducted and Problems Identified:

Family 1:

Family 2:

Family 3:

Action taken for the problems:

Family 1:

Family 2:

Family 3:

Student's Reflection for the Visit:

Supervisor's Grading and Signature with Date:

SECOND PROFESSIONAL YEAR

Visit number:

Date of Visit:

Objective of Visit:

Activities conducted and Problems Identified:

Family 1:

Family 2:

Family 3:

Action taken for the problems:

Family 1:

Family 2:

Family 3:

Student's Reflection for the Visit:

Supervisor's Grading and Signature with Date:

SECOND PROFESSIONAL YEAR

Visit number:

Date of Visit:

Objective of Visit:

Activities conducted and Problems Identified:

Family 1:

Family 2:

Family 3:

Action taken for the problems:

Family 1:

Family 2:

Family 3:

Student's Reflection for the Visit:

Supervisor's Grading and Signature with Date:

SECOND PROFESSIONAL YEAR

Visit number:

Date of Visit:

Objective of Visit:

Activities conducted and Problems Identified:

Family 1:

Family 2:

Family 3:

Action taken for the problems:

Family 1:

Family 2:

Family 3:

Student's Reflection for the Visit:

Supervisor's Grading and Signature with Date:

SECOND PROFESSIONAL YEAR

Visit number:

Date of Visit:

Objective of Visit:

Activities conducted and Problems Identified:

Family 1:

Family 2:

Family 3:

Action taken for the problems:

Family 1:

Family 2:

Family 3:

Student's Reflection for the Visit:

Supervisor's Grading and Signature with Date:

THIRD PROFESSIONAL YEAR

Visit number:

Date of Visit:

Objective of Visit:

Activities conducted and Problems Identified:

Family 1:

Family 2:

Family 3:

Action taken for the problems:

Family 1:

Family 2:

Family 3:

Student's Reflection for the Visit:

Supervisor's Grading and Signature with Date:

THIRD PROFESSIONAL YEAR

Visit number:

Date of Visit:

Objective of Visit:

Activities conducted and Problems Identified:

Family 1:

Family 2:

Family 3:

Action taken for the problems:

Family 1:

Family 2:

Family 3:

Student's Reflection for the Visit:

Supervisor's Grading and Signature with Date:

THIRD PROFESSIONAL YEAR

Visit number:

Date of Visit:

Objective of Visit:

Activities conducted and Problems Identified:

Family 1:

Family 2:

Family 3:

Action taken for the problems:

Family 1:

Family 2:

Family 3:

Student's Reflection for the Visit:

Supervisor's Grading and Signature with Date:

THIRD PROFESSIONAL YEAR

Visit number:

Date of Visit:

Objective of Visit:

Activities conducted and Problems Identified:

Family 1:

Family 2:

Family 3:

Action taken for the problems:

Family 1:

Family 2:

Family 3:

Student's Reflection for the Visit:

Supervisor's Grading and Signature with Date:

THIRD PROFESSIONAL YEAR

Visit number:

Date of Visit:

Objective of Visit:

Activities conducted and Problems Identified:

Family 1:

Family 2:

Family 3:

Action taken for the problems:

Family 1:

Family 2:

Family 3:

Student's Reflection for the Visit:

Supervisor's Grading and Signature with Date:

THIRD PROFESSIONAL YEAR

Visit number:

Date of Visit:

Objective of Visit:

Activities conducted and Problems Identified:

Family 1:

Family 2:

Family 3:

Action taken for the problems:

Family 1:

Family 2:

Family 3:

Student's Reflection for the Visit:

Supervisor's Grading and Signature with Date:

FOURTH PROFESSIONAL YEAR

Visit number:

Date of Visit:

Objective of Visit:

Activities conducted and Problems Identified:

Family 1:

Family 2:

Family 3:

Action taken for the problems:

Family 1:

Family 2:

Family 3:

Student's Reflection for the Visit:

Supervisor's Grading and Signature with Date:

FOURTH PROFESSIONAL YEAR

Visit number:

Date of Visit:

Objective of Visit:

Activities conducted and Problems Identified:

Family 1:

Family 2:

Family 3:

Action taken for the problems:

Family 1:

Family 2:

Family 3:

Student's Reflection for the Visit:

Supervisor's Grading and Signature with Date:

FOURTH PROFESSIONAL YEAR

Visit number:

Date of Visit:

Objective of Visit:

Activities conducted and Problems Identified:

Family 1:

Family 2:

Family 3:

Action taken for the problems:

Family 1:

Family 2:

Family 3:

Student's Reflection for the Visit:

Supervisor's Grading and Signature with Date:

STUDENT'S NOTES

An Overview of Field Practice Area

Date:______________

Specific learning objectives: At the end of the session, Phase III (Part-1) student will be able to:

1. Collect data in order to create a map of community assets and resources within a defined area.
2. Record vital statistics of the field practice area.

A community map highlights people, physical structures and institutions that can be utilized to discover strengths and resources of a community and can help to uncover solutions to community problems.

KEY VOCABULARY

- Community: People with common interests living in a particular area.
- Institution: An established organization—such as a park, library, police station, or hospital—designed to benefit the overall community.

Draw a Community Spot Map

Vital Statistics of the Field Practice Area

Total Population:

Male:

Female:

Total Number of Eligible Couples:

Crude Birth Rate:

Crude Death Rate:

Maternal Mortality Rate:

Infant Mortality Rate:

Couple Protection Rate:

Supervisor's Signature

Family Number 1

CHAPTER 1

Identification and Demographic Data

Date:______________

Specific learning objectives: At the end of the session, Phase III (Part-1) student will be able to:

1. Develop effective communication skills.
2. Describe the significance of each discussed variable in relation to health.
3. Discuss the role of family in health and disease.

Identification data

- Name of the Head of the Family ______________ Age ________ (in completed years)
- Gender ______________ Address ______________
- Setting: Urban/Rural
- Family Type: Joint/Nuclear/Three generation
- Total number of family members ______________
- Religion: Hindu/ Muslim/ Sikh/ Christian/ Other (specify) ______________
- Whether migrants–Yes/No
- If yes, State of Origin ______________

Demographic Data

S. No.	Name	Relation-ship with the head of family	Age	Sex	Marital status	Educational status	Occupation	Income	Remarks

***Exact date of birth of under-five.**

- Identify persons in the family belonging to vulnerable group:
- Any vital events in the family in last one year (Birth/Death/Marriage/Divorce/Adoption/Migration):

____

____

- Any history of neonatal death/maternal death/under-5 death/accidental death:

____

____

- History of diabetes, hypertension, tuberculosis or any other chronic illness:

____

____

- Any consanguinity in the family with its degree (second/third):

Inference

- Family size

____

____

- Dependency ratio

____

____

- Unemployment

____

____

Supervisor's Signature

CHAPTER 2

Socio-Economic Data

Date:____________

Specific learning objectives: At the end of the session, Phase III (Part-1) student will be able to:

1. Demonstrate the steps of assessment of socio-economic status and application of various socioeconomic status scales in different settings.
2. Apply the concept of poverty line
3. Illustrate the role of socio-economic status in health and disease.

Income source and expenditure pattern

- House: Rented / Owned
- Total Family Income / month Rs.:
- Total Expenditure/month Rs.:
- Per capita Income / month (total family income divided by total family members) Rs.:

Sources ofIncome

Land	House	Shop	Wages/salary of all members	Cottage Industry/ Farm Stock	Others	Total

Average expenditure per month (in rupees)

Rent	Food	Clothing	Education	Fuel	Electricity	Recreation	Transport	Smoking	Alcohol	Medicine	Doctor's fee	*Social customs	Health insurance	Others	Total

*Social customs e.g Marriage, Child birth, Mundan, Birthday, Gauna etc. calculate average per month from annual expenditure.

Assessment

SES Score: Socioeconomic Class:

(Based on Modified BG Prasad/Modified Kuppuswamy scale in urban and Modified BG Prasad/ Modified Udai Pareek in rural area (refer to Annexure 3):

- Does the family belong to "Below poverty line" category: Yes/No

  (If yes, confirm this by asking for BPL card/ color of the ration card)
- Any benefit received by the family from the government or NGO: pension/coverage under government health insurance scheme/benefits under ration card, any other)

Advice given: ______________________________

____

____

____

____

Supervisor's Signature

CHAPTER 3

Environmental Data

Date:____________

Specific learning objective: At the end of the session, Phase III (Part-1) student will be able to:

1. Assess the Environmental conditions of the family
2. Demonstrate the influence of environmental factors on health of the family.
3. Suggest suitable modifications in the environment to alleviate/ prevent health problems in the family within the given constraints.

Physical Environment

A. External Environment (Surroundings of the house)

- Pucca roads outside house: Present/Absent
- Lighting on roads or in the area: Adequate/Inadequate
- Accidental hazards: Construction sites/Open wells/Pits/Others(specify)
- Source of noise pollution (major roads, factory, railway track etc.): Present/Absent
- Waste disposal area: Nearby/Far
- Open drains outside house: Yes/No

B. Internal Environment (Inside the house)

General details

- Ownership of the house: Owned/Rented
- Approximate total plot area of the house (sq. ft.):
- Set-back: Present/Absent, if present, specify what % of total area ____________

Type of construction

- Floor: Pucca / Kutcha / Pucca Kutcha
- Wall: Kutcha / Bricked/Cemented
- Roofing: Pucca / Kutcha / Tiled
- No. of living rooms:
- No. of occupants:

Overcrowding: Present/ Absent

If present; specify the criteria: Persons per room/ Area/Gender separation (Refer to Appendix 4)

Light: Adequate / Inadequate

Source of light: Natural / Artificial

Accident prone areas in the house (slippery floors, roof without boundary wall, steps without railings/ inadequate lighting, others if any specify): Present/Absent

Dampness in the house: Present/Absent

Source of Indoor air pollution (smoking, wood burning, chulha without chimney): Present/Absent

Measurement of the house

Rooms Measurement (in feet)		Ventilators (in feet)		Windows (in feet)		Doors (in feet)		Ventilation
S. No.	Size (lxbxh)	No.	Size (lxb)	No.	Size (lxb)	No.	Size (lxb)	Satisfactory / Not Satisfactory

Ventilation: Adequate/ Inadequate

- Source of ventilation: Natural/ Artificial (Fans/Exhaust fans/AC/Coolers)
- Cross Ventilation: Present / Absent

Kitchen

- Location: Separate / Veranda / Open / Living Room
- Cleanliness: Clean / Dirty
- Floor: Pucca / Kutcha
- Storage of cooked and raw food: Covered /Uncovered containers
- Storage of vegetables, fruits and leftover cooked food: In refrigerator/ Outside
- Lighting (Natural): Adequate / Inadequate
- Lighting (Artificial): Adequate / Inadequate

- Fuel used: Kerosene / Cooking Gas / Coal / Firewood / Others
- Smoke outlet: Present / Absent
- Presence of soot particles on kitchen walls (indicator of indoor air pollution): Yes/No
- Sullage disposal: Closed drain/Open drain/No drain (stagnant water collection)

Water Supply

- Source: Piped Water Supply / Boring / Hand Pump / Tanker / Other (specify)
- Supply: Intermittent /Continuous
- Method of Storage of drinking water:
- Type of container used: Covered /Uncovered
- Method of drawing drinking water: Mug/Ladle/Steel Glass / Tumbler / Other specify
- Methods of purification used at household level: Boiling / Filtration / Chlorination / Reverse osmosis/ None / Any other (Specify)

Refuse Collection/Disposal

- Collection Inside house: Heaps / Open bins / Closed bins
- Waste segregation in biodegradable and nonbiodegradable bins: Yes/No
- Frequency of refuse disposal (Specify):
- Waste disposal method: Burning/Open ground dumping/Collection by municipality/any other specify

Privy (Lavatory)

- Own/ Community / Shared / None
- If shared;Approx. no. of families using toilet:
- Type: Flush type / Open field defecation
- Sewage system: Present/Absent
- Septic Tank: Present/Absent

Bathroom

- Separate in House / Not Separate / Community Bathroom
- Drainage: Open/Closed

Biological Environment

- Potential Mosquito Breeding sites: Absent / Present
- Mosquito breeding: Present / Absent (Specify places)
- Potential housefly breeding places: absent/present
- Housefly breeding: Present / Absent
- Cattle in the family: Yes / No If yes; distance from living room ____________________
- Rodents seen in the house: Yes / No
- Pets in the house: Yes / No; If yes, which Pets:
- Community Dogs: Present / Absent

House Map (Transverse Section - Draw to Scale; Depict kitchen/Toilet/Room/Floor Clearly) Note: - In case of more than one floor, please attach additional sheet.

Psychological Environment

Reasons for Psychological stress

- Unemployed adult: Yes / No
- Poverty: Yes/No
- Overcrowding: Yes/No
- Any addiction in the family, specify ____________________

- Gambling: Yes/No
- Marital conflicts / Abuse / Divorce or Separation: Yes/No
- Sibling rivalry- Y/N
- Family conflict- Y/N, if yes, identify the factors leading to it ____________
- Any unmarried daughter: Yes/No
- Orphans in the family: Yes/No
- Children >6 years, not going to school: Yes/No
- If yes, state the reason ____________
- Children <14 years, working (Child Labor): Yes/No
- If yes, place of work ____________
- Any Delinquent Child in the Family: Yes/No
- Child marriage/ Dowry/Non-involvement of women in decision making: Yes/No
- Chronic Illness in the family: Yes/No

Emotional problems

- Is there any case of mental illness in the family- yes/no; if Yes, give details ____________
____
____
- Is there any evidence of any diagnosed case of mental retardation in family: Y/N?

Personality disorders

Any family member suffering from personality disorder: Y/N

In case of any psychological/mental problem, state the effect of illness on:

(a) Individual Patient: Psychosocial level ____________,

Economic level ____________

(b) Family: Psychosocial level ____________,

Economic level ____________

(c) Attitude of family members: Positive and Caring / Sympathetic / Empathetic / Indifferent / Non-Co-operative.

Family status from its community's viewpoint

- Is the family generally accepted by the Community-Yes / No?
- In the case of rejection, identify the reasons ____________

Assessment of environmental status

Environmental factors conducive to health:

1.

2.

3.

4.

5.

Environmental factors detrimental to health:

1.

2.

3.

4.

5.

Supervisor's Signature

CHAPTER 4

Socio-Cultural Environment

Date:__________

Specific learning objectives: At the end of the session, Phase III (Part-1) student will be able to:

1. Describe knowledge, attitude, customs, beliefs and practices of the family in health and disease.
2. Impart health education to promote healthy practices.

Information regarding customs and health practices

Name of the respondent: ____________________

Menstruation

- Menstruation is a normal physiological process: Yes/No
- Any restrictions during menstruation (Custom/Religious): Yes/No; If Yes specify ____________________

Marriage and Childbearing

- System of marriage: Within Religion / Caste / Kinship Group
- What is the legal age for marriage in India for boys: __________, for girls? __________
- At what age you were married? ____________________
- Average expenditure on marriage ____________________
- Practice of dowry: Prevalent/Non-prevalent
- Pardah System: Prevalent/Non-prevalent
- Preference for a male child: Yes/No
- Age at first pregnancy of the respondent (if applicable) ____________________
- Number of children born (if applicable): ____________________
- Any spacing methods used: Y/N; if yes, specify ____________________

Detail regarding the last pregnancy and its outcome

- Registered in antenatal Clinic: Yes/No; period of gestation at the time of registration in weeks ____________
- Diet during pregnancy:
  - Any additions:
  - Any restrictions:
- Physical activity:
- Whether antenatal care received from a health facility: Yes/No.
  - Number of antenatal visits ____________
- Delivery: Institutional/Home; Delivered by: Doctor/Nurse/Trained Dai/Untrained Dai/Relatives or Neighbors
- Cord applicant: None/Ash/Cow dung/Ghee/Antiseptic/Other
- Isolation during puerperium: Yes/No, if yes specify the number of days ____________

Prevalent beliefs/practices in the family regarding child rearing. (To be asked to the lady who has borne children, if not available, ask in general).

- Is there any special practice regarding child rearing in your family (e.g., Oil bath, hygiene etc.)? If yes, please specify:
- Is there a practice of giving pre-lacteal feed to the baby? If yes, please specify:
- Is colostrum (thick yellow milk) given to the new born baby? Yes/No
- When do you start giving breast milk to the new-born baby? (specify hours after delivery)
- For how long a baby is given only breast milk?
- Is water given to the baby during the first 6 months of age? Yes/No
- Usually in your family for how long a child is breast fed?
- Is milk other than breast milk given to the child in your family? Yes/No
- If yes, please specify What is given? What age it is started? How it is given? Is it diluted with water?

  ____

  ____

- When is complementary feeding usually started (age in months):
- What food is usually given for complementary feeding (specify):

  ____

- Is your child registered with any Well Baby Clinic/ Anganwadi Yes/No;
  - If No, reason: don't know about it / no clinic available/no need /other
- Do you visit the clinic regularly with the baby: Yes/No.
  - If No, specify why?
- Do you/other family members take your child for immunization? Yes/No;
  - If Yes, Where: Hospital /Health Centre/Private Doctor /Dispensary/Others(specify)
- Whom do you consult in the event of child's illness? Government / Private facility

- Which kind of system of medicine do you usually follow for child's illness? Allopathic / Homeopathic / Ayurvedic / Yunani / Others (specify)

Other child rearing practices

- Application of kajal: Y/N; if yes, with common applicator: Y/N
- Exposure to sunlight: Y/N
- Food prohibited during fever: Y/N
- Restriction of fluids during diarrhea: Y/N

Health seeking behavior

- What is the belief of family regarding causation of disease: Past sins/ Gods will /Evil eye/ Scientific reasons (Specify)
- Does your family believe in faith healing: Yes/No; If yes, specify ____________________
- Does the family attend any health center/ clinic in case of illness: Yes/No; If no, why ____________________
____
- Who is your first point of contact in case any member of your family is ill: Home remedy/ Health centre/Hospital /Local doctor (Specify)/Other (Specify) ____________________
- What type of treatment does your family seek at the time of illness: Allopathic / Ayurvedic / Homeopathic / Yunani / Siddha / Puja /Other rituals (specify) ____________________
- What is the usual source of medical care, if somebody is ill in your family: Govt. Hospital / Govt. Dispensary / MCH Centre / Private Practitioner/Any Other (Specify) ____________________

Knowledge and Practices in some common diseases

Knowledge

Are you aware of	Y/N	Can you enumerate mode of transmission?	Do you know how it can be prevented?	Is social stigma attached to the disease? Y/N
Tuberculosis				
Measles				
Dengue				
Diarrhea				
Hypertension				
Diabetes				

Practice: Respond if any of the family members have suffered any of the following diseases in the past one year

Diseases	Which system you are following for treatment of these diseases (Allopathy/Homeopathy/Yunani/Siddha/ Aayurveda/self-medication/any other)	Compliance to medications (Y/N)
Tuberculosis		
Measles		
Dengue		
Diarrhea		
Hypertension		
Diabetes		

Personal hygiene: Satisfactory/Unsatisfactory; If unsatisfactory, specify ____________

Analysis and Interpretation

Social problems existing in the family: ____________

Customs and practices conducive to health: ____________

Customs and practices harmful for health: ____________

Supervisor's Signature

CHAPTER 5

Dietary Assessment

Date:_______________

Specific learning objectives: At the end of the session, Phase III (Part 1) student will be able to:

1. Describe the concept of balanced diet.
2. Demonstrate steps of dietary survey.
3. Collect the accurate information regarding food consumption of both the household and individual member.
4. Detect deficiencies/ excess of various nutrients and correlate them to the nutritional status of the family members.
5. Advise the family regarding desired change in diet in case of any nutritional disorder/ deficiency/ excess.

Dietary habits of family members

- Food habits: Vegetarian/Non-vegetarian/Egg-Vegetarian
- Meals consumed: bed tea, breakfast, mid-morning snack, lunch, evening tea/ snack, dinner, bedtime drink (milk/tea etc.)/post-dinner snack

Assess the nutritional requirements of each family

Depending upon age, gender, type of work (sedentary, moderate, heavy) and physiological state (pregnancy, lactation etc.), requirements of calories and proteins can be determined from ICMR- NIN, 2020 reference charts (Annexure 5)

Name of family Member	Calorie requirement (kcal/day)	Protein Requirement (g/day)	Fat Requirement (g/day)	Dietary Fiber Requirement (g/day)	Any special needs

Dietary assessment

There are various methods for dietary assessment of an individual and a family (Annexure 5). Two commonly used methods are discussed below.

Method I - Diet survey based on 24-hour recall method.

Step 1. Calculate the food intake for the family by asking the quantities of various food items including beverages consumed by each family member and summing them to obtain diet consumed by the family in last 24 hours.

Daily diet consumption by the family (24-hour Recall Method)

S. No.	Member Name	Meal	Name of food items	Quantity (ml/g/ number)	Calories (kcal)	Protein (g)	Fat (g)	Dietary Fiber (g)
1.		Breakfast Mid-morning snack Lunch Evening tea/ snack Dinner Post- dinner drinks/snack						
2.		Breakfast Mid-morning snack Lunch Evening tea/ snack Dinner Post- dinner drinks/snack						
3.		Breakfast Mid-morning snack Lunch Evening tea/ snack Dinner Post- dinner drinks/snack						
4.		Breakfast Mid-morning snack Lunch Evening tea/ snack Dinner Post- dinner drinks/snack						

Contd.

Contd.

5.		Breakfast Mid-morning snack Lunch Evening tea/ snack Dinner Post- dinner drinks/snack						
6.		Breakfast Mid-morning snack Lunch Evening tea/ snack Dinner Post- dinner drinks/snack						
7.		Breakfast Mid-morning snack Lunch Evening tea / snack Dinner Post- dinner drinks/snack						
8.		Breakfast Mid-morning snack Lunch Evening tea/ snack Dinner Post- dinner drinks/snack						
9.		Breakfast Mid-morning snack Lunch Evening tea/ snack Dinner Post- dinner drinks/snack						
10.		Breakfast Mid-morning snack Lunch Evening tea/ snack Dinner Post- dinner drinks/snack						
Total intake								

Note – Calorie, Protein, Fat and Dietary Fiber content of each food item can be calculated directly using reference tables for cooked food items or through estimation of raw food materials contained in them.

Step 2. Calculation of the caloric and nutrients requirements for the family:

Requirement for an individual is assessed as per referenced recommendations given by ICMR- NIN, 2020 (Appendix 5) and total family requirement is calculated by summating requirements of all family members .

Total Family requirement of Calories =

Total Family requirement of Proteins =

Total Family requirement of Fats=

Total Family requirement of Dietary fiber=

Step 3: Find the difference between intake and requirement and interpret:

- Calorie excess / deficit:

  {(Calorie intake – Caloric requirement)/ Calorie requirement)} × 100
- Protein excess/deficiency for family (%):

  {(Protein intake – Protein requirement)/Protein requirement}x100
- Fat excess/deficiency for family (%):
- Dietary Fiber excess/deficiency for family (%):

Method II- Diet Survey based on inventory method

Step 1: Enquire about the quantity of different raw food stuffs used for cooking by the family per day. Method for assessment of average daily consumption of raw food:

- Find out fortnightly/monthly consumption for items procured fortnightly/monthly, e.g. rice, wheat, pulses, oil etc. and calculate average daily consumption.
- Find out weekly consumption for items such as fish, meat, eggs, fruits etc. and calculate average daily consumption.
- Find out daily consumption of regularly used items such as milk, vegetables etc.
- Find out consumption of any occasionally used item during last 24 hours e.g., biscuits, sweets, ice-cream etc.
- Deduct the consumption of food by guest, if any
- Take into account if any member has not taken meal(s) during last 24 hours.
- Calculate average daily consumption of quantity of each item and thereby deduce the calorie and protein intake per day by the family.

Step 2: Calculation of the caloric and protein requirements for the family (EAR, RDA Tables, ICMR-NIN,2020 in Annexure 5)

Step 3: Find the difference between intake and requirement and interpret

- Calorie excess / deficit:

  {(Calorie intake – Caloric requirement)/ Calorie requirement)} × 100

- Protein excess/deficiency for family (%):

  {(Protein intake- protein requirement)/Protein requirement} ×100

1. Comment on food items consumed by the family

____

____

____

____

2. Comment on nutrients consumed by the family

____

____

____

____

Nutritional status of family

Sr. No.	Name	Age	Nutritional assessment based on anthropometry/clinical examination*	Dietary deficiency	Action taken

*Mention values for anthropometry and clinical findings and diagnosis based on these.

Supervisor's Signature

Chapter 6

Immunization

Date:__________

Specific learning objectives: At the end of the session, Phase III (Part 1) student will be able to:

1. Describe steps of eliciting information about immunization status of individuals.
2. Enlist vaccines used under Universal Immunization Programme, age of administration, dosage schedule, contraindications and advantages.
3. Impart education about vaccine preventable diseases to the community.

Immunization Data (for pregnant mothers and under five children)

Name of child						
Age/ date of birth						
Vaccines received						
6 weeks						
10 weeks						
14 weeks						
9 months						
16-24 months						
5 years						
10 years						
Pregnant woman						
TT1						
TT2						
TT- Booster						
Immunization status						

(#) Immunization status: mark 'F' for fully immunized, 'P' for partly immunized and 'U' for unimmunized.

Other vaccines (specify: Name of the individual immunized, name of the vaccine, doses and dates)

Vaccines not given by due date

Name of the individual	Due vaccine (dose) not given	Reasons for delay/ failure	Advice given/action taken

Adverse Events Following Immunization (AEFI); (if any):

Action taken in case of AEFI:

Supervisor's Signature

Chapter 7

Health Records of Vulnerable Groups

Date:____________

Specific learning objectives: At the end of the session, Phase III (Part 1) student will be able to:
- Describe the concept of high risk and screening.
- Illustrate the significance of screening/preventive check- up in relation to health status.
- Demonstrate the importance of early diagnosis of risk factors and health problems, timely referral, management in various target groups.

A. Antenatal / Postnatal Check-up: (Tick appropriate)

Identification details

Name:	Age:	Education:	Occupation:
Husband Name:	Age:	Education:	Occupation:
Income:	SES:		

Presenting complaints

Amenorrhea (details):

Any other associated complaints:

Marital History

Age at marriage: Age at cohabit: Consanguinity and its degree (if applicable):

Present Antenatal history

- L.M.P:
- Expected date of delivery:
- Time of confirmation of pregnancy (weeks):
- Test for confirmation of pregnancy: Done/not done; if yes, specify
- Registered in ANC Clinic: Yes/No; if yes, time of registration- I/2nd/3rd trimester
- Number of ANC Visits: Where visited: hospital/ health center/ home visit by a Health Care Worker

Trimester History

Trimester 1	Trimester 2	Trimester 3
Excessive Vomiting: Y/N	Quickening: Y/N; specify weeks of gestation	Pain abdomen: Y/N
Bleeding p/v: Y/N	Blurring of vision: Y/N	Headache/ seizures: Y/N
Fever with rash: Y/N	Epigastric pain: Y/N	Reduced fetal movements: Y/N
Drug intake: Y/N	Pedal edema: Y/N	Leaking or Bleeding p/v: Y/N
X-ray exposure: Y/N; If yes reason ______	Headache: Y/N	Iron and Folic acid supplementation: Y/N; No. of days ______ Calcium supplementation: Y/N
Folic acid supplementation: Y/N; No. of days	Iron and Folic acid supplementation: Y/N; No. of days ______	Weight gain (Min. 5Kg): Y/N
	Calcium supplementation: Y/N	
	Albendazole: Y/N	
TT immunization: Y/N	TT immunization: Y/N	Investigation USG:
Weight gain (Min. 1 Kg): Y/N	Weight gain (Min. 5 Kg): Y/N	
Investigations Hb: Y/N Blood group (wife and husband): Y/N; Compatible: Yes/No RBS: Y/N VDRL: Y/N Hep-B: Y/N HIV: Y/N Urine for albumin and sugar: Y/N	Investigations HB: Y/N USG: Y/N	

Menstrual History

Age at menarche: ______; Cycle; ______; Duration: ______;

Frequency: ______; Soaking ______ Pads per day; ______

Passage of clots: ______; Dysmenorrhea: ______

Any associated problem: ______

Obstetric History

Gravida ______ Para ______ Live ______ Abortion ______

Age at first pregnancy:

Interval between current and previous pregnancy:

Record of previous pregnancies, if any

	Antenatal period		Intra natal period			Postnatal period	Newborn			Family Planning status	Remarks
Order of pregnancy	Normal/ High Risk; specify	ANC by a skilled health care worker (Yes/No)	Type of delivery (Full Term/ Pre-Term)	Normal vaginal/C-Section	Conducted By whom (skilled HCW/ Untrained worker) and where (Home/Hosp.)	Normal/ Eventful; specify	Sex	Alive/ dead	If dead age and cause of death		

Past History

Hypertension: Y/N, Diabetes: Y/N, TB: Y/N, Blood transfusion: Y/N; Major surgery: Y/N; Prolonged hospitalization: Y/N; COPD: Y/N; Seizure disorder: Y/N; Chronic medication intake: Y/N

Family History

History of Twins: Y/N, Preterm: Y/N, Recurrent Abortion: Y/N; Diabetes: Y/N

Nutritional History/ Problems including nutritional deficiencies in ANC/ PNC Period:

Assess the diet of the antenatal / postnatal / lactating woman by 24-hour recall method

Meal	Food Items consumed	Calorie intake (Kcal)	Protein intake (gm)
Breakfast			
Mid-morning snack			
Lunch			
Evening snacks			
Dinner			
Any Other			
Total			

- Calorie requirement: (kcal)
- Excess/Deficit: (kcal)
- Protein requirement: (gm)
- Excess/deficit: (gm)

Housing and environment: ______________________________

____

____

____

____

Accidental hazards: ______________________________

____

____

____

Socio-cultural Practices: ______________________________

____

____

____

Physical examination

1. **General examination**
   - Anemia/ Pallor: Yes/No, if yes, severity: Mild/ Moderate/Severe
   - Any Icterus/JVP/Clubbing/Cyanosis/Lymphadenopathy/Pedal Oedema
   - Present weight (kg.):

- Gain in weight (as per gestation): Less/More/Normal
- Pre-pregnancy weight (if available):
- B.P:___________/___________mm Hg: Comment on status: ___________

2. Abdominal examination

On inspection	On Palpation	On Auscultation
Shape of the abdomen:	Abdominal girth	Fetal heart sound:___________/min.
Symmetry:	Fundal height	
Fullness of Flanks:	Fundal grip	
Striae gravidarum:	Lateral grip	
Striae nigra:	1st pelvic grip	
Scar:	2nd pelvic grip	

If ANC Case registered, then the information from the card should be transferred.

Treatment taken, if any:

____

____

____

____

High risk/ Normal pregnancy, if high risk, criteria present:

Preparation for delivery: Money, vehicle, place of delivery, awareness about JSY

Plan for family planning: Yes/No

Plan to continue IFA and Calcium for 6months post-natal: Yes/No

Plan to adopt postpartum contraceptive: Y/N; If yes: PPIUCD/PoP/Condoms/Conventional methods

Assessment for breast feeding:

Follow up Notes

Date	Weight	BP	Fundal Height	Lie and Presentation	Fetal Heart Sound	Lab Reports (Hb, Urine for Sugar and Albumin)	Dietary or Any Other Advice Given	Signature of Faculty

Supervisor's Signature

B. In Postnatal Case, in Addition to the Antenatal Work-up Following History Needs to be Taken

Date:____________

Natal History

Place of delivery: Institutional/Home

Person conducted delivery: Doctor/ Health staff/ TBA/Untrained dai

Type of delivery: normal vaginal/C-section/vaginal-assisted delivery

Delivery was uneventful/eventful; if complication happened, specify: postpartum hemorrhage, obstructed labor, malpresentation, others

Neonatal history

General	Feeding
Birth order: Gender: M/F Birth weight: ; LBW: Y/N	Initiation of breastfeeding: hrs. of delivery Colostrum given: Y/N Pre-lacteal feed given: Y/N; if yes, specify
Cried immediately after birth: Y/N	Breastfeeding is on demand: Y/N
Anything applied to umbilical cord: Y/N	Frequency of breastfeeding in a day:
When did the child pass first stool?	Burping is done after breastfeeding: Y/N
When did the child urinate for the first time?	• Is artificial feeding being done: Y/N; if yes • When was it started: • Reason for its initiation: • What formula/artificial feed is being given: • Given with the help of: cup and spoon/bottle/palade
When was the first bath given to the child?	
Prophylactic Vit.K injection given at birth: Y/N	
Immunization at birth: OPV, HepB, BCG, any other; specify	
Application of kajal to eyes:	

Postnatal history of the mother

- Status of vaginal bleeding: normal/excessive
- Any complication during postpartum period:
- Breast pain/tenderness: Y/N

- Pain/burning micturition: Y/N
- Foul smelling lochia: Y/N
- Pain in abdomen: Y/N
- Fever: Y/N
- Any other problem; specify:
- Postnatal visits: institutional/home; number of visits ______

Physical Examination

<table>
<tr><th colspan="2">Neonate</th><th>Mother</th></tr>
<tr><td colspan="2">Congenital malformations/defects/deformities: Y/N</td><td rowspan="3">General Physical Examination:</td></tr>
<tr><td colspan="2">Anterior fontanelle; any abnormality</td></tr>
<tr><td>Eyes-</td><td>Discharge: Y/N
Redness: Y/N
Icterus: Y/N</td></tr>
<tr><td>Abdomen-</td><td>Soft/hard
Hernia: Y/N</td><td rowspan="2">Breast examination:</td></tr>
<tr><td>Umbilicus-</td><td>Fallen off: Y/N
Redness: Y/N
Discharge: Y/N</td></tr>
<tr><td>Primitive reflexes-</td><td>Rooting: Y/N
Suckling: Y/N</td><td rowspan="2">Abdomen:</td></tr>
<tr><td>Anthropometry-</td><td>Weight:
Length:
Head circumference:
Chest circumference:</td></tr>
</table>

Supervisor's Signature

C. Under-Five Child

Use separate sheets for more than one under-five in the family.

Date:________

Identification details

Name: Gender: Age / Date of birth:

Informant:

Education of mother: Occupation of mother: Income:

Education of father: Occupation of father: Income:

SES:

Presenting complaints

Chief complaints:

Elaborate the chief complaints in chronological order:

Specifically ask for symptoms of nutrient deficiency:

Past history

History of similar as well as common conditions (diarrhoea, malnutrition, ARI etc.):

Undergoing any treatment for any chronic condition: Y/N; if yes, specify: ________

History of recurrent hospitalization: Y/N; specify reason ________

Personal history: Pica/bed wetting/ nail biting/thumb sucking

Birth history

Birth order: Living order:

Any significant antenatal history:

Preterm/ Full term; Normal /Abnormal (specify):

Delivered by Doctor/Midwife/Trained Dai/Untrained Dai/Other (specify) ________ Place of delivery: Home/ Hospital

Birth weight: kgs; Normal/LBW

Child registered with under-five/ well baby clinic: Y/N

Immunization status: Vaccines given appropriate for age: Yes/No; if yes, specify ________

Vaccination status: Unimmunized/Partially immunized /Completely Immunized for age

Nutrition history:

Feeding: Breastfed/Non breastfed

Exclusive Breast feeding up to ________________ months; breast feeding continued up to/stopped at the age of ________________ months

Details of bottle feeding/artificial feeding if any: ________________

____

Details of complimentary feeding:

When was started: ; Which food items were given: ________________

____

Details of present nutrition

Meal	Food items	Quantity of Food items	Calorie intake (Kcal/d)	Protein intake (g/d)
Breakfast Mid-morning snack Lunch Evening Snacks Dinner Any Other				

- Total calorie intake: Total calorie requirement:
- Total protein intake: Total protein requirement:
- Any excess/deficit:

Details of any supplementary nutrition if received at Anganwadi:

Growth monitoring at Anganwadi center is being done: Y/N

Any food items disliked by the child:

Does the mother wash her hands before cooking food: Y/N

Does the mother wash her hands before feeding food: Y/N

Growth and development milestones

For growth, ask mother to show growth chart, analyze and interpret the growth chart (Annexure 6):

____

____

For development, rule out deafness and dumbness in the child followed by assessment of developmental milestones (Annexure 7)

Major developmental milestones

Milestone	Age at which it was achieved	Appropriate age for achievement of the milestone (in completed months)	Inference (Normal/Delayed development)
Social smile		2	
Head holding		4	
Can speak monosyllables (ma,ba,da etc.)		6	
Sits without support		9	
Crawls		9	
Stands without support		12	
Runs		24	

Sibling history

Age difference between the child and his/her immediate elder sibling:

Any gender bias in the family:

Psychosocial history:

Housing and environment:

Accidental Hazards:

Physical examination

Clinical examination from head to toe

Organ/System to be examined	Observation
General appearance	Normal built/thin/edematous
Hair	Normal/lusterless/thin and sparse/flag sign
Face	Normal/pigmentation/moon face
Eyes (Conjunctiva) (Cornea)	Normal/pallor/dry and wrinkled/bitot's spot Normal/dry/keratomalacia
Lips	Normal/cheilosis/angular stomatitis
Tongue	Normal/pale/red and raw, geographic
Teeth	Normal/mottled enamel/caries
Gums	Normal/swollen/bleeding
Glands	Normal/ thyroid enlargement/parotid enlargement
Skin	Normal/dry/follicular hyperkeratosis/flaky paint dermatosis
Nails	Normal/koilonychia
Knees	Normal/knock knee/epiphyseal enlargement
Feet	Normal/pedal edema
Other systems	Hepatomegaly/muscle weakness/sensory loss/delayed reflexes/ cardiac enlargement

Anthropometric measurements

Weight:

Length/Height:

Head circumference:

Chest circumference:

Mid-arm circumference:

Is she/he a high-risk child? Y/N, If yes why? ____________________

Complete diagnosis

____

____

____

____

Action taken / advice given

____

____

____

____

Follow up Notes:

Date	Age	Height	Weight	Follow up Notes	Signature of Faculty

Supervisor's Signature

D. Adolescent Health Record (10-19 Years)

Use separate sheets for more than one adolescent in the family.

Date of Visit:____________

Identification details

Name:

Age:

Sex:

Date of Birth:

Presenting complaints with history of present illness (Indicate positive findings only):

Past History (Indicate significant events only):

Menstrual History (in case of adolescent girls) :

Psychosocial Assessment (This assessment should be done for all adolescents irrespective of the presenting complaints/issues).

Education

- Whether attended school: Y/N; if yes, age of joining:
- Age of leaving school:
- Reasons for leaving school:
- Are you studying? Y /N; If yes, how is your performance at school / college?

____

Employment

- Are you employed somewhere? Yes / No;
- If yes, reason for the same __________________________________
- Vocational Training received if any: Y/N

Nutrition

- Food habits: Vegetarian/Non-vegetarian/Eggs and Vegetarian
- Like/dislike for any specific food items:
- On a normal day how may meals do you have:
- How many times a week do you eat outside:

Nutritional Assessment

Meal	Food items	Quantity of Food items	Calorie intake (Kcal/d)	Protein intake (g/d)
Breakfast Lunch Evening Snacks Dinner Any Other				

Total calorie intake: Calorie requirement: Excess/Deficit:

Total protein intake: Protein requirement: Excess/Deficit:

Activity

What do you do in your free time: Watching TV/Internet/Yoga/Sports/Music/Others; specify ___________

____

____

Substance abuse

Have you ever used: Tobacco / Alcohol / Other substances? Yes / No

If yes, are you using them currently? Yes / No

Sexuality

Have you ever had sex? Yes / No

If yes; With consent / forced

Are you aware of safe sex practices: Yes/No

Are you sexually active now? Yes / No

Safety

Do you feel safe at home? Yes / No

Do you feel safe in your school/workplace? Yes / No

Mental Health

Do you feel able to cope with your situation? Yes / No

Have you ever thought of ending your life? Yes / No

Personal Hygiene ____________________

____

Examination Physical Appearance (including signs of any physical assault): ____________________

____

Mental State (encircle in finding)

Alert / Drowsy   Well Oriented / Not Well oriented   Coherent / Incoherent

General Physical Examination:

Weight __________ Kg. Height __________ cm BMI __________

Blood Pressure __________ mm Hg Pulse / Heart rate__________/ min

Respiratory rate __________ / min.

Pallor: Jaundice: Clubbing:

Lymphadenopathy: Thyroid swelling: Teeth cavities:

Gum Bleeding: Others:

Systemic Examination (Do complete systemic examination and note relevant findings)

____

____

____

____

Laboratory investigations

____

____

____

____

Diagnosis and Advice

____

____

____

____

Follow up Record

Date	Follow up Notes	Signature of Faculty

Supervisor's Signature

E. Eligible Couple Health Record

Use separate sheets for more than one eligible couple

Date:____________

Identification details

Name: Age: Education: Occupation:

Spouse Name: Age: Education: Occupation:

Income: SES:

Religion: Setting: Rural/Urban

Age at marriage:

Age at first pregnancy:

Was the first pregnancy planned: Yes /No

Knowledge, attitude and Practices

Knowledge	Attitude	Practices
Do you know that child birth can be planned: Y/N	Attitude towards utilization of contraceptive methods: positive/negative	Are you using any contraceptive method: Y/N;If yes, type of contraceptive used: ________ duration of use ________ If No; specify reasons
When did you come to know: Before marriage/after marriage	Are you willing to undergo sterilization (in case of fulfilling eligibility): Y/N	Usage of contraceptives: Regular/ Irregular
Source of information: Spouse/Friends/neighbors/HCWs/ Mass media/Other		
Do you have knowledge about methods of family planning: Y/N; If yes, name them:		
1. 2. 3. 4. 5.		
What should be the ideal gap between two children:		
Where youcan get family welfare services: Govt. Hospital / Govt. dispensary / MCH Centre / Private Practitioner /Anganwadi / ASHA / Any other		

Inference

Unregulated fertility / Spacing method / Permanent method

Advice given:

Agency suggested for supply of contraceptives:

Any other suggestion given:

Follow up record

Date	Follow up notes	Signature of faculty

Supervisor's Signature

F. Geriatric Health Record (60 Years and Above)

Add extra sheets in case of more than one geriatric case in the family

Date:____________

Identification details

Name:

Age:

Gender:

Education:

Occupation:

Income:

SES:

Present history of illness (in chronological order)

Symptom	Onset of symptoms (sudden/gradual)	Duration	Description of symptoms

Past history

H/o Diabetes mellitus/Hypertension/CAD/TB/COPD/Asthma/Other

Duration of illness:

Place of seeking treatment: Compliance with the treatment:

Do you face restriction in activity of daily living: Y/N; if yes, which activities ____________

Immunization history

History of vaccine received: Pneumococcal/Influenza/COVID-19/Others

Social history

Interpersonal relationship with other family members and neighbors:

Receiving care and affection by family members: Y/N

Is he/she socially active:

Is he/she socially dependent: Y/N

Is he/she availing any old age pension: Y/N

Nutrition

Housing (rule out any accident-prone area in the house):

Physical examination

General appearance:

Height: Weight: BMI:

Blood pressure:

Any sign of malnutrition:

Dentition: edentulous/ artificial teething/any other

Systemic examination: ______

Follow up record

Date	Follow up notes	Signature of faculty

Supervisor's Signature

Preventive checkup of other family members

Enter the relevant information in the format given below for all family members (One page per family member) Add additional pages if required

Date of Examination	Name	Age/ Sex	Significant Findings on History	Significant Findings on Examination	Height	Weight	BMI	Blood Pressure	Hemoglobin	Diagnosis	Action Taken	Follow up

Preventive checkup of other family members

Enter the relevant information in the format given below for all family members (One page per family member) Add additional pages if required

Date of Examination	Name	Age/ Sex	Significant Findings on History	Significant Findings on Examination	Height	Weight	BMI	Blood Pressure	Hemoglobin	Diagnosis	Action Taken	Follow up

Preventive checkup of other family members

Enter the relevant information in the format given below for all family members (One page per family member) Add additional pages if required

Date of Examination	Name	Age/ Sex	Significant Findings on History	Significant Findings on Examination	Height	Weight	BMI	Blood Pressure	Hemoglobin	Diagnosis	Action Taken	Follow up

Preventive checkup of other family members

Enter the relevant information in the format given below for all family members (One page per family member) Add additional pages if required

Date of Examination	Name	Age/ Sex	Significant Findings on History	Significant Findings on Examination	Height	Weight	BMI	Blood Pressure	Hemoglobin	Diagnosis	Action Taken	Follow up

Chapter 8

Summary, Conclusion and Recommendations

Date:______________

FAMILY DIAGNOSIS:

SOCIAL PATHOLOGY:

POSITIVE AND NEGATIVE FACTORS IDENTIFIED

S No.	Positive factors	Negative factors
1.		
2.		
3.		
4.		
5.		

MEDICAL AND SOCIAL PROBLEMS IDENTIFIED

Medical Problems

S No.	Medical Problems	Action Taken
1.		
2.		
3.		
4.		
5.		

Social Problems

S No.	Medical Problems	Action Taken
1.		
2.		
3.		
4.		
5.		

OBJECTIVES OF THE FAMILY HEALTH CARE PROGRAMME

S No.	Name the objectives that has been achieved	State how
1.		
2.		
3.		
4.		
5.		

S No.	Name the objectives that has not beenachieved	Reason for non- achievement
1.		
2.		
3.		
4.		
5.		

Supervisor's Signature

Family Number 2

CHAPTER 1

Identification and Demographic Data

Date:__________

Specific learning objectives: At the end of the session, Phase III (Part-1) student will be able to:

1. Develop effective communication skills.
2. Describe the significance of each discussed variable in relation to health.
3. Discuss the role of family in health and disease.

Identification data

- Name of the Head of the Family __________ Age _____ (in completed years)
- Gender ________ Address __________
- Setting: Urban/Rural
- Family Type: Joint/Nuclear/Three generation
- Total number of family members __________
- Religion: Hindu/ Muslim/ Sikh/ Christian/ Other (specify) __________
- Whether migrants–Yes/No
- If yes, State of Origin __________

Demographic Data

S. No.	Name	Relation-ship with the head of family	Age	Sex	Marital status	Educational status	Occupation	Income	Remarks

***Exact date of birth of under-five.**

- Identify persons in the family belonging to vulnerable group:
- Any vital events in the family in last one year (Birth/Death/Marriage/Divorce/Adoption/Migration):

  ____

  ____

- Any history of neonatal death/maternal death/under-5 death/accidental death:

  ____

  ____

- History of diabetes, hypertension, tuberculosis or any other chronic illness:

  ____

  ____

- Any consanguinity in the family with its degree (second/third):

Inference

- Family size

  ____

  ____

- Dependency ratio

  ____

  ____

- Unemployment

  ____

  ____

Supervisor's Signature

CHAPTER 2

Socio-Economic Data

Date:__________

Specific learning objectives: At the end of the session, Phase III (Part-1) student will be able to:

1. Demonstrate the steps of assessment of socio-economic status and application of various socioeconomic status scales in different settings.
2. Apply the concept of poverty line
3. Illustrate the role of socio-economic status in health and disease.

Income source and expenditure pattern

- House: Rented / Owned
- Total Family Income / month Rs.:
- Total Expenditure/month Rs.:
- Per capita Income / month (total family income divided by total family members) Rs.:

Sources ofIncome

Land	House	Shop	Wages/salary of all members	Cottage Industry/ Farm Stock	Others	Total

Average expenditure per month (in rupees)

Rent	Food	Clothing	Education	Fuel	Electricity	Recreation	Transport	Smoking	Alcohol	Medicine	Doctor's fee	*Social customs	Health insurance	Others	Total

*Social customs e.g Marriage, Child birth, Mundan, Birthday, Gauna etc. calculate average per month from annual expenditure.

Assessment

SES Score: Socioeconomic Class:

(Based on Modified BG Prasad/Modified Kuppuswamy scale in urban and Modified BG Prasad/ Modified Udai Pareek in rural area (refer to Annexure 3):

- Does the family belong to "Below poverty line" category: Yes/No

  (If yes, confirm this by asking for BPL card/ color of the ration card)
- Any benefit received by the family from the government or NGO: pension/coverage under government health insurance scheme/benefits under ration card, any other)

Advice given: ______________________________

____

____

____

____

Supervisor's Signature

Chapter 3

Environmental Data

Date:____________

Specific learning objective: At the end of the session, Phase III (Part-1) student will be able to:

1. Assess the Environmental conditions of the family
2. Demonstrate the influence of environmental factors on health of the family.
3. Suggest suitable modifications in the environment to alleviate/ prevent health problems in the family within the given constraints.

Physical Environment

A. External Environment (Surroundings of the house)

- Pucca roads outside house: Present/Absent
- Lighting on roads or in the area: Adequate/Inadequate
- Accidental hazards: Construction sites/Open wells/Pits/Others(specify)
- Source of noise pollution (major roads, factory, railway track etc.): Present/Absent
- Waste disposal area: Nearby/Far
- Open drains outside house: Yes/No

B. Internal Environment (Inside the house)

General details

- Ownership of the house: Owned/Rented
- Approximate total plot area of the house (sq. ft.):
- Set-back: Present/Absent, if present, specify what % of total area ________________________

Type of construction

- Floor: Pucca / Kutcha / Pucca Kutcha
- Wall: Kutcha / Bricked/Cemented
- Roofing: Pucca / Kutcha / Tiled
- No. of living rooms:
- No. of occupants:

Overcrowding: Present/ Absent

If present; specify the criteria: Persons per room/ Area/Gender separation (Refer to Appendix 4)

Light: Adequate / Inadequate

Source of light: Natural / Artificial

Accident prone areas in the house (slippery floors, roof without boundary wall, steps without railings/ inadequate lighting, others if any specify): Present/Absent

Dampness in the house: Present/Absent

Source of Indoor air pollution (smoking, wood burning, chulha without chimney): Present/Absent

Measurement of the house

Rooms Measurement (in feet)		Ventilators (in feet)		Windows (in feet)		Doors (in feet)		Ventilation
S. No.	Size (lxbxh)	No.	Size (lxb)	No.	Size (lxb)	No.	Size (lxb)	Satisfactory / Not Satisfactory

Ventilation: Adequate/ Inadequate

- Source of ventilation: Natural/ Artificial (Fans/Exhaust fans/AC/Coolers)
- Cross Ventilation: Present / Absent

Kitchen

- Location: Separate / Veranda / Open / Living Room
- Cleanliness: Clean / Dirty
- Floor: Pucca / Kutcha
- Storage of cooked and raw food: Covered /Uncovered containers
- Storage of vegetables, fruits and leftover cooked food: In refrigerator/ Outside
- Lighting (Natural): Adequate / Inadequate
- Lighting (Artificial): Adequate / Inadequate

- Fuel used: Kerosene / Cooking Gas / Coal / Firewood / Others
- Smoke outlet: Present / Absent
- Presence of soot particles on kitchen walls (indicator of indoor air pollution): Yes/No
- Sullage disposal: Closed drain/Open drain/No drain (stagnant water collection)

Water Supply

- Source: Piped Water Supply / Boring / Hand Pump / Tanker / Other (specify)
- Supply: Intermittent /Continuous
- Method of Storage of drinking water:
- Type of container used: Covered /Uncovered
- Method of drawing drinking water: Mug/Ladle/Steel Glass / Tumbler / Other specify
- Methods of purification used at household level: Boiling / Filtration / Chlorination / Reverse osmosis/ None / Any other (Specify)

Refuse Collection/Disposal

- Collection Inside house: Heaps / Open bins / Closed bins
- Waste segregation in biodegradable and nonbiodegradable bins: Yes/No
- Frequency of refuse disposal (Specify):
- Waste disposal method: Burning/Open ground dumping/Collection by municipality/any other specify

Privy (Lavatory)

- Own/ Community / Shared / None
- If shared;Approx. no. of families using toilet:
- Type: Flush type / Open field defecation
- Sewage system: Present/Absent
- Septic Tank: Present/Absent

Bathroom

- Separate in House / Not Separate / Community Bathroom
- Drainage: Open/Closed

Biological Environment

- Potential Mosquito Breeding sites: Absent / Present
- Mosquito breeding: Present / Absent (Specify places)
- Potential housefly breeding places: absent/present
- Housefly breeding: Present / Absent
- Cattle in the family: Yes / No   If yes; distance from living room ______________________
- Rodents seen in the house: Yes / No
- Pets in the house: Yes / No; If yes, which Pets:
- Community Dogs: Present / Absent

House Map (Transverse Section - Draw to Scale; Depict kitchen/Toilet/Room/Floor Clearly) Note: - In case of more than one floor, please attach additional sheet.

Psychological Environment

Reasons for Psychological stress

- Unemployed adult: Yes / No
- Poverty: Yes/No
- Overcrowding: Yes/No
- Any addiction in the family, specify ______________________________

- Gambling: Yes/No
- Marital conflicts / Abuse / Divorce or Separation: Yes/No
- Sibling rivalry- Y/N
- Family conflict- Y/N, if yes, identify the factors leading to it ______
- Any unmarried daughter: Yes/No
- Orphans in the family: Yes/No
- Children >6 years, not going to school: Yes/No
- If yes, state the reason ______
- Children <14 years, working (Child Labor): Yes/No
- If yes, place of work ______
- Any Delinquent Child in the Family: Yes/No
- Child marriage/ Dowry/Non-involvement of women in decision making: Yes/No
- Chronic Illness in the family: Yes/No

Emotional problems

- Is there any case of mental illness in the family- yes/no; if Yes, give details ______
  ______
  ______
- Is there any evidence of any diagnosed case of mental retardation in family: Y/N?

Personality disorders

Any family member suffering from personality disorder: Y/N

In case of any psychological/mental problem, state the effect of illness on:

(a) Individual Patient: Psychosocial level ______,

Economic level ______

(b) Family: Psychosocial level ______,

Economic level ______

(c) Attitude of family members: Positive and Caring / Sympathetic / Empathetic / Indifferent / Non-Co-operative.

Family status from its community's viewpoint

- Is the family generally accepted by the Community-Yes / No?
- In the case of rejection, identify the reasons ______

Assessment of environmental status

Environmental factors conducive to health:

1.

2.

3.

4.

5.

Environmental factors detrimental to health:

1.

2.

3.

4.

5.

Supervisor's Signature

CHAPTER 4

Socio-Cultural Environment

Date:__________

Specific learning objectives: At the end of the session, Phase III (Part-1) student will be able to:

1. Describe knowledge, attitude, customs, beliefs and practices of the family in health and disease.
2. Impart health education to promote healthy practices.

Information regarding customs and health practices

Name of the respondent: __________

Menstruation

- Menstruation is a normal physiological process: Yes/No
- Any restrictions during menstruation (Custom/Religious): Yes/No; If Yes specify __________

Marriage and Childbearing

- System of marriage: Within Religion / Caste / Kinship Group
- What is the legal age for marriage in India for boys: __________ , for girls? __________
- At what age you were married? __________
- Average expenditure on marriage __________
- Practice of dowry: Prevalent/Non-prevalent
- Pardah System: Prevalent/Non-prevalent
- Preference for a male child: Yes/No
- Age at first pregnancy of the respondent (if applicable) __________
- Number of children born (if applicable): __________
- Any spacing methods used: Y/N; if yes, specify __________

Detail regarding the last pregnancy and its outcome

- Registered in antenatal Clinic: Yes/No; period of gestation at the time of registration in weeks ________________
- Diet during pregnancy:
  - Any additions:
  - Any restrictions:
- Physical activity:
- Whether antenatal care received from a health facility: Yes/No.
  - Number of antenatal visits ________________
- Delivery: Institutional/Home; Delivered by: Doctor/Nurse/Trained Dai/Untrained Dai/Relatives or Neighbors
- Cord applicant: None/Ash/Cow dung/Ghee/Antiseptic/Other
- Isolation during puerperium: Yes/No, if yes specify the number of days ________________

Prevalent beliefs/practices in the family regarding child rearing. (To be asked to the lady who has borne children, if not available, ask in general).

- Is there any special practice regarding child rearing in your family (e.g., Oil bath, hygiene etc.)? If yes, please specify:
- Is there a practice of giving pre-lacteal feed to the baby? If yes, please specify:
- Is colostrum (thick yellow milk) given to the new born baby? Yes/No
- When do you start giving breast milk to the new-born baby? (specify hours after delivery)
- For how long a baby is given only breast milk?
- Is water given to the baby during the first 6 months of age? Yes/No
- Usually in your family for how long a child is breast fed?
- Is milk other than breast milk given to the child in your family? Yes/No
- If yes, please specify What is given? What age it is started? How it is given? Is it diluted with water?

  ____

  ____
- When is complementary feeding usually started (age in months):
- What food is usually given for complementary feeding (specify):

  ____
- Is your child registered with any Well Baby Clinic/ Anganwadi Yes/No;
  - If No, reason: don't know about it / no clinic available/no need /other
- Do you visit the clinic regularly with the baby: Yes/No.
  - If No, specify why?
- Do you/other family members take your child for immunization? Yes/No;
  - If Yes, Where: Hospital /Health Centre/Private Doctor /Dispensary/Others(specify)
- Whom do you consult in the event of child's illness? Government / Private facility

- Which kind of system of medicine do you usually follow for child's illness? Allopathic / Homeopathic / Ayurvedic / Yunani / Others (specify)

Other child rearing practices

- Application of kajal: Y/N; if yes, with common applicator: Y/N
- Exposure to sunlight: Y/N
- Food prohibited during fever: Y/N
- Restriction of fluids during diarrhea: Y/N

Health seeking behavior

- What is the belief of family regarding causation of disease: Past sins/ Gods will /Evil eye/ Scientific reasons (Specify)
- Does your family believe in faith healing: Yes/No; If yes, specify ____________
- Does the family attend any health center/ clinic in case of illness: Yes/No; If no, why ____________
- Who is your first point of contact in case any member of your family is ill: Home remedy/ Health centre/Hospital /Local doctor (Specify)/Other (Specify) ____________
- What type of treatment does your family seek at the time of illness: Allopathic / Ayurvedic / Homeopathic / Yunani / Siddha / Puja /Other rituals (specify) ____________
- What is the usual source of medical care, if somebody is ill in your family: Govt. Hospital / Govt. Dispensary / MCH Centre / Private Practitioner/Any Other (Specify) ____________

Knowledge and Practices in some common diseases

Knowledge

Are you aware of	Y/N	Can you enumerate mode of transmission?	Do you know how it can be prevented?	Is social stigma attached to the disease? Y/N
Tuberculosis				
Measles				
Dengue				
Diarrhea				
Hypertension				
Diabetes				

Practice: Respond if any of the family members have suffered any of the following diseases in the past one year

Diseases	Which system you are following for treatment of these diseases (Allopathy/Homeopathy/Yunani/Siddha/ Aayurveda/self-medication/any other)	Compliance to medications (Y/N)
Tuberculosis		
Measles		
Dengue		
Diarrhea		
Hypertension		
Diabetes		

Personal hygiene: Satisfactory/Unsatisfactory; If unsatisfactory, specify ____________________

Analysis and Interpretation

Social problems existing in the family: ____________________

____

____

____

Customs and practices conducive to health: ____________________

____

____

____

____

Customs and practices harmful for health: ____________________

____

____

____

____

Supervisor's Signature

CHAPTER 5

Dietary Assessment

Date:______________

Specific learning objectives: At the end of the session, Phase III (Part 1) student will be able to:

1. Describe the concept of balanced diet.
2. Demonstrate steps of dietary survey.
3. Collect the accurate information regarding food consumption of both the household and individual member.
4. Detect deficiencies/ excess of various nutrients and correlate them to the nutritional status of the family members.
5. Advise the family regarding desired change in diet in case of any nutritional disorder/ deficiency/ excess.

Dietary habits of family members

- Food habits: Vegetarian/Non-vegetarian/Egg-Vegetarian
- Meals consumed: bed tea, breakfast, mid-morning snack, lunch, evening tea/ snack, dinner, bedtime drink (milk/tea etc.)/post-dinner snack

Assess the nutritional requirements of each family

Depending upon age, gender, type of work (sedentary, moderate, heavy) and physiological state (pregnancy, lactation etc.), requirements of calories and proteins can be determined from ICMR- NIN, 2020 reference charts (Annexure 5)

Name of family Member	Calorie requirement (kcal/day)	Protein Requirement (g/day)	Fat Requirement (g/day)	Dietary Fiber Requirement (g/day)	Any special needs

Dietary assessment

There are various methods for dietary assessment of an individual and a family (Annexure 5). Two commonly used methods are discussed below.

Method I - Diet survey based on 24-hour recall method.

Step 1. Calculate the food intake for the family by asking the quantities of various food items including beverages consumed by each family member and summing them to obtain diet consumed by the family in last 24 hours.

Daily diet consumption by the family (24-hour Recall Method)

S. No.	Member Name	Meal	Name of food items	Quantity (ml/g/ number)	Calories (kcal)	Protein (g)	Fat (g)	Dietary Fiber (g)
1.		Breakfast Mid-morning snack Lunch Evening tea/ snack Dinner Post- dinner drinks/snack						
2.		Breakfast Mid-morning snack Lunch Evening tea/ snack Dinner Post- dinner drinks/snack						
3.		Breakfast Mid-morning snack Lunch Evening tea/ snack Dinner Post- dinner drinks/snack						
4.		Breakfast Mid-morning snack Lunch Evening tea/ snack Dinner Post- dinner drinks/snack						

Contd.

Contd.

5.		Breakfast Mid-morning snack Lunch Evening tea/ snack Dinner Post- dinner drinks/snack						
6.		Breakfast Mid-morning snack Lunch Evening tea/ snack Dinner Post- dinner drinks/snack						
7.		Breakfast Mid-morning snack Lunch Evening tea / snack Dinner Post- dinner drinks/snack						
8.		Breakfast Mid-morning snack Lunch Evening tea/ snack Dinner Post- dinner drinks/snack						
9.		Breakfast Mid-morning snack Lunch Evening tea/ snack Dinner Post- dinner drinks/snack						
10.		Breakfast Mid-morning snack Lunch Evening tea/ snack Dinner Post- dinner drinks/snack						
Total intake								

Note – Calorie, Protein, Fat and Dietary Fiber content of each food item can be calculated directly using reference tables for cooked food items or through estimation of raw food materials contained in them.

Step 2. Calculation of the caloric and nutrients requirements for the family:

Requirement for an individual is assessed as per referenced recommendations given by ICMR- NIN, 2020 (Appendix 5) and total family requirement is calculated by summating requirements of all family members .

Total Family requirement of Calories =

Total Family requirement of Proteins =

Total Family requirement of Fats=

Total Family requirement of Dietary fiber=

Step 3: Find the difference between intake and requirement and interpret:

- Calorie excess / deficit:

  {(Calorie intake – Caloric requirement)/ Calorie requirement)} × 100
- Protein excess/deficiency for family (%):

  {(Protein intake – Protein requirement)/Protein requirement}x100
- Fat excess/deficiency for family (%):
- Dietary Fiber excess/deficiency for family (%):

Method II- Diet Survey based on inventory method

Step 1: Enquire about the quantity of different raw food stuffs used for cooking by the family per day. Method for assessment of average daily consumption of raw food:

- Find out fortnightly/monthly consumption for items procured fortnightly/monthly, e.g. rice, wheat, pulses, oil etc. and calculate average daily consumption.
- Find out weekly consumption for items such as fish, meat, eggs, fruits etc. and calculate average daily consumption.
- Find out daily consumption of regularly used items such as milk, vegetables etc.
- Find out consumption of any occasionally used item during last 24 hours e.g., biscuits, sweets, ice-cream etc.
- Deduct the consumption of food by guest, if any
- Take into account if any member has not taken meal(s) during last 24 hours.
- Calculate average daily consumption of quantity of each item and thereby deduce the calorie and protein intake per day by the family.

Step 2: Calculation of the caloric and protein requirements for the family (EAR, RDA Tables, ICMR-NIN,2020 in Annexure 5)

Step 3: Find the difference between intake and requirement and interpret

- Calorie excess / deficit:

  {(Calorie intake – Caloric requirement)/ Calorie requirement)} × 100

- Protein excess/deficiency for family (%):

  {(Protein intake- protein requirement)/Protein requirement} ×100

1. Comment on food items consumed by the family

____

____

____

____

2. Comment on nutrients consumed by the family

____

____

____

____

Nutritional status of family

Sr. No.	**Name**	**Age**	**Nutritional assessment based on anthropometry/clinical examination***	**Dietary deficiency**	**Action taken**

*Mention values for anthropometry and clinical findings and diagnosis based on these.

Supervisor's Signature

CHAPTER 6

Immunization

Date:__________

Specific learning objectives: At the end of the session, Phase III (Part 1) student will be able to:

1. Describe steps of eliciting information about immunization status of individuals.
2. Enlist vaccines used under Universal Immunization Programme, age of administration, dosage schedule, contraindications and advantages.
3. Impart education about vaccine preventable diseases to the community.

Immunization Data (for pregnant mothers and under five children)

Name of child						
Age/ date of birth						
Vaccines received						
6 weeks						
10 weeks						
14 weeks						
9 months						
16-24 months						
5 years						
10 years						
Pregnant woman						
TT1						
TT2						
TT- Booster						
Immunization status						

(#) Immunization status: mark 'F' for fully immunized, 'P' for partly immunized and 'U' for unimmunized.

Other vaccines (specify: Name of the individual immunized, name of the vaccine, doses and dates)
Vaccines not given by due date

Name of the individual	Due vaccine (dose) not given	Reasons for delay/ failure	Advice given/action taken

Adverse Events Following Immunization (AEFI); (if any):
Action taken in case of AEFI:

Supervisor's Signature

CHAPTER 7

Health Records of Vulnerable Groups

Date:______________

Specific learning objectives: At the end of the session, Phase III (Part 1) student will be able to:

- Describe the concept of high risk and screening.
- Illustrate the significance of screening/preventive check- up in relation to health status.
- Demonstrate the importance of early diagnosis of risk factors and health problems, timely referral, management in various target groups.

A. Antenatal / Postnatal Check-up: (Tick appropriate)

Identification details

Name:	Age:	Education:	Occupation:
Husband Name:	Age:	Education:	Occupation:
Income:	SES:		

Presenting complaints

Amenorrhea (details):

Any other associated complaints:

Marital History

Age at marriage: Age at cohabit: Consanguinity and its degree (if applicable):

Present Antenatal history

- L.M.P:
- Expected date of delivery:
- Time of confirmation of pregnancy (weeks):
- Test for confirmation of pregnancy: Done/not done; if yes, specify
- Registered in ANC Clinic: Yes/No; if yes, time of registration- I/2nd/3rd trimester
- Number of ANC Visits: Where visited: hospital/ health center/ home visit by a Health Care Worker

Trimester History

Trimester 1	Trimester 2	Trimester 3
Excessive Vomiting: Y/N	Quickening: Y/N; specify weeks of gestation	Pain abdomen: Y/N
Bleeding p/v: Y/N	Blurring of vision: Y/N	Headache/ seizures: Y/N
Fever with rash: Y/N	Epigastric pain: Y/N	Reduced fetal movements: Y/N
Drug intake: Y/N	Pedal edema: Y/N	Leaking or Bleeding p/v: Y/N
X-ray exposure: Y/N; If yes reason ____________	Headache: Y/N	Iron and Folic acid supplementation: Y/N; No. of days ____________ Calcium supplementation: Y/N
Folic acid supplementation: Y/N; No. of days	Iron and Folic acid supplementation: Y/N; No. of days ____________ Calcium supplementation: Y/N Albendazole: Y/N	Weight gain (Min. 5Kg): Y/N
TT immunization: Y/N	TT immunization: Y/N	Investigation USG:
Weight gain (Min. 1 Kg): Y/N	Weight gain (Min. 5 Kg): Y/N	
Investigations Hb: Y/N Blood group (wife and husband): Y/N; Compatible: Yes/No RBS: Y/N VDRL: Y/N Hep-B: Y/N HIV: Y/N Urine for albumin and sugar: Y/N	Investigations HB: Y/N USG: Y/N	

Menstrual History

Age at menarche: ____________; Cycle; ____________; Duration: ____________;

Frequency: ____________; Soaking ____________ Pads per day; ____________

Passage of clots: ____________; Dysmenorrhea: ____________

Any associated problem: ____________

Obstetric History

Gravida ____________ Para ____________ Live ____________ Abortion ____________

Age at first pregnancy:

Interval between current and previous pregnancy:

Record of previous pregnancies, if any

	Antenatal period		Intra natal period			Postnatal period	Newborn			Family Planning status	Remarks
Order of pregnancy	Normal/ High Risk; specify	ANC by a skilled health care worker (Yes/No)	Type of delivery (Full Term/ Pre-Term)	Normal vaginal/C-Section	Conducted By whom (skilled HCW/ Untrained worker) and where (Home/Hosp.)	Normal/ Eventful; specify	Sex	Alive/ dead	If dead age and cause of death		

Past History

Hypertension: Y/N, Diabetes: Y/N, TB: Y/N, Blood transfusion: Y/N; Major surgery: Y/N; Prolonged hospitalization: Y/N; COPD: Y/N; Seizure disorder: Y/N; Chronic medication intake: Y/N

Family History

History of Twins: Y/N, Preterm: Y/N, Recurrent Abortion: Y/N; Diabetes: Y/N

Nutritional History/ Problems including nutritional deficiencies in ANC/ PNC Period:

Assess the diet of the antenatal / postnatal / lactating woman by 24-hour recall method

Meal	Food Items consumed	Calorie intake (Kcal)	Protein intake (gm)
Breakfast			
Mid-morning snack			
Lunch			
Evening snacks			
Dinner			
Any Other			
Total			

- Calorie requirement: (kcal)
- Excess/Deficit: (kcal)
- Protein requirement: (gm)
- Excess/deficit: (gm)

Housing and environment: ______________________________

____

____

____

____

Accidental hazards: ______________________________

____

____

____

Socio-cultural Practices: ______________________________

____

____

____

Physical examination

1. General examination

- Anemia/ Pallor: Yes/No, if yes, severity: Mild/ Moderate/Severe
- Any Icterus/JVP/Clubbing/Cyanosis/Lymphadenopathy/Pedal Oedema
- Present weight (kg.):

- Gain in weight (as per gestation): Less/More/Normal
- Pre-pregnancy weight (if available):
- B.P:__________/__________mm Hg: Comment on status: ____________________

2. Abdominal examination

On inspection	On Palpation	On Auscultation
Shape of the abdomen:	Abdominal girth	Fetal heart sound:__________/min.
Symmetry:	Fundal height	
Fullness of Flanks:	Fundal grip	
Striae gravidarum:	Lateral grip	
Striae nigra:	1st pelvic grip	
Scar:	2nd pelvic grip	

If ANC Case registered, then the information from the card should be transferred.

Treatment taken, if any:

____

____

____

____

High risk/ Normal pregnancy, if high risk, criteria present:

Preparation for delivery: Money, vehicle, place of delivery, awareness about JSY

Plan for family planning: Yes/No

Plan to continue IFA and Calcium for 6months post-natal: Yes/No

Plan to adopt postpartum contraceptive: Y/N; If yes: PPIUCD/PoP/Condoms/Conventional methods

Assessment for breast feeding:

Follow up Notes

Date	Weight	BP	Fundal Height	Lie and Presentation	Fetal Heart Sound	Lab Reports (Hb, Urine for Sugar and Albumin)	Dietary or Any Other Advice Given	Signature of Faculty

Supervisor's Signature

B. In Postnatal Case, in Addition to the Antenatal Work-up Following History Needs to be Taken

Date:____________

Natal History

Place of delivery: Institutional/Home

Person conducted delivery: Doctor/ Health staff/ TBA/Untrained dai

Type of delivery: normal vaginal/C-section/vaginal-assisted delivery

Delivery was uneventful/eventful; if complication happened, specify: postpartum hemorrhage, obstructed labor, malpresentation, others

Neonatal history

General	Feeding
Birth order: Gender: M/F Birth weight: ; LBW: Y/N	Initiation of breastfeeding: hrs. of delivery Colostrum given: Y/N Pre-lacteal feed given: Y/N; if yes, specify
Cried immediately after birth: Y/N	Breastfeeding is on demand: Y/N
Anything applied to umbilical cord: Y/N	Frequency of breastfeeding in a day:
When did the child pass first stool?	Burping is done after breastfeeding: Y/N
When did the child urinate for the first time?	• Is artificial feeding being done: Y/N; if yes • When was it started: • Reason for its initiation: • What formula/artificial feed is being given: • Given with the help of: cup and spoon/bottle/palade
When was the first bath given to the child?	
Prophylactic Vit.K injection given at birth: Y/N	
Immunization at birth: OPV, HepB, BCG, any other; specify	
Application of kajal to eyes:	

Postnatal history of the mother

- Status of vaginal bleeding: normal/excessive
- Any complication during postpartum period:
- Breast pain/tenderness: Y/N

- Pain/burning micturition: Y/N
- Foul smelling lochia: Y/N
- Pain in abdomen: Y/N
- Fever: Y/N
- Any other problem; specify:
- Postnatal visits: institutional/home; number of visits ____________

Physical Examination

Neonate		Mother
Congenital malformations/defects/deformities: Y/N		General Physical Examination:
Anterior fontanelle; any abnormality		
Eyes-	Discharge: Y/N Redness: Y/N Icterus: Y/N	
Abdomen-	Soft/hard Hernia: Y/N	Breast examination:
Umbilicus-	Fallen off: Y/N Redness: Y/N Discharge: Y/N	
Primitive reflexes-	Rooting: Y/N Suckling: Y/N	Abdomen:
Anthropometry-	Weight: Length: Head circumference: Chest circumference:	

Supervisor's Signature

C. Under-Five Child

Use separate sheets for more than one under-five in the family.

Date:______________

Identification details

Name: Gender: Age / Date of birth:

Informant:

Education of mother: Occupation of mother: Income:

Education of father: Occupation of father: Income:

SES:

Presenting complaints

Chief complaints:

Elaborate the chief complaints in chronological order:

Specifically ask for symptoms of nutrient deficiency:

Past history

History of similar as well as common conditions (diarrhoea, malnutrition, ARI etc.):

Undergoing any treatment for any chronic condition: Y/N; if yes, specify: ____________________

History of recurrent hospitalization: Y/N; specify reason ______________________________

Personal history: Pica/bed wetting/ nail biting/thumb sucking

Birth history

Birth order: Living order:

Any significant antenatal history:

Preterm/ Full term; Normal /Abnormal (specify):

Delivered by Doctor/Midwife/Trained Dai/Untrained Dai/Other (specify) __________________ Place of delivery: Home/ Hospital

Birth weight: kgs; Normal/LBW

Child registered with under-five/ well baby clinic: Y/N

Immunization status: Vaccines given appropriate for age: Yes/No; if yes, specify ______________

Vaccination status: Unimmunized/Partially immunized /Completely Immunized for age

Nutrition history:

Feeding: Breastfed/Non breastfed

Exclusive Breast feeding up to ________________ months; breast feeding continued up to/stopped at the age of ________________ months

Details of bottle feeding/artificial feeding if any: ____

____

Details of complimentary feeding:

When was started: ; Which food items were given: ________________________________

____

Details of present nutrition

Meal	**Food items**	**Quantity of Food items**	**Calorie intake (Kcal/d)**	**Protein intake (g/d)**
Breakfast Mid-morning snack Lunch Evening Snacks Dinner Any Other				

- Total calorie intake: Total calorie requirement:
- Total protein intake: Total protein requirement:
- Any excess/deficit:

Details of any supplementary nutrition if received at Anganwadi:

Growth monitoring at Anganwadi center is being done: Y/N

Any food items disliked by the child:

Does the mother wash her hands before cooking food: Y/N

Does the mother wash her hands before feeding food: Y/N

Growth and development milestones

For growth, ask mother to show growth chart, analyze and interpret the growth chart (Annexure 6):

____

____

For development, rule out deafness and dumbness in the child followed by assessment of developmental milestones (Annexure 7)

Major developmental milestones

Milestone	Age at which it was achieved	Appropriate age for achievement of the milestone (in completed months)	Inference (Normal/Delayed development)
Social smile		2	
Head holding		4	
Can speak monosyllables (ma,ba,da etc.)		6	
Sits without support		9	
Crawls		9	
Stands without support		12	
Runs		24	

Sibling history

Age difference between the child and his/her immediate elder sibling:

Any gender bias in the family:

Psychosocial history:

Housing and environment:

Accidental Hazards:

Physical examination

Clinical examination from head to toe

Organ/System to be examined	Observation
General appearance	Normal built/thin/edematous
Hair	Normal/lusterless/thin and sparse/flag sign
Face	Normal/pigmentation/moon face
Eyes (Conjunctiva) (Cornea)	Normal/pallor/dry and wrinkled/bitot's spot Normal/dry/keratomalacia
Lips	Normal/cheilosis/angular stomatitis
Tongue	Normal/pale/red and raw, geographic
Teeth	Normal/mottled enamel/caries
Gums	Normal/swollen/bleeding
Glands	Normal/ thyroid enlargement/parotid enlargement
Skin	Normal/dry/follicular hyperkeratosis/flaky paint dermatosis
Nails	Normal/koilonychia
Knees	Normal/knock knee/epiphyseal enlargement
Feet	Normal/pedal edema
Other systems	Hepatomegaly/muscle weakness/sensory loss/delayed reflexes/ cardiac enlargement

Anthropometric measurements

Weight:

Length/Height:

Head circumference:

Chest circumference:

Mid-arm circumference:

Is she/he a high-risk child? Y/N, If yes why? ____________________

Complete diagnosis

____

____

____

____

Action taken / advice given

____

____

____

____

Follow up Notes:

Date	Age	Height	Weight	Follow up Notes	Signature of Faculty

Supervisor's Signature

D. Adolescent Health Record (10-19 Years)

Use separate sheets for more than one adolescent in the family.

Date of Visit:____________

Identification details

Name:

Age:

Sex:

Date of Birth:

Presenting complaints with history of present illness (Indicate positive findings only):

Past History (Indicate significant events only):

Menstrual History (in case of adolescent girls) :

Psychosocial Assessment (This assessment should be done for all adolescents irrespective of the presenting complaints/issues).

Education

- Whether attended school: Y/N; if yes, age of joining:
- Age of leaving school:
- Reasons for leaving school:
- Are you studying? Y /N; If yes, how is your performance at school / college?

____

Employment

- Are you employed somewhere? Yes / No;
- If yes, reason for the same ____________________________
- Vocational Training received if any: Y/N

Nutrition

- Food habits: Vegetarian/Non-vegetarian/Eggs and Vegetarian
- Like/dislike for any specific food items:
- On a normal day how may meals do you have:
- How many times a week do you eat outside:

Nutritional Assessment

Meal	Food items	Quantity of Food items	Calorie intake (Kcal/d)	Protein intake (g/d)
Breakfast Lunch Evening Snacks Dinner Any Other				

Total calorie intake: Calorie requirement: Excess/Deficit:

Total protein intake: Protein requirement: Excess/Deficit:

Activity

What do you do in your free time: Watching TV/Internet/Yoga/Sports/Music/Others; specify ______________

____

____

Substance abuse

Have you ever used: Tobacco / Alcohol / Other substances? Yes / No

If yes, are you using them currently? Yes / No

Sexuality

Have you ever had sex? Yes / No

If yes; With consent / forced

Are you aware of safe sex practices: Yes/No

Are you sexually active now? Yes / No

Safety

Do you feel safe at home? Yes / No

Do you feel safe in your school/workplace? Yes / No

Mental Health

Do you feel able to cope with your situation? Yes / No

Have you ever thought of ending your life? Yes / No

Personal Hygiene ______________________________

____

Examination Physical Appearance (including signs of any physical assault): ______________

____

Mental State (encircle in finding)

Alert / Drowsy   Well Oriented / Not Well oriented   Coherent / Incoherent

General Physical Examination:

Weight ____________ Kg. Height ____________ cm BMI ______________

Blood Pressure ______________ mm Hg Pulse / Heart rate______________/ min

Respiratory rate ____________ / min.

Pallor: Jaundice: Clubbing:

Lymphadenopathy: Thyroid swelling: Teeth cavities:

Gum Bleeding: Others:

Systemic Examination (Do complete systemic examination and note relevant findings)

____

____

____

____

Laboratory investigations

____

____

____

____

Diagnosis and Advice

____

____

____

____

Follow up Record

Date	Follow up Notes	Signature of Faculty

Supervisor's Signature

E. Eligible Couple Health Record

Use separate sheets for more than one eligible couple

Date:____________

Identification details

Name:	Age:	Education:	Occupation:
Spouse Name:	Age:	Education:	Occupation:
Income:	SES:		
Religion:	Setting: Rural/Urban		

Age at marriage:

Age at first pregnancy:

Was the first pregnancy planned: Yes /No

Knowledge, attitude and Practices

Knowledge	Attitude	Practices
Do you know that child birth can be planned: Y/N	Attitude towards utilization of contraceptive methods: positive/negative	Are you using any contraceptive method: Y/N;If yes, type of contraceptive used: ________ duration of use ________ If No; specify reasons
When did you come to know: Before marriage/after marriage	Are you willing to undergo sterilization (in case of fulfilling eligibility): Y/N	Usage of contraceptives: Regular/ Irregular
Source of information: Spouse/Friends/neighbors/HCWs/ Mass media/Other		
Do you have knowledge about methods of family planning: Y/N; If yes, name them:		
1. 2. 3. 4. 5.		
What should be the ideal gap between two children:		
Where youcan get family welfare services: Govt. Hospital / Govt. dispensary / MCH Centre / Private Practitioner /Anganwadi / ASHA / Any other		

Inference

Unregulated fertility / Spacing method / Permanent method

Advice given:

Agency suggested for supply of contraceptives:

Any other suggestion given:

Follow up record

Date	Follow up notes	Signature of faculty

Supervisor's Signature

F. Geriatric Health Record (60 Years and Above)

Add extra sheets in case of more than one geriatric case in the family

Date:______________

Identification details

Name:

Age:

Gender:

Education:

Occupation:

Income:

SES:

Present history of illness (in chronological order)

Symptom	Onset of symptoms (sudden/gradual)	Duration	Description of symptoms

Past history

H/o Diabetes mellitus/Hypertension/CAD/TB/COPD/Asthma/Other

Duration of illness:

Place of seeking treatment: Compliance with the treatment:

Do you face restriction in activity of daily living: Y/N; if yes, which activities ____________________

Immunization history

History of vaccine received: Pneumococcal/Influenza/COVID-19/Others

Social history

Interpersonal relationship with other family members and neighbors:

Receiving care and affection by family members: Y/N

Is he/she socially active:

Is he/she socially dependent: Y/N

Is he/she availing any old age pension: Y/N

Nutrition

____

____

____

Housing (rule out any accident-prone area in the house):

____

____

____

Physical examination

General appearance:

Height: Weight: BMI:

Blood pressure:

Any sign of malnutrition:

Dentition: edentulous/ artificial teething/any other

Systemic examination: ____

____

____

Follow up record

Date	Follow up notes	Signature of faculty

Supervisor's Signature

Preventive checkup of other family members

Enter the relevant information in the format given below for all family members (One page per family member) Add additional pages if required

Date of Examination	Name	Age/ Sex	Significant Findings on History	Significant Findings on Examination	Height	Weight	BMI	Blood Pressure	Hemoglobin	Diagnosis	Action Taken	Follow up

Preventive checkup of other family members

Enter the relevant information in the format given below for all family members (One page per family member) Add additional pages if required

Date of Examination	Name	Age/ Sex	Significant Findings on History	Significant Findings on Examination	Height	Weight	BMI	Blood Pressure	Hemoglobin	Diagnosis	Action Taken	Follow up

Preventive checkup of other family members

Enter the relevant information in the format given below for all family members (One page per family member) Add additional pages if required

Date of Examination	Name	Age/ Sex	Significant Findings on History	Significant Findings on Examination	Height	Weight	BMI	Blood Pressure	Hemoglobin	Diagnosis	Action Taken	Follow up

Preventive checkup of other family members

Enter the relevant information in the format given below for all family members (One page per family member) Add additional pages if required

Date of Examination	Name	Age/ Sex	Significant Findings on History	Significant Findings on Examination	Height	Weight	BMI	Blood Pressure	Hemoglobin	Diagnosis	Action Taken	Follow up

CHAPTER 8

Summary, Conclusion and Recommendations

Date:______________

FAMILY DIAGNOSIS:

SOCIAL PATHOLOGY:

POSITIVE AND NEGATIVE FACTORS IDENTIFIED

S No.	Positive factors	Negative factors
1.		
2.		
3.		
4.		
5.		

MEDICAL AND SOCIAL PROBLEMS IDENTIFIED

Medical Problems

S No.	Medical Problems	Action Taken
1.		
2.		
3.		
4.		
5.		

Social Problems

S No.	Medical Problems	Action Taken
1.		
2.		
3.		
4.		
5.		

OBJECTIVES OF THE FAMILY HEALTH CARE PROGRAMME

S No.	Name the objectives that has been achieved	State how
1.		
2.		
3.		
4.		
5.		

S No.	Name the objectives that has not beenachieved	Reason for non- achievement
1.		
2.		
3.		
4.		
5.		

Supervisor's Signature

Family Number 3

CHAPTER 1

Identification and Demographic Data

Date:__________

Specific learning objectives: At the end of the session, Phase III (Part-1) student will be able to:

1. Develop effective communication skills.
2. Describe the significance of each discussed variable in relation to health.
3. Discuss the role of family in health and disease.

Identification data

- Name of the Head of the Family __________ Age _____ (in completed years)
- Gender ________ Address __________
- Setting: Urban/Rural
- Family Type: Joint/Nuclear/Three generation
- Total number of family members __________
- Religion: Hindu/ Muslim/ Sikh/ Christian/ Other (specify) __________
- Whether migrants–Yes/No
- If yes, State of Origin __________

Demographic Data

S. No.	Name	Relation-ship with the head of family	Age	Sex	Marital status	Educational status	Occupation	Income	Remarks

***Exact date of birth of under-five.**

- Identify persons in the family belonging to vulnerable group:
- Any vital events in the family in last one year (Birth/Death/Marriage/Divorce/Adoption/Migration):

- Any history of neonatal death/maternal death/under-5 death/accidental death:

- History of diabetes, hypertension, tuberculosis or any other chronic illness:

- Any consanguinity in the family with its degree (second/third):

Inference

- Family size

- Dependency ratio

- Unemployment

Supervisor's Signature

Chapter 2

Socio-Economic Data

Date:__________

Specific learning objectives: At the end of the session, Phase III (Part-1) student will be able to:

1. Demonstrate the steps of assessment of socio-economic status and application of various socioeconomic status scales in different settings.
2. Apply the concept of poverty line
3. Illustrate the role of socio-economic status in health and disease.

Income source and expenditure pattern

- House: Rented / Owned
- Total Family Income / month Rs.:
- Total Expenditure/month Rs.:
- Per capita Income / month (total family income divided by total family members) Rs.:

Sources ofIncome

Land	House	Shop	Wages/salary of all members	Cottage Industry/ Farm Stock	Others	Total

Average expenditure per month (in rupees)

Rent	Food	Clothing	Education	Fuel	Electricity	Recreation	Transport	Smoking	Alcohol	Medicine	Doctor's fee	*Social customs	Health insurance	Others	Total

*Social customs e.g Marriage, Child birth, Mundan, Birthday, Gauna etc. calculate average per month from annual expenditure.

Assessment

SES Score: Socioeconomic Class:

(Based on Modified BG Prasad/Modified Kuppuswamy scale in urban and Modified BG Prasad/ Modified Udai Pareek in rural area (refer to Annexure 3):

- Does the family belong to "Below poverty line" category: Yes/No

  (If yes, confirm this by asking for BPL card/ color of the ration card)
- Any benefit received by the family from the government or NGO: pension/coverage under government health insurance scheme/benefits under ration card, any other)

Advice given: ____

____

____

____

____

Supervisor's Signature

CHAPTER 3

Environmental Data

Date:__________

Specific learning objective: At the end of the session, Phase III (Part-1) student will be able to:

1. Assess the Environmental conditions of the family
2. Demonstrate the influence of environmental factors on health of the family.
3. Suggest suitable modifications in the environment to alleviate/ prevent health problems in the family within the given constraints.

Physical Environment

A. External Environment (Surroundings of the house)

- Pucca roads outside house: Present/Absent
- Lighting on roads or in the area: Adequate/Inadequate
- Accidental hazards: Construction sites/Open wells/Pits/Others(specify)
- Source of noise pollution (major roads, factory, railway track etc.): Present/Absent
- Waste disposal area: Nearby/Far
- Open drains outside house: Yes/No

B. Internal Environment (Inside the house)

General details

- Ownership of the house: Owned/Rented
- Approximate total plot area of the house (sq. ft.):
- Set-back: Present/Absent, if present, specify what % of total area __________

Type of construction

- Floor: Pucca / Kutcha / Pucca Kutcha
- Wall: Kutcha / Bricked/Cemented
- Roofing: Pucca / Kutcha / Tiled
- No. of living rooms:
- No. of occupants:

Overcrowding: Present/ Absent

If present; specify the criteria: Persons per room/ Area/Gender separation (Refer to Appendix 4)

Light: Adequate / Inadequate

Source of light: Natural / Artificial

Accident prone areas in the house (slippery floors, roof without boundary wall, steps without railings/ inadequate lighting, others if any specify): Present/Absent

Dampness in the house: Present/Absent

Source of Indoor air pollution (smoking, wood burning, chulha without chimney): Present/Absent

Measurement of the house

Rooms Measurement (in feet)		Ventilators (in feet)		Windows (in feet)		Doors (in feet)		Ventilation
S. No.	Size (lxbxh)	No.	Size (lxb)	No.	Size (lxb)	No.	Size (lxb)	Satisfatory / Not Satisfatory

Ventilation: Adequate/ Inadequate

- Source of ventilation: Natural/ Artificial (Fans/Exhaust fans/AC/Coolers)
- Cross Ventilation: Present / Absent

Kitchen

- Location: Separate / Veranda / Open / Living Room
- Cleanliness: Clean / Dirty
- Floor: Pucca / Kutcha
- Storage of cooked and raw food: Covered /Uncovered containers
- Storage of vegetables, fruits and leftover cooked food: In refrigerator/ Outside
- Lighting (Natural): Adequate / Inadequate
- Lighting (Artificial): Adequate / Inadequate

- Fuel used: Kerosene / Cooking Gas / Coal / Firewood / Others
- Smoke outlet: Present / Absent
- Presence of soot particles on kitchen walls (indicator of indoor air pollution): Yes/No
- Sullage disposal: Closed drain/Open drain/No drain (stagnant water collection)

Water Supply

- Source: Piped Water Supply / Boring / Hand Pump / Tanker / Other (specify)
- Supply: Intermittent /Continuous
- Method of Storage of drinking water:
- Type of container used: Covered /Uncovered
- Method of drawing drinking water: Mug/Ladle/Steel Glass / Tumbler / Other specify
- Methods of purification used at household level: Boiling / Filtration / Chlorination / Reverse osmosis/ None / Any other (Specify)

Refuse Collection/Disposal

- Collection Inside house: Heaps / Open bins / Closed bins
- Waste segregation in biodegradable and nonbiodegradable bins: Yes/No
- Frequency of refuse disposal (Specify):
- Waste disposal method: Burning/Open ground dumping/Collection by municipality/any other specify

Privy (Lavatory)

- Own/ Community / Shared / None
- If shared;Approx. no. of families using toilet:
- Type: Flush type / Open field defecation
- Sewage system: Present/Absent
- Septic Tank: Present/Absent

Bathroom

- Separate in House / Not Separate / Community Bathroom
- Drainage: Open/Closed

Biological Environment

- Potential Mosquito Breeding sites: Absent / Present
- Mosquito breeding: Present / Absent (Specify places)
- Potential housefly breeding places: absent/present
- Housefly breeding: Present / Absent
- Cattle in the family: Yes / No If yes; distance from living room ____________________
- Rodents seen in the house: Yes / No
- Pets in the house: Yes / No; If yes, which Pets:
- Community Dogs: Present / Absent

House Map (Transverse Section - Draw to Scale; Depict kitchen/Toilet/Room/Floor Clearly) Note: - In case of more than one floor, please attach additional sheet.

Psychological Environment

Reasons for Psychological stress

- Unemployed adult: Yes / No
- Poverty: Yes/No
- Overcrowding: Yes/No
- Any addiction in the family, specify ____________________

- Gambling: Yes/No
- Marital conflicts / Abuse / Divorce or Separation: Yes/No
- Sibling rivalry- Y/N
- Family conflict- Y/N, if yes, identify the factors leading to it ____________________
- Any unmarried daughter: Yes/No
- Orphans in the family: Yes/No
- Children >6 years, not going to school: Yes/No
- If yes, state the reason ____________________
- Children <14 years, working (Child Labor): Yes/No
- If yes, place of work ____________________
- Any Delinquent Child in the Family: Yes/No
- Child marriage/ Dowry/Non-involvement of women in decision making: Yes/No
- Chronic Illness in the family: Yes/No

Emotional problems

- Is there any case of mental illness in the family- yes/no; if Yes, give details ____________________
  ____
  ____
- Is there any evidence of any diagnosed case of mental retardation in family: Y/N?

Personality disorders

Any family member suffering from personality disorder: Y/N

In case of any psychological/mental problem, state the effect of illness on:

(a) Individual Patient: Psychosocial level ____________________,

Economic level ____________________

(b) Family: Psychosocial level ____________________,

Economic level ____________________

(c) Attitude of family members: Positive and Caring / Sympathetic / Empathetic / Indifferent / Non-Co-operative.

Family status from its community's viewpoint

- Is the family generally accepted by the Community-Yes / No?
- In the case of rejection, identify the reasons ____________________

Assessment of environmental status

Environmental factors conducive to health:

1.

2.

3.

4.

5.

Environmental factors detrimental to health:

1.

2.

3.

4.

5.

Supervisor's Signature

CHAPTER 4

Socio-Cultural Environment

Date: ____________

Specific learning objectives: At the end of the session, Phase III (Part-1) student will be able to:

1. Describe knowledge, attitude, customs, beliefs and practices of the family in health and disease.
2. Impart health education to promote healthy practices.

Information regarding customs and health practices

Name of the respondent: ____________

Menstruation

- Menstruation is a normal physiological process: Yes/No
- Any restrictions during menstruation (Custom/Religious): Yes/No; If Yes specify ____________
____

Marriage and Childbearing

- System of marriage: Within Religion / Caste / Kinship Group
- What is the legal age for marriage in India for boys: ____________ , for girls? ____________
- At what age you were married? ____________
- Average expenditure on marriage ____________
- Practice of dowry: Prevalent/Non-prevalent
- Pardah System: Prevalent/Non-prevalent
- Preference for a male child: Yes/No
- Age at first pregnancy of the respondent (if applicable) ____________
- Number of children born (if applicable): ____________
- Any spacing methods used: Y/N; if yes, specify ____________

Detail regarding the last pregnancy and its outcome

- Registered in antenatal Clinic: Yes/No; period of gestation at the time of registration in weeks ______________
- Diet during pregnancy:
  - Any additions:
  - Any restrictions:
- Physical activity:
- Whether antenatal care received from a health facility: Yes/No.
  - Number of antenatal visits ______________
- Delivery: Institutional/Home; Delivered by: Doctor/Nurse/Trained Dai/Untrained Dai/Relatives or Neighbors
- Cord applicant: None/Ash/Cow dung/Ghee/Antiseptic/Other
- Isolation during puerperium: Yes/No, if yes specify the number of days ______________

Prevalent beliefs/practices in the family regarding child rearing. (To be asked to the lady who has borne children, if not available, ask in general).

- Is there any special practice regarding child rearing in your family (e.g., Oil bath, hygiene etc.)? If yes, please specify:
- Is there a practice of giving pre-lacteal feed to the baby? If yes, please specify:
- Is colostrum (thick yellow milk) given to the new born baby? Yes/No
- When do you start giving breast milk to the new-born baby? (specify hours after delivery)
- For how long a baby is given only breast milk?
- Is water given to the baby during the first 6 months of age? Yes/No
- Usually in your family for how long a child is breast fed?
- Is milk other than breast milk given to the child in your family? Yes/No
- If yes, please specify What is given? What age it is started? How it is given? Is it diluted with water?

  ____

  ____

- When is complementary feeding usually started (age in months):
- What food is usually given for complementary feeding (specify):

  ____

- Is your child registered with any Well Baby Clinic/ Anganwadi Yes/No;
  - If No, reason: don't know about it / no clinic available/no need /other
- Do you visit the clinic regularly with the baby: Yes/No.
  - If No, specify why?
- Do you/other family members take your child for immunization? Yes/No;
  - If Yes, Where: Hospital /Health Centre/Private Doctor /Dispensary/Others(specify)
- Whom do you consult in the event of child's illness? Government / Private facility

- Which kind of system of medicine do you usually follow for child's illness? Allopathic / Homeopathic / Ayurvedic / Yunani / Others (specify)

Other child rearing practices

- Application of kajal: Y/N; if yes, with common applicator: Y/N
- Exposure to sunlight: Y/N
- Food prohibited during fever: Y/N
- Restriction of fluids during diarrhea: Y/N

Health seeking behavior

- What is the belief of family regarding causation of disease: Past sins/ Gods will /Evil eye/ Scientific reasons (Specify)
- Does your family believe in faith healing: Yes/No; If yes, specify ____________
- Does the family attend any health center/ clinic in case of illness: Yes/No; If no, why ____________
____
- Who is your first point of contact in case any member of your family is ill: Home remedy/ Health centre/Hospital /Local doctor (Specify)/Other (Specify) ____________
- What type of treatment does your family seek at the time of illness: Allopathic / Ayurvedic / Homeopathic / Yunani / Siddha / Puja /Other rituals (specify) ____________
- What is the usual source of medical care, if somebody is ill in your family: Govt. Hospital / Govt. Dispensary / MCH Centre / Private Practitioner/Any Other (Specify) ____________

Knowledge and Practices in some common diseases

Knowledge

Are you aware of	Y/N	Can you enumerate mode of transmission?	Do you know how it can be prevented?	Is social stigma attached to the disease? Y/N
Tuberculosis				
Measles				
Dengue				
Diarrhea				
Hypertension				
Diabetes				

Practice: Respond if any of the family members have suffered any of the following diseases in the past one year

Diseases	Which system you are following for treatment of these diseases (Allopathy/Homeopathy/Yunani/Siddha/ Aayurveda/self-medication/any other)	Compliance to medications (Y/N)
Tuberculosis		
Measles		
Dengue		
Diarrhea		
Hypertension		
Diabetes		

Personal hygiene: Satisfactory/Unsatisfactory; If unsatisfactory, specify ____________________

Analysis and Interpretation

Social problems existing in the family: ____________________

Customs and practices conducive to health: ____________________

Customs and practices harmful for health: ____________________

Supervisor's Signature

CHAPTER 5

Dietary Assessment

Date:__________

Specific learning objectives: At the end of the session, Phase III (Part 1) student will be able to:

1. Describe the concept of balanced diet.
2. Demonstrate steps of dietary survey.
3. Collect the accurate information regarding food consumption of both the household and individual member.
4. Detect deficiencies/ excess of various nutrients and correlate them to the nutritional status of the family members.
5. Advise the family regarding desired change in diet in case of any nutritional disorder/ deficiency/ excess.

Dietary habits of family members

- Food habits: Vegetarian/Non-vegetarian/Egg-Vegetarian
- Meals consumed: bed tea, breakfast, mid-morning snack, lunch, evening tea/ snack, dinner, bedtime drink (milk/tea etc.)/post-dinner snack

Assess the nutritional requirements of each family

Depending upon age, gender, type of work (sedentary, moderate, heavy) and physiological state (pregnancy, lactation etc.), requirements of calories and proteins can be determined from ICMR- NIN, 2020 reference charts (Annexure 5)

Name of family Member	Calorie requirement (kcal/day)	Protein Requirement (g/day)	Fat Requirement (g/day)	Dietary Fiber Requirement (g/day)	Any special needs

Dietary assessment

There are various methods for dietary assessment of an individual and a family (Annexure 5). Two commonly used methods are discussed below.

Method I - Diet survey based on 24-hour recall method.

Step 1. Calculate the food intake for the family by asking the quantities of various food items including beverages consumed by each family member and summing them to obtain diet consumed by the family in last 24 hours.

Daily diet consumption by the family (24-hour Recall Method)

S. No.	Member Name	Meal	Name of food items	Quantity (ml/g/ number)	Calories (kcal)	Protein (g)	Fat (g)	Dietary Fiber (g)
1.		Breakfast Mid-morning snack Lunch Evening tea/ snack Dinner Post- dinner drinks/snack						
2.		Breakfast Mid-morning snack Lunch Evening tea/ snack Dinner Post- dinner drinks/snack						
3.		Breakfast Mid-morning snack Lunch Evening tea/ snack Dinner Post- dinner drinks/snack						
4.		Breakfast Mid-morning snack Lunch Evening tea/ snack Dinner Post- dinner drinks/snack						

Contd.

Contd.

5.		Breakfast Mid-morning snack Lunch Evening tea/ snack Dinner Post- dinner drinks/snack						
6.		Breakfast Mid-morning snack Lunch Evening tea/ snack Dinner Post- dinner drinks/snack						
7.		Breakfast Mid-morning snack Lunch Evening tea / snack Dinner Post- dinner drinks/snack						
8.		Breakfast Mid-morning snack Lunch Evening tea/ snack Dinner Post- dinner drinks/snack						
9.		Breakfast Mid-morning snack Lunch Evening tea/ snack Dinner Post- dinner drinks/snack						
10.		Breakfast Mid-morning snack Lunch Evening tea/ snack Dinner Post- dinner drinks/snack						
Total intake								

Note – Calorie, Protein, Fat and Dietary Fiber content of each food item can be calculated directly using reference tables for cooked food items or through estimation of raw food materials contained in them.

Step 2. Calculation of the caloric and nutrients requirements for the family:

Requirement for an individual is assessed as per referenced recommendations given by ICMR- NIN, 2020 (Appendix 5) and total family requirement is calculated by summating requirements of all family members .

Total Family requirement of Calories =

Total Family requirement of Proteins =

Total Family requirement of Fats=

Total Family requirement of Dietary fiber=

Step 3: Find the difference between intake and requirement and interpret:

- Calorie excess / deficit:

  {(Calorie intake – Caloric requirement)/ Calorie requirement)} × 100
- Protein excess/deficiency for family (%):

  {(Protein intake – Protein requirement)/Protein requirement}x100
- Fat excess/deficiency for family (%):
- Dietary Fiber excess/deficiency for family (%):

Method II- Diet Survey based on inventory method

Step 1: Enquire about the quantity of different raw food stuffs used for cooking by the family per day. Method for assessment of average daily consumption of raw food:

- Find out fortnightly/monthly consumption for items procured fortnightly/monthly, e.g. rice, wheat, pulses, oil etc. and calculate average daily consumption.
- Find out weekly consumption for items such as fish, meat, eggs, fruits etc. and calculate average daily consumption.
- Find out daily consumption of regularly used items such as milk, vegetables etc.
- Find out consumption of any occasionally used item during last 24 hours e.g., biscuits, sweets, ice-cream etc.
- Deduct the consumption of food by guest, if any
- Take into account if any member has not taken meal(s) during last 24 hours.
- Calculate average daily consumption of quantity of each item and thereby deduce the calorie and protein intake per day by the family.

Step 2: Calculation of the caloric and protein requirements for the family (EAR, RDA Tables, ICMR-NIN,2020 in Annexure 5)

Step 3: Find the difference between intake and requirement and interpret

- Calorie excess / deficit:

  {(Calorie intake – Caloric requirement)/ Calorie requirement)} × 100

- Protein excess/deficiency for family (%):

  {(Protein intake- protein requirement)/Protein requirement} ×100

1. Comment on food items consumed by the family

___

___

___

___

2. Comment on nutrients consumed by the family

___

___

___

___

Nutritional status of family

Sr. No.	Name	Age	Nutritional assessment based on anthropometry/clinical examination*	Dietary deficiency	Action taken

*Mention values for anthropometry and clinical findings and diagnosis based on these.

Supervisor's Signature

CHAPTER 6

Immunization

Date:_____________

Specific learning objectives: At the end of the session, Phase III (Part 1) student will be able to:

1. Describe steps of eliciting information about immunization status of individuals.
2. Enlist vaccines used under Universal Immunization Programme, age of administration, dosage schedule, contraindications and advantages.
3. Impart education about vaccine preventable diseases to the community.

Immunization Data (for pregnant mothers and under five children)

Name of child						
Age/ date of birth						
Vaccines received						
6 weeks						
10 weeks						
14 weeks						
9 months						
16-24 months						
5 years						
10 years						
Pregnant woman						
TT1						
TT2						
TT- Booster						
Immunization status						

(#) Immunization status: mark 'F' for fully immunized, 'P' for partly immunized and 'U' for unimmunized.

Other vaccines (specify: Name of the individual immunized, name of the vaccine, doses and dates)
Vaccines not given by due date

Name of the individual	Due vaccine (dose) not given	Reasons for delay/ failure	Advice given/action taken

Adverse Events Following Immunization (AEFI); (if any):
Action taken in case of AEFI:

Supervisor's Signature

CHAPTER 7

Health Records of Vulnerable Groups

Date:__________

Specific learning objectives: At the end of the session, Phase III (Part 1) student will be able to:

- Describe the concept of high risk and screening.
- Illustrate the significance of screening/preventive check- up in relation to health status.
- Demonstrate the importance of early diagnosis of risk factors and health problems, timely referral, management in various target groups.

A. Antenatal / Postnatal Check-up: (Tick appropriate)

Identification details

Name:	Age:	Education:	Occupation:
Husband Name:	Age:	Education:	Occupation:
Income:	SES:		

Presenting complaints

Amenorrhea (details):

Any other associated complaints:

Marital History

Age at marriage: Age at cohabit: Consanguinity and its degree (if applicable):

Present Antenatal history

- L.M.P:
- Expected date of delivery:
- Time of confirmation of pregnancy (weeks):
- Test for confirmation of pregnancy: Done/not done; if yes, specify
- Registered in ANC Clinic: Yes/No; if yes, time of registration- I/2nd/3rd trimester
- Number of ANC Visits: Where visited: hospital/ health center/ home visit by a Health Care Worker

Trimester History

Trimester 1	Trimester 2	Trimester 3
Excessive Vomiting: Y/N	Quickening: Y/N; specify weeks of gestation	Pain abdomen: Y/N
Bleeding p/v: Y/N	Blurring of vision: Y/N	Headache/ seizures: Y/N
Fever with rash: Y/N	Epigastric pain: Y/N	Reduced fetal movements: Y/N
Drug intake: Y/N	Pedal edema: Y/N	Leaking or Bleeding p/v: Y/N
X-ray exposure: Y/N; If yes reason ______________	Headache: Y/N	Iron and Folic acid supplementation: Y/N; No. of days ______________ Calcium supplementation: Y/N
Folic acid supplementation: Y/N; No. of days	Iron and Folic acid supplementation: Y/N; No. of days ______________	Weight gain (Min. 5Kg): Y/N
	Calcium supplementation: Y/N	
	Albendazole: Y/N	
TT immunization: Y/N	TT immunization: Y/N	Investigation USG:
Weight gain (Min. 1 Kg): Y/N	Weight gain (Min. 5 Kg): Y/N	
Investigations Hb: Y/N Blood group (wife and husband): Y/N; Compatible: Yes/No RBS: Y/N VDRL: Y/N Hep-B: Y/N HIV: Y/N Urine for albumin and sugar: Y/N	Investigations HB: Y/N USG: Y/N	

Menstrual History

Age at menarche: ______________; Cycle; ______________; Duration: ______________;

Frequency: ______________; Soaking ______________ Pads per day; ______________

Passage of clots: ______________; Dysmenorrhea: ______________

Any associated problem: ______________

Obstetric History

Gravida ______________ Para ______________ Live ______________ Abortion ______________

Age at first pregnancy:

Interval between current and previous pregnancy:

Record of previous pregnancies, if any

	Antenatal period		Intra natal period			Postnatal period	Newborn			Family Planning status	Remarks
Order of pregnancy	Normal/ High Risk; specify	ANC by a skilled health care worker (Yes/No)	Type of delivery (Full Term/ Pre-Term)	Normal vaginal/C-Section	Conducted By whom (skilled HCW/ Untrained worker) and where (Home/Hosp.)	Normal/ Eventful; specify	Sex	Alive/ dead	If dead age and cause of death		

Past History

Hypertension: Y/N, Diabetes: Y/N, TB: Y/N, Blood transfusion: Y/N; Major surgery: Y/N; Prolonged hospitalization: Y/N; COPD: Y/N; Seizure disorder: Y/N; Chronic medication intake: Y/N

Family History

History of Twins: Y/N, Preterm: Y/N, Recurrent Abortion: Y/N; Diabetes: Y/N

Nutritional History/ Problems including nutritional deficiencies in ANC/ PNC Period:

Assess the diet of the antenatal / postnatal / lactating woman by 24-hour recall method

Meal	Food Items consumed	Calorie intake (Kcal)	Protein intake (gm)
Breakfast			
Mid-morning snack			
Lunch			
Evening snacks			
Dinner			
Any Other			
Total			

- Calorie requirement: (kcal)
- Excess/Deficit: (kcal)
- Protein requirement: (gm)
- Excess/deficit: (gm)

Housing and environment: ____________________

Accidental hazards: ____________________

Socio-cultural Practices: ____________________

Physical examination

1. **General examination**
   - Anemia/ Pallor: Yes/No, if yes, severity: Mild/ Moderate/Severe
   - Any Icterus/JVP/Clubbing/Cyanosis/Lymphadenopathy/Pedal Oedema
   - Present weight (kg.):

- Gain in weight (as per gestation): Less/More/Normal
- Pre-pregnancy weight (if available):
- B.P:__________/__________mm Hg: Comment on status: __________

2. Abdominal examination

On inspection	On Palpation	On Auscultation
Shape of the abdomen:	Abdominal girth	Fetal heart sound:__________/min.
Symmetry:	Fundal height	
Fullness of Flanks:	Fundal grip	
Striae gravidarum:	Lateral grip	
Striae nigra:	1st pelvic grip	
Scar:	2nd pelvic grip	

If ANC Case registered, then the information from the card should be transferred.

Treatment taken, if any:

____

____

____

____

High risk/ Normal pregnancy, if high risk, criteria present:

Preparation for delivery: Money, vehicle, place of delivery, awareness about JSY

Plan for family planning: Yes/No

Plan to continue IFA and Calcium for 6months post-natal: Yes/No

Plan to adopt postpartum contraceptive: Y/N; If yes: PPIUCD/PoP/Condoms/Conventional methods

Assessment for breast feeding:

Follow up Notes

Date	Weight	BP	Fundal Height	Lie and Presentation	Fetal Heart Sound	Lab Reports (Hb, Urine for Sugar and Albumin)	Dietary or Any Other Advice Given	Signature of Faculty

Supervisor's Signature

B. In Postnatal Case, in Addition to the Antenatal Work-up Following History Needs to be Taken

Date:______________

Natal History

Place of delivery: Institutional/Home

Person conducted delivery: Doctor/ Health staff/ TBA/Untrained dai

Type of delivery: normal vaginal/C-section/vaginal-assisted delivery

Delivery was uneventful/eventful; if complication happened, specify: postpartum hemorrhage, obstructed labor, malpresentation, others

Neonatal history

General	Feeding
Birth order: Gender: M/F Birth weight: ; LBW: Y/N	Initiation of breastfeeding: hrs. of delivery Colostrum given: Y/N Pre-lacteal feed given: Y/N; if yes, specify
Cried immediately after birth: Y/N	Breastfeeding is on demand: Y/N
Anything applied to umbilical cord: Y/N	Frequency of breastfeeding in a day:
When did the child pass first stool?	Burping is done after breastfeeding: Y/N
When did the child urinate for the first time?	• Is artificial feeding being done: Y/N; if yes • When was it started: • Reason for its initiation: • What formula/artificial feed is being given: • Given with the help of: cup and spoon/bottle/palade
When was the first bath given to the child?	
Prophylactic Vit.K injection given at birth: Y/N	
Immunization at birth: OPV, HepB, BCG, any other; specify	
Application of kajal to eyes:	

Postnatal history of the mother

- Status of vaginal bleeding: normal/excessive
- Any complication during postpartum period:
- Breast pain/tenderness: Y/N

- Pain/burning micturition: Y/N
- Foul smelling lochia: Y/N
- Pain in abdomen: Y/N
- Fever: Y/N
- Any other problem; specify:
- Postnatal visits: institutional/home; number of visits ____________

Physical Examination

Neonate		**Mother**
Congenital malformations/defects/deformities: Y/N		General Physical Examination:
Anterior fontanelle; any abnormality		
Eyes-	Discharge: Y/N Redness: Y/N Icterus: Y/N	
Abdomen-	Soft/hard Hernia: Y/N	Breast examination:
Umbilicus-	Fallen off: Y/N Redness: Y/N Discharge: Y/N	
Primitive reflexes-	Rooting: Y/N Suckling: Y/N	Abdomen:
Anthropometry-	Weight: Length: Head circumference: Chest circumference:	

Supervisor's Signature

C. Under-Five Child

Use separate sheets for more than one under-five in the family.

Date:____________

Identification details

Name: Gender: Age / Date of birth:

Informant:

Education of mother: Occupation of mother: Income:

Education of father: Occupation of father: Income:

SES:

Presenting complaints

Chief complaints:

Elaborate the chief complaints in chronological order:

Specifically ask for symptoms of nutrient deficiency:

Past history

History of similar as well as common conditions (diarrhoea, malnutrition, ARI etc.):

Undergoing any treatment for any chronic condition: Y/N; if yes, specify: ____________

History of recurrent hospitalization: Y/N; specify reason ____________

Personal history: Pica/bed wetting/ nail biting/thumb sucking

Birth history

Birth order: Living order:

Any significant antenatal history:

Preterm/ Full term; Normal /Abnormal (specify):

Delivered by Doctor/Midwife/Trained Dai/Untrained Dai/Other (specify) ____________ Place of delivery: Home/ Hospital

Birth weight: kgs; Normal/LBW

Child registered with under-five/ well baby clinic: Y/N

Immunization status: Vaccines given appropriate for age: Yes/No; if yes, specify ____________

Vaccination status: Unimmunized/Partially immunized /Completely Immunized for age

Nutrition history:

Feeding: Breastfed/Non breastfed

Exclusive Breast feeding up to ______________ months; breast feeding continued up to/stopped at the age of ______________ months

Details of bottle feeding/artificial feeding if any: ______________________________

____

Details of complimentary feeding:

When was started: ; Which food items were given: ______________________

____

Details of present nutrition

Meal	Food items	Quantity of Food items	Calorie intake (Kcal/d)	Protein intake (g/d)
Breakfast Mid-morning snack Lunch Evening Snacks Dinner Any Other				

- Total calorie intake: Total calorie requirement:
- Total protein intake: Total protein requirement:
- Any excess/deficit:

Details of any supplementary nutrition if received at Anganwadi:

Growth monitoring at Anganwadi center is being done: Y/N

Any food items disliked by the child:

Does the mother wash her hands before cooking food: Y/N

Does the mother wash her hands before feeding food: Y/N

Growth and development milestones

For growth, ask mother to show growth chart, analyze and interpret the growth chart (Annexure 6):

____

____

For development, rule out deafness and dumbness in the child followed by assessment of developmental milestones (Annexure 7)

Major developmental milestones

Milestone	Age at which it was achieved	Appropriate age for achievement of the milestone (in completed months)	Inference (Normal/Delayed development)
Social smile		2	
Head holding		4	
Can speak monosyllables (ma,ba,da etc.)		6	
Sits without support		9	
Crawls		9	
Stands without support		12	
Runs		24	

Sibling history

Age difference between the child and his/her immediate elder sibling:

Any gender bias in the family:

Psychosocial history:

Housing and environment:

Accidental Hazards:

Physical examination

Clinical examination from head to toe

Organ/System to be examined	Observation
General appearance	Normal built/thin/edematous
Hair	Normal/lusterless/thin and sparse/flag sign
Face	Normal/pigmentation/moon face
Eyes (Conjunctiva)	Normal/pallor/dry and wrinkled/bitot's spot
(Cornea)	Normal/dry/keratomalacia
Lips	Normal/cheilosis/angular stomatitis
Tongue	Normal/pale/red and raw, geographic
Teeth	Normal/mottled enamel/caries
Gums	Normal/swollen/bleeding
Glands	Normal/ thyroid enlargement/parotid enlargement
Skin	Normal/dry/follicular hyperkeratosis/flaky paint dermatosis
Nails	Normal/koilonychia
Knees	Normal/knock knee/epiphyseal enlargement
Feet	Normal/pedal edema
Other systems	Hepatomegaly/muscle weakness/sensory loss/delayed reflexes/ cardiac enlargement

Anthropometric measurements

Weight:

Length/Height:

Head circumference:

Chest circumference:

Mid-arm circumference:

Is she/he a high-risk child? Y/N, If yes why? ____________________

Complete diagnosis

____

____

____

____

Action taken / advice given

____

____

____

____

Follow up Notes:

Date	Age	Height	Weight	Follow up Notes	Signature of Faculty

Supervisor's Signature

D. Adolescent Health Record (10-19 Years)

Use separate sheets for more than one adolescent in the family.

Date of Visit:____________

Identification details

Name:

Age:

Sex:

Date of Birth:

Presenting complaints with history of present illness (Indicate positive findings only):

Past History (Indicate significant events only):

Menstrual History (in case of adolescent girls) :

Psychosocial Assessment (This assessment should be done for all adolescents irrespective of the presenting complaints/issues).

Education

- Whether attended school: Y/N; if yes, age of joining:
- Age of leaving school:
- Reasons for leaving school:
- Are you studying? Y /N; If yes, how is your performance at school / college?

  ____

Employment

- Are you employed somewhere? Yes / No;
- If yes, reason for the same ____________________________
- Vocational Training received if any: Y/N

Nutrition

- Food habits: Vegetarian/Non-vegetarian/Eggs and Vegetarian
- Like/dislike for any specific food items:
- On a normal day how may meals do you have:
- How many times a week do you eat outside:

Nutritional Assessment

Meal	Food items	Quantity of Food items	Calorie intake (Kcal/d)	Protein intake (g/d)
Breakfast Lunch Evening Snacks Dinner Any Other				

Total calorie intake: Calorie requirement: Excess/Deficit:

Total protein intake: Protein requirement: Excess/Deficit:

Activity

What do you do in your free time: Watching TV/Internet/Yoga/Sports/Music/Others; specify ___________

____

____

Substance abuse

Have you ever used: Tobacco / Alcohol / Other substances? Yes / No

If yes, are you using them currently? Yes / No

Sexuality

Have you ever had sex? Yes / No

If yes; With consent / forced

Are you aware of safe sex practices: Yes/No

Are you sexually active now? Yes / No

Safety

Do you feel safe at home? Yes / No

Do you feel safe in your school/workplace? Yes / No

Mental Health

Do you feel able to cope with your situation? Yes / No

Have you ever thought of ending your life? Yes / No

Personal Hygiene ______________________________

____

Examination Physical Appearance (including signs of any physical assault): ______________________________

____

Mental State (encircle in finding)

Alert / Drowsy   Well Oriented / Not Well oriented   Coherent / Incoherent

General Physical Examination:

Weight ______________ Kg. Height ______________ cm BMI ______________

Blood Pressure ______________ mm Hg Pulse / Heart rate______________/ min

Respiratory rate ______________ / min.

Pallor: Jaundice: Clubbing:

Lymphadenopathy: Thyroid swelling: Teeth cavities:

Gum Bleeding: Others:

Systemic Examination (Do complete systemic examination and note relevant findings)

____

____

____

____

Laboratory investigations

____

____

____

____

Diagnosis and Advice

____

____

____

____

Follow up Record

Date	Follow up Notes	Signature of Faculty

Supervisor's Signature

E. Eligible Couple Health Record

Use separate sheets for more than one eligible couple

Date:__________

Identification details

Name: Age: Education: Occupation:

Spouse Name: Age: Education: Occupation:

Income: SES:

Religion: Setting: Rural/Urban

Age at marriage:

Age at first pregnancy:

Was the first pregnancy planned: Yes /No

Knowledge, attitude and Practices

Knowledge	Attitude	Practices
Do you know that child birth can be planned: Y/N	Attitude towards utilization of contraceptive methods: positive/negative	Are you using any contraceptive method: Y/N;If yes, type of contraceptive used: __________ duration of use __________ If No; specify reasons
When did you come to know: Before marriage/after marriage	Are you willing to undergo sterilization (in case of fulfilling eligibility): Y/N	Usage of contraceptives: Regular/ Irregular
Source of information: Spouse/Friends/neighbors/HCWs/ Mass media/Other		
Do you have knowledge about methods of family planning: Y/N; If yes, name them:		
1. 2. 3. 4. 5.		
What should be the ideal gap between two children:		
Where youcan get family welfare services: Govt. Hospital / Govt. dispensary / MCH Centre / Private Practitioner /Anganwadi / ASHA / Any other		

Inference

Unregulated fertility / Spacing method / Permanent method

Advice given:

Agency suggested for supply of contraceptives:

Any other suggestion given:

Follow up record

Date	Follow up notes	Signature of faculty

Supervisor's Signature

F. Geriatric Health Record (60 Years and Above)

Add extra sheets in case of more than one geriatric case in the family

Date:______________

Identification details

Name:

Age:

Gender:

Education:

Occupation:

Income:

SES:

Present history of illness (in chronological order)

Symptom	Onset of symptoms (sudden/gradual)	Duration	Description of symptoms

Past history

H/o Diabetes mellitus/Hypertension/CAD/TB/COPD/Asthma/Other

Duration of illness:

Place of seeking treatment: Compliance with the treatment:

Do you face restriction in activity of daily living: Y/N; if yes, which activities ____________________

Immunization history

History of vaccine received: Pneumococcal/Influenza/COVID-19/Others

Social history

Interpersonal relationship with other family members and neighbors:

Receiving care and affection by family members: Y/N

Is he/she socially active:

Is he/she socially dependent: Y/N

Is he/she availing any old age pension: Y/N

Nutrition

____

____

____

Housing (rule out any accident-prone area in the house):

____

____

____

Physical examination

General appearance:

Height: Weight: BMI:

Blood pressure:

Any sign of malnutrition:

Dentition: edentulous/ artificial teething/any other

Systemic examination: ______________________________

____

____

Follow up record

Date	Follow up notes	Signature of faculty

Supervisor's Signature

Preventive checkup of other family members

Enter the relevant information in the format given below for all family members (One page per family member) Add additional pages if required

Date of Examination	Name	Age/ Sex	Significant Findings on History	Significant Findings on Examination	Height	Weight	BMI	Blood Pressure	Hemoglobin	Diagnosis	Action Taken	Follow up

Preventive checkup of other family members

Enter the relevant information in the format given below for all family members (One page per family member) Add additional pages if required

Date of Examination	Name	Age/ Sex	Significant Findings on History	Significant Findings on Examination	Height	Weight	BMI	Blood Pressure	Hemoglobin	Diagnosis	Action Taken	Follow up

Preventive checkup of other family members

Enter the relevant information in the format given below for all family members (One page per family member) Add additional pages if required

Date of Examination	Name	Age/ Sex	Significant Findings on History	Significant Findings on Examination	Height	Weight	BMI	Blood Pressure	Hemoglobin	Diagnosis	Action Taken	Follow up

Preventive checkup of other family members

Enter the relevant information in the format given below for all family members (One page per family member) Add additional pages if required

Date of Examination	Name	Age/ Sex	Significant Findings on History	Significant Findings on Examination	Height	Weight	BMI	Blood Pressure	Hemoglobin	Diagnosis	Action Taken	Follow up

CHAPTER 8

Summary, Conclusion and Recommendations

Date:____________

FAMILY DIAGNOSIS:

SOCIAL PATHOLOGY:

POSITIVE AND NEGATIVE FACTORS IDENTIFIED

S No.	Positive factors	Negative factors
1.		
2.		
3.		
4.		
5.		

MEDICAL AND SOCIAL PROBLEMS IDENTIFIED

Medical Problems

S No.	Medical Problems	Action Taken
1.		
2.		
3.		
4.		
5.		

Social Problems

S No.	Medical Problems	Action Taken
1.		
2.		
3.		
4.		
5.		

OBJECTIVES OF THE FAMILY HEALTH CARE PROGRAMME

S No.	Name the objectives that has been achieved	State how
1.		
2.		
3.		
4.		
5.		

S No.	Name the objectives that has not beenachieved	Reason for non- achievement
1.		
2.		
3.		
4.		
5.		

Supervisor's Signature

Chapter 9

Community Diagnosis

Date:______________

Specific learning objectives: At the end of the session, Phase III (Part-1) students will be able to:

1. Describe socio-demography, economic status, environment and socio-culture practices prevalent in the community.
2. Diagnose community health problems, make community diagnosis and suggest measures to improve community health.

Name of Village/Ward/ Urban Colony:

Study area: Urban /Peri-Urban /Urban Slums/Rural

Predominant religion represented in the population: Sikhs/ Hindus/ Muslims/ Christians/ Others

Important Community / Social organizations

Govt.: 1. ________________. 2. ________________. 3. ________________.

NGOs: 1.________________. 2. ________________. 3. ________________.

Principal means of livelihood: Agriculture/ Small scale industries/ Large scale industries/ Salaried jobs/ Self employed

Name of local governing body: Gram Panchayat/Zila Parishad/Municipal Corporation

Births and deaths recorded by: Gram Pradhan/Panchayat /Chowkidar/ANM/TBA/Any other

Educational facilities available:

No. of Schools: Govt.________________ Private ________________

No. of Colleges: Govt.________________ Private ________________

Health facilities available: Govt/Private/Charitable

Medical Care

Medical system utilized by the community members: Allopathy/ Homeopathy/ Ayurveda/ Siddha/Unani/ Others specify________________________________

____

Medical manpower/Health care workers available

Allopathic doctors ________________, AAYUSH Practitioners ________________, Unregistered Medical

Practitioners/Quacks ______

TBAs: ______ AWS/AWW/AWH ______ VHG ______

Water Supply: Tap/Well/Other Specify ______

Excreta disposal: Community Sanitary Latrine/Personal/Any other, specify______

Waste water disposal: Open drain/Closed drain

Refuse disposal: Dumping/Composting/ Bins (Municipal Corporation)

Disposal of dead: Ritual burning/Crematorium/Other, specify ______.

Communication facilities: Mobile phone/ Landline phone/Telephone booths

Major transport in the area: Bus/ Taxi/ Auto/ Rickshaw/ Own vehicle

General facilities: Bank/Post office/Ration shop/School/College

Recreation facilities in the area: Park/ Playground/ Gym/ Club

Social problems in the community: Alcoholism/Drug abuse/Gambling/Violence/Other specify ______

______

Main health problems in community (Interview opinion leaders/ Panchayat members)

1. ______
2. ______
3. ______
4. ______

Community Diagnosis:

______

______

______

______

______

Supervisor's Signature

Morbidity Status of Family Members

(Who are presently sick or sick during last one year)

Name of family member					
Present complaints					
Findings of clinical examination					
Probable diagnosis					
Action Taken					
Description of illnesses during last one year with no. of attacks					
Action Taken					

Annexure-1

Symbols Used in Family Tree

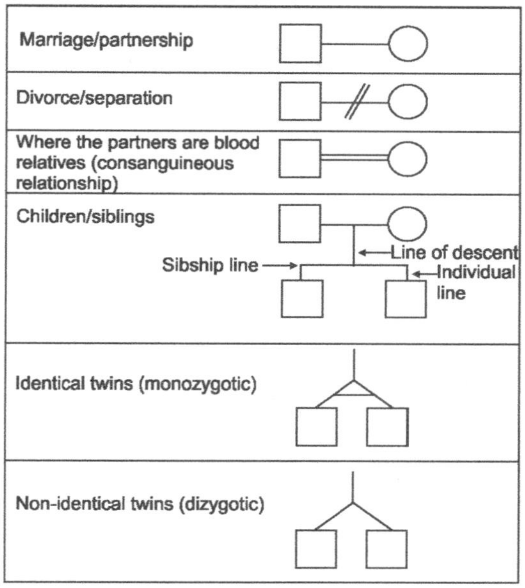

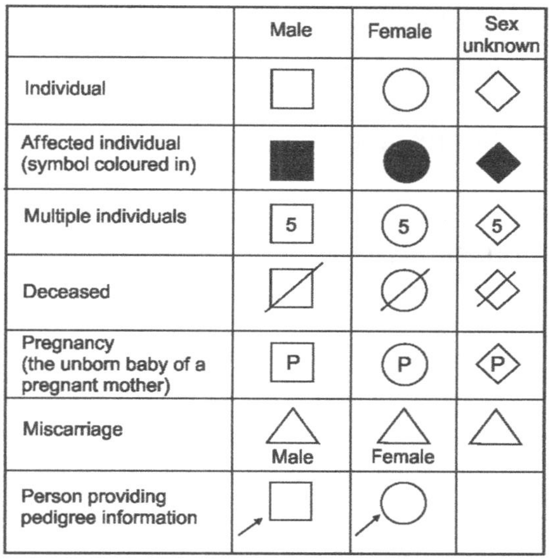

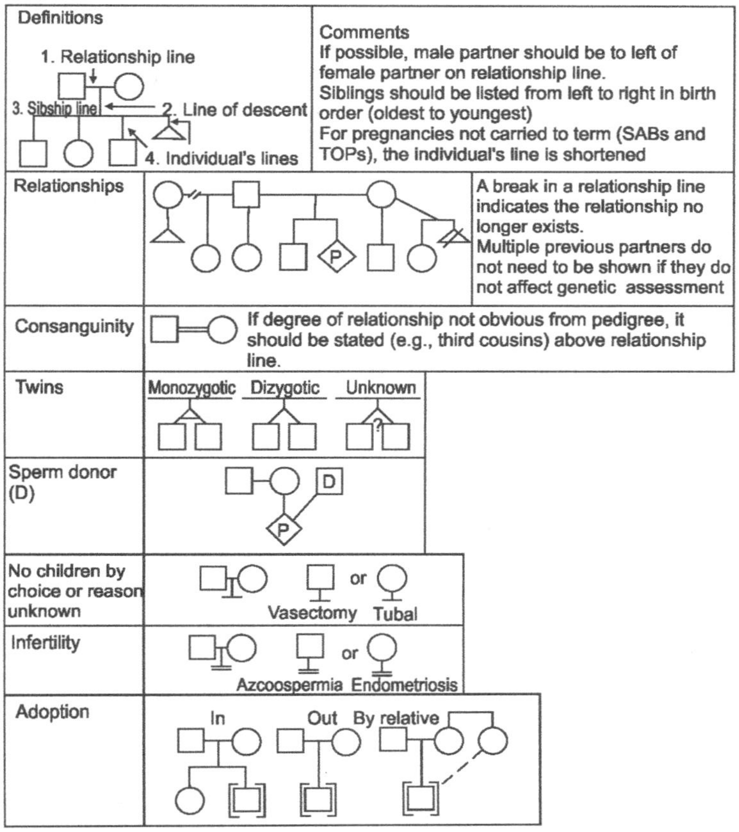

ANNEXURE-2

2A. EDUCATIONAL STATUS

ILLITERATE

LITERATE-A person above the age of 7 years who is able to read and write in any language with understanding

PRIMARY SCHOOL- A person whose education is up to 5th standard only. i.e. He/she has passed only 5th standard in school

MIDDLE SCHOOL- A person whose education is up to 8th standard only. i.e. He/she has passed only 8th standard in school.

SECONDARY SCHOOL- A person whose education is upto10th standard only. i.e. He/she has only passed 10th standard in school.

SENIOR SECONDARY- A person whose education is upto 12th standard only. i.e. He/she has only passed 12th standard in school.

GRADUATE- A person who has a graduate degree

POST – GRADUATE - A person who has completed his post-graduation from college.

2B. OCCUPATION

UNSKILLED work requiring neither education nor training eg coolie, peon, watchman, domestic helpers, etc.

SEMI-SKILLED work requiring some training eg. factory labourer, lab attendee, petty shopkeeper

SKILLED complicated work requiring long training, eg. carpenter, mason, mechanic, car driver, telephone operator, mechanics, etc.

CLERICAL training in arithmetic, reading and writing. Essentially repetitive nature of work, eg. clerk, typist, accountant, shopkeeper, sales man farm owner, etc.

SEMI-PROFESSIONAL occupation requiring post high school or college education Eg.. lecturers, insurance inspectors, musicians, etc.

PROFESSIONAL involved in decision making process, policy, execution eg. doctors, senior administrative officers, senior lecturers, readers and professors, college principles, advocates, engineers, estate planters , auditors, newspaper editors, expert musicians , architect, managing directors of industrial and business firms, managers

2C. CLASSIFICATION OF AN INDIVIDUAL BASED ON OCCUPATION AND PHYSICAL ACTIVITY

Activity based on occupations	Male	Female
Sedentary (not > an hour in an activity with HR PR increase)	Teacher, tailor, barber, executive, shoemaker, priest, peon, postman, retired personnel, etc	Teacher, tailor, executive, housewife, nurses
Moderate	Fisherman, basket maker, potter, agricultural labour, carpenter, electrician, weaver, driver, mason, fitter, turner,industrial labour, goldsmith, coolie, welder, weaver	Maid, coolie, weaver, agricultural labour, beedi maker, basket maker
Heavy	Stonecutter, black smith, mine worker wood cutter, gang-man	Woodcutter, stone cutter

Annexure- 3

Scales Used for Classification of Socioeconomic Class

3A. MODIFIED KUPPUSWAMY'S CLASSIFICATION, 2021 (USED FOR URBAN AREAS)

Initially, the scale formulated by Kuppuswamy (1976) was used for determining SES of an individual, but later on, it was modified to determine SES of a family rather than an individual. The Kuppuswamy SES has included 3 parameters, and each parameter is further classified into subgroups and scores have been allotted to each subgroup. The total score of Kuppuswamy SES ranges from 3 to 29 and it classifies families into 5 groups. The scale has been revised repeatedly over the past years because the parameter of overall income of the family from all the sources scale loses its pertinence following the devaluation in the worth of Indian rupee.

Kuppuswamy SES is revised, "as per changes in the consumer price index (CPI) for industrial workers as projected by the central ministry of statistics and programme implementation on their website." The values of the CPI are "explicated in reference to a base year". As per the Labour Bureau, Government of India, "the current base year to be considered is 2012".

For calculation of CPI (for the scale updated for the Year 2021), the current inflation rate of January 2021 i.e.: 4.06 has been taken into account. If we multiply the generated income scale values of the year 2012 with the conversion factor of 4.06 that will update the Kuppuswamy SES scale for January 2021.

The inflation rate is calculated using the formula [(b-a/a) x 100], where 'b' is the CPI of current year and 'a' is the CPI of last year.

S. No.	Updated Monthly Family Income in Rupees (2012)	Updated Monthly Family Income in Rupees (2018)	Updated Monthly Family Income in Rupees (2020)	Updated Monthly Family Income in Rupees (2021)	Score
1.	≥ 30,375	≥ 126,360	≥ 199,862	≥123,322	12
2.	15,188–30,374	63,182–126,359	99,931–199,861	61,663-123,321	10
3.	11,362–15,187	47,266–63,181	74,755 –99,930	46129-61,662	6
4.	7594–11,361	31,591–47,265	49,962–74,755	30,831-46,128	4
5.	4556–7593	18,953–31,590	29,973– 49,961	18,497-30,830	3
6.	1521–4555	6327–18,952	10,002–29,972	6,175-18,496	2
7.	≤ 1520	≤ 6326	≤ 10,001	≤ 6174	1

3A. MODIFIED KUPPUSWAMY'S SOCIOECONOMIC STATUS SCALE, 2021 (USED FOR URBAN AREAS)

S No.	Occupation of the Head	Score
1.	Legislators, Senior Officials and Managers	10
2.	Professionals	9
3.	Technicians and Associate Professionals	8
4.	Clerks	7
5.	Skilled Workers and Shop and Market Sales Workers	6
6.	Skilled Agricultural and Fishery Workers	5
7.	Craft and Related Trade Workers	4
8.	Plant and Machine Operators and Assemblers	3
9.	Elementary Occupation	2
10.	Unemployed	1

S No	Education of the Head	Score
1.	Profession or Honours	7
2.	Graduate	6
3.	Intermediate or diploma	5
4.	High school certificate	4
5.	Middle school certificate	3
6.	Primary school certificate	2
7.	Illiterate	1

S No	Income of the Head (Monthly Income in Rs)	Score
1.	≥123,322	12
2.	61,663-123,321	10
3.	46129-61,662	6
4.	30,831-46,128	4
5.	18,497-30,830	3
6.	6,175-18,496	2
7.	≤ 6174	1

S. No.	Score	Socioeconomic Class
1	26–29	Upper (I)
2	16–25	Upper Middle (II)
3	11–15	Lower Middle (III)
4	5–10	Upper Lower (IV)
5	< 5	Lower (V)

Source: Saleem SM, Jan SS. Modified Kuppuswamy socioeconomic scale updated for the year 2021. Indian J Forensic Community Med 2021; 8(1): 1-3

3B. MODIFIED UDAI PAREEK SCALE FOR SOCIAL CLASSIFICATION (USED IN RURAL AREAS)

Components	Score	Components	Score
Caste		**Social participation**	
Scheduled caste	1	None	0
Lower caste	2	Member of one organization	1
Artisan caste	3	Member of more than one organization	2
Agriculture caste	4	Office holder in such an organization	3
Prestige caste	5	Wide public leader	4
Dominant caste	6	**House**	
Occupation		No house	0
None	0	Hut	1
Labourer	1	Kutcha house	2
Caste occupation	2	Mixed house	3
Business	3	Pucca house	4
Independent profession	4	Mansion	5
Cultivation	5	**Farm power**	
Service	6	No draught animals	1
Education		1-2 draught animals	2
Illiterate	0	3-4 draught animals	4
Can read only	1	5-6 draught animals	6
Can read and write	2	**Material possessions**	
Primary	3	Bullock cart	0
Middle	4	Cycle	1
High school	5	Radio	2
Graduate	6	Chairs	3
And above	7	Mobile phone	4
Land		Television	5
No land	0	Refrigerators	6
<1 acre	1	**Family member**	
1-5 acre	2	Up to 5	2
5-10 acre	3	>5	1
10-15 acre	4		
15-20 acre	5		
≥20	6		

Grade	Category	Score on scale
I	Upper class	>43
II	Upper middle class	33-42
III	Middle class	24-32
IV	Lower middle class	13-23
V	Lower class	<13

3C. MODIFIED BG PRASAD'S CLASSIFICATION UPDATED FOR THE YEAR 2020 (CAN BE USED FOR BOTH URBAN AND RURAL AREAS OF THE COUNTRY)

	Social Class	Monthly per capita income in Rs (Revised for 2020)
I	Upper class	7533 and above
II	Upper middle	3766-7532
III	Lower middle	2260-3765
IV	Upper lower	1130-2259
V	Lower	1129 and below

ANNEXURE-4

Housing and Environment

4A. TYPE OF HOUSE

Pucca	Kutcha	Semi pucca/Mixed
Floor- paved	Floor- mud	Any combination of pucca and kutcha house
Walls- stone/brick	Walls- mud/thached	
Roof- tin/asbestos/concrete	Roof- thatched/slate/other stones	

4B. SET-BACK

Open space around the house is called set-back. It should be minimum one third of the total area in (33.3%) in urban areas and two thirds of the total area (66.7%) in rural areas.

4C. CRITERIA FOR OVERCROWDING

<table>
<tr><th>Person per room</th><th>Floor space</th><th>Sex separation</th></tr>
<tr>
<td>The criteria for counting of persons are as follows:
• An infant (a child under 12 months of age) is not counted.
• Children aged 1–10 years are counted as half a person each.
• All those above the age of 10 years are counted as one person each.
Taking above into consideration, person per room criteria is as below:</td>
<td>Measure the length (L) and breadth (B) of all the rooms and calculate the floor area by the formula:
Floor area = L × B
• Add up all the room area to calculate the total area.
• Calculate the number of occupants in the same manner as in persons per room.
• Divide the total area by the number of persons residing in the house.
• This will give the floor space per person.
Assess overcrowding using standards given below:</td>
<td>Overcrowding is considered to exist if 2 persons over 9 years of age not husband and wife and of opposite sex are obliged to sleep in the same room.</td>
</tr>
<tr>
<td><table>
<tr><th>No. of rooms</th><th>Max no. of persons recommended</th></tr>
<tr><td>1</td><td>Two</td></tr>
<tr><td>2</td><td>Three</td></tr>
<tr><td>3</td><td>Five</td></tr>
<tr><td>4</td><td>Seven</td></tr>
<tr><td>5</td><td>Ten</td></tr>
</table>
Additional 2 persons for each further room after 5 rooms.</td>
<td><table>
<tr><th>Area (sq.ft.)</th><th>Max no. of persons recommended</th></tr>
<tr><td>50-70</td><td>Half</td></tr>
<tr><td>70-90</td><td>One</td></tr>
<tr><td>90-100</td><td>One andhalf</td></tr>
<tr><td>110 and above</td><td>Two</td></tr>
</table></td>
<td></td>
</tr>
</table>

Note: Rooms used as bedroom, sitting room, prayer room, dining room, servant's room - all are considered as living rooms and therefore counted and measured for assessing overcrowding. Kitchen, bathroom, latrine, store, garage etc. are not considered as living rooms. However, a room used in common for living purpose and as kitchen or store is also considered as living room.

4D. CRITERIA FOR ADEQUATE LIGHTNING

A person should be able to read the fine print of newspaper in the four corners and centre of room. In case of illiteracy, a person should be able to perform an intricate task like separating husk from rice etc. There should be no sharp shadows, no glare. The source of light should be steady without any flickering and the distribution of light should be uniform. These criteria hold true for natural as well as artificial lighting.

4E. CRITERIA FOR ADEQUATE VENTILATION

The window area should be 1/5th of the floor area. Doors and windows combined should have 2/5th of floor area. Every room should be provided with at least two windows, and at least one of them should open directly to an open space. There should be cross ventilation. The windows should be placed at a height of 3 feet (1 metre) above the ground in living rooms. It is considered that a space of 1,000 to 1200 cubic feet per person is quite sufficient.

4F. CATTLE SHED

It should be minimum 25 feet away from a house.

ANNEXURE-5

Nutritional Assessment

5A. DIETARY SURVEY METHODS

Two types of dietary surveys

1. Qualitative survey

Food items consumed, their frequency (daily, weekly or once a while/occasionally), food preferred and food avoided. Dietary beliefs and practices of interest (dietary practices during infancy, childhood, pregnancy and lactational) are also taken into consideration.

2. Quantitative survey

Amount or quantities of food items consumed are recorded and nutrient composition are determined from tables of food consumption

METHODS OF DIET SURVEY (Source: Recommended Dietary Allowances and RDA of Indians (ICMR 2010) and Their Uses in Planning Diets)

National level	Institutional level (Used for Hostel, Hospital, Canteen, Jail, Orphanages etc.)	Family/Household Level	Individual Level
Food Balance Sheet (FBS)	• Inventory Method • Weighment Method	• Inventory Method • Weighment Method • Consumption Expenditure Survey	• Food Record or Diary • Diet history • 24-hour dietary recall • Food Frequency Questionnaire

1. **Food balance sheet**
   - Total food available or produced in the country.
   - Expressed as Per person per day of food availability.
2. **Inventory method list (log book method)**
   - Average intake of food per person per day
     (Stock at the beginning of week – stocks at the end of the week) / total number of inmates partaking the meal x numbers of days of survey
3. **Weighment methods**
   - Weighing of raw food and cooked food.
   - More accurate but difficult and least practical method.

- Raw foods weighed consecutively for one week (one dietary cycle).
- Only edible portions of raw food are weighed before cooking.
- Expressed as intake per person per day.

4. **Duplicate samples**
   - What is consumed in the family, the same amount of each food item is kept separately per day as duplicate sample.
   - The samples collected are weighed or sent to laboratory for analysis.

5. **Food frequency questionnaire**
   - List of foods and asked how often each is consumed per day/week/month. It gives an idea about the usual diet of the individual/family.

6. **24hrs recall method**
   - Most popular, practical, easy and low-cost method.
   - Participants are asked to recall all food and drink they have consumed in the previous 24 hours.
   - Most accurate when administered more than once for each individual
   - Avoid festival, fast and feast days into consideration.

5B. STANDARDIZED CUP OR BOWL OR GLASS TO BE USED FOR MEASUREMENT

Size of Teaspoon, Tablespoon and Cup

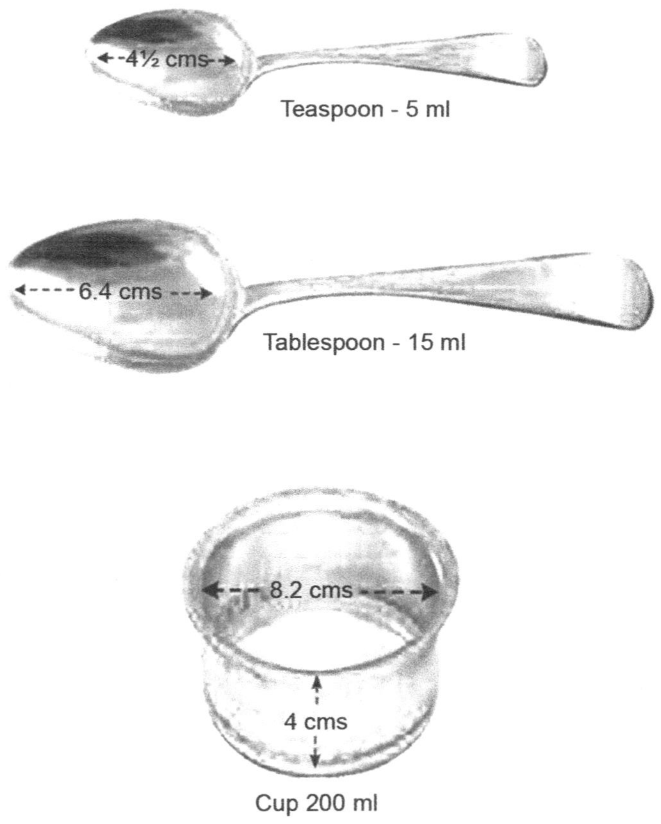

(Source: Dietary Guidelines for Indians- a Manual. 2nd ed.Hyderabad: NIN, ICMR; 2011)

5C. APPROXIMATE NUTRITIVE VALUE OF COMMON FOOD ITEMS (COOKED) IN INDIA

Food Item (Cooked)	Quantity for one serving (g/ml)	Calories (kcal)	Carbo-hydrate (g)	Protein (g)	Fat (g)	Dietary Fiber (g)
Lunch/Dinner						
Rice: basmati	140g	172	36.5	4.1	0.5	1.3
Rice:Cooked	200g	260	57.2	4.8	0.4	0.6
parboiled	340g	304	55.7	10.1	4.6	5.2
Sambar Rice	210g	327	48	5.4	12	3.1
Rice: Fried/Pulao	205g	317	52.9	9.1	8.4	4.8
Khichdi	75g	136	21.2	3.4	4.3	1.1
Pongal	30g	77	15.6	2.7	0.5	2.8
Phulka	55g	158	27.3	4.8	3.5	4.9
Paratha plain	150g	441	76.3	10.9	10.8	11.4
Paratha-aaloo	55g	166	25.8	4.8	5.1	5.1
Paratha -methi	20g	72	8.1	1.3	3.8	0.7
Poori	40g	78	16.1	2.3	1.1	2.2
Roti-Jowar	65g	130	24.4	4.2	1.8	4.1
Roti- Bajra	125g	294	43.3	5.4	11.0	7.8
Roti- Ragi	205g	97	19.7	2.4	2.1	3.1
Porridge- Ragi	290g	201	45.8	3.7	0.6	0.5
Porridge -Cereals	180g	214	47.1	4.8	0.9	7.5
Gruel						
Breakfast						
Idli	55g	90	19.4	2.8	0.3	0.9
Vada	20g	56	6.6	2.2	1.9	1.7
Vegetablesandwich	90g	134	20.4	3.0	5.2	2.4
Samosa	60g	196	24.6	3.9	9.2	2.2
Kachori	40g	152	19.0	3.9	6.8	2.1
Wheat dalia	25g	31	5.3	1	0.6	1.0
Vermicelli Upma	70g	141	19.8	2.8	5.5	0.8
Rava Upma	150g	242	34.3	5.3	9.3	2.5
Poha	130g	249	43.1	6.0	5.5	2.5
Sabudana Khichdi	105g	318	65.0	1.3	6.2	1.3
Coconut chutney	25g	55	4.4	1.7	2.9	0.9
Tomato chutney	30g	31	3.2	0.7	1.6	0.9
Puffed rice	20g	65	14.7	1.5	0.2	0.3
Chocos (without milk)	50g	192	45.8	2.3	1.3	0.3
Cornflakes (without milk	30g	107	25.2	2.3	0.1	1.0
Bread-White	25g	61	13.0	2.0	0.8	0.7
Bread- Brown	25g	61	12.3	2.2	0.8	0.9
Thepla (Gujrat)	30g	86	11.5	2.9	3.2	2.3
Dhokla	20g	34	4.4	1.6	1.1	0.8
Plain Dosa	80g	159	28.1	4.1	3.0	1.1
Aappam (Kerala)	95g	170	31.2	3.8	3.0	1.6
Adai (Tamilnadu)	80g	186	27.4	5.1	6.2	4.4

Contd.

Contd.

Vegetables/Pulses						
Greens with dal (eg. Dal palak)	160g	127	18.6	7.5	2.5	4.5
Palak paneer	95g	78	7.6	3.7	3.4	5.4
Legumes with gravy (Rajma/Chana)	170g	186	23.4	6.4	6.9	10.9
Kadi	135g	77	6.3	2.5	4.2	1.2
Pickle (all)	15g	19	1.4	0.3	1.6	0.2
Ladyfinger	20g	29	2.7	0.8	1.5	1.0
Dal fry	155g	137	20.7	7.4	2.3	4.3
Kurma	65g	91	7.3	2.0	5.3	2.8
Potato masal sabji	45g	52	8.3	0.7	1.7	0.8
Sambar	180g	123	18.5	6.1	2.6	4.2
Non Vegetarian						
Boiled egg	45g	70	0.5	5.7	4.8	0
Ommelette (1 egg)	80g	127	4.1	6.1	7.6	1.0
Chicken curry	130g	202	4.2	17.6	14.7	0.6
Fish deep fried	30g	74	0.8	8.5	4.6	0.1
Mutton biryani	140g	167	19.7	5.1	7.1	1.6
Mutton curry	145g	181	5.9	8.9	14.3	0.5
Prawn deep fry	145g	447	25.5	18.3	29.9	1.4
Chicken biryani	140g	206	30.6	9.1	5.2	1.6
Sweets						
Besan burfi	20g	98	11.9	2.7	4.4	1.3
Chikki	10g	42	5	0.7	2.3	0.4
Jalebi	20g	92	11	1.0	5.0	0.2
Gulabjamun	60g	224	28	6.4	9.9	0.5
Rasgulla	35g	87	4.5	5.0	1.2	0.2
Beverages						
Tea with milk	210ml	128	14.4	4.9	4.6	0.2
Coffee with milk	210ml	134	13.7	5.3	5.3	0
Milk with 1 teaspoonfull sugar Buttermilk	210ml	146	9.9	6.7	6.3	0
Lassi sweet	155ml	23	0.8	1.2	1.7	0
Curd	280ml	257	33.8	8.1	8.5	0
Coconut milk	120g	72	3.6	3.7	3.9	0
Tender coconut	50ml	215	6.0	1.7	20.5	0.6
Water	330ml	79	14.5	4.6	0.7	0
Soft drink, cola, aerated	250ml	110	27.5	0	0	0
Soft drink, noncola, aerated	250ml	130	32.5	0	0	0

Source: Dr Mohan's Atlas of Indian Foods. Authors– Sudha V, Mohan V, Anjana RM, Krishnaswamy K. ed 1, 2013

5D. DEFINITIONS OF REFERENCE MAN AND WOMAN

Reference Indian adult man: An Indian reference man is between 19 and 39 years of age and weighs 65 kg. He is free from disease and physically fit for active work. On each working day he is employed for 8 hours in occupation that usually involves moderate activity. While not at work he spends 8 hours in bed, 4 to 6 hours sitting and moving around and 2 hours in walking and in active recreation or household duties (ICMR-NIN Expert Group on Nutrition Requirements for Indians, Recommended Dietary Allowances (RDA) and Estimated Average Requirements (EAR)-2020).

Reference Indian adult woman: An Indian reference woman is between 19 and 39 years of age, healthy and weighs 55 kg. She may be engaged for 8 hours in general household work, in light industry or in other moderately active work. Apart from 8 hours in bed, she spends 4 to 6 hours sitting or moving around only through light activity, and 2 hours in walking or in active recreation or in household duties (ICMR-NIN Expert Group on Nutrition Requirements for Indians, Recommended Dietary Allowances (RDA) and Estimated Average Requirements (EAR)-2020).

EAR (Estimated Average Requirement): The EAR is the nutrient requirement used in public health nutrition, to evaluate the nutrition intake of a population.

RDA (Recommended Dietary Allowance): The RDA is for healthy individuals and may be prescribed to satisfy the nutritional needs of specific nutrients in specific life stage and gender group and ensures that there is a very small risk of nutrient intake being inadequate.

TUL (Toxic Upper Limit of Intake): Nutrients are toxic when ingested at very high doses. Intake of nutrients more than TUL invites the risk of toxicity.

Source: ICMR-NIN Expert Group on Nutrient Requirement for Indians, Recommended Dietary Allowances (RDA) and Estimated Average Requirements (EAR)-2020)

5E. SUMMARY OF EAR FOR INDIANS—ICMR-NIN, 2020

Age Group	Category of work	Body Wt	Energy (**)	Pro-tein	Cal-cium	Magne-sium	Iron	Zinc	Iodine	Thia-mine	Ribo-flavin	Niacin	Vit B_6	Folate	Vit B_{12}	Vit C	Vit A	Vit D
		(kg)	(Kcal/d)	(g/d)	(mg/d)	(mg/d)	(mg/d)	(mg/d)	(µg/day)	(mg/d)	(mg/d)	(mg/d)	(mg/d)	(µg/d)	(µg/d)	(mg/d)	(µg/d)	(IU/d)
Men	Sedentary	65	2110	43.0	800	370	11	14.1	95	1.2	1.6	12	1.6	250	2	65	460	400
	Moderate		2710							1.5	2.1	15	2.1					
	Heavy		3470							1.9	2.7	19	2.6					
Women	Sedentary	55	1660	36.0	800	310	15	11.0	95	1.1	1.6	9	1.6	180	2	55	390	400
	Moderate		2130							1.4	2.0	12	1.6					
	Heavy		2720							1.8	2.6	15	2.1					
	Pregnant woman	55 + 10	+350	+7.6 (2nd trimester) +17.6 (3rd trimester)	800	370	21	12.0	160	1.6	2.3	+2	1.9	480	+0.2	+10	406	400
	Lactation																	
	0-6 m	–	+600	+13.6	1000	335	16	11.8	200	1.7	2.5	+4	+0.22	280	+0.8	+40	720	400
	7-12 m		+520	+10.6							2.4		+0.16					
Infants	0-6 m*	5.8	530	7.0	–	–	–	–	–	–	–	–	–	–	–	–	–	–
	6-12 m	8.5	680	9.0	–	–	2	2.1	–	–	–	–	0.5	71	1	–	170	–
Children	1-3 y	12.9	1110	10.0	400	73	6	2.8	65	0.6	0.8	6	0.8	97	1	24	180	400
	4-6 y	18.3	1360	13.0	450	104	8	3.7	65	0.8	1.1	8	1.0	111	2	27	240	
	7-9 y	25.3	1700	19.0	500	144	10	4.9	65	1.0	1.3	10	1.3	142	2	36	290	
Boys	10-12 y	34.9	2220	27.0	650	199	12	7.0	70	1.3	1.7	12	1.7	180	2	45	360	400
Girls	10-12 y	36.4	2060	27.0	650	207	16	7.1	70	1.2	1.6	12	1.6	186	2	44	370	400
Boys	13-15 y	50.5	2860	36.0	800	287	15	11.9	100	1.6	2.2	16	2.2	238	2	60	430	400
Girls	13-15 y	49.6	2400	35.0	800	282	17	10.7	100	1.3	1.9	13	1.8	204	2	55	420	400
Boys	16-18 y	64.4	3320	45.0	850	367	18	14.7	100	1.9	2.5	19	2.5	286	2	70	480	400
Girls	16-18 y	55.7	2500	37.0	850	317	18	11.8	100	1.4	1.9	14	1.9	223	2	57	400	400

*Adequate Intake (AI)

**There is no RDA for energy, the EAR for energy is equivalent to the Estimated Energy Requirement (EER)

Note: For adequate intake of Biotin and Pantothenic acid, refer to the text on summary of recommendations

5F. SUMMARY OF RDA FOR INDIANS—ICMR-NIN, 2020

Age Group	Category of work	Body Wt	Protein	Dietary Fiber*	Calcium	Magne-sium	Iron	Zinc	Iod-ine	Thia-mine	Ribo-flavin	Niacin	Vit B_6	Folate	Vit B_{12}	Vit C	Vit A	Vit D
		(kg)	(g/d)	(g/d)	(mg/d)	(mg/d)	(mg/d)	(mg/d)	(µg/day)	(mg/d)	(mg/d)	(mg/d)	(mg/d)	(µg/d)	(µg/d)	(mg/d)	(µg/d)	(IU/d)
Men	Sedentary			30						1.4	2.0	14	1.9	300	2.2	80	1000	600
	Moderate	65	54.0	40	1000	440	19	17	140	1.8	2.5	18	2.4					
	Heavy			50						2.3	3.2	23	3.1					
Women	Sedentary	55	46.0	25	1000	370	29	13.2	140	1.4	1.9	11	1.9	220	2.2	65	840	600
	Moderate			30						1.7	2.4	14	1.9					
	Heavy			40						2.2	3.1	18	2.4					
	Pregnant woman	55 + 10	+9.5 (2nd trimester) +22.0 (3rd trimester)	–	1000	440	27	14.5	220	2.0	2.7	+2	2.3	570	+0.25	+15	900	600
	Lactation 0-6m		+17.0	–	1200	400	23	14.1	280	2.1	3.0	+5	+0.26	330	+1.0	+5.0	950	600
	7-12m		+13.0								2.9		+0.17					
Infants	0-6m*	5.8	8.0	–	300	30	–	–	100	0.2	0.4	2	0.1	25	1.2	20	350	400
	6-12m	8.5	10.5	–	300	75	3	2.5	130	0.4	0.6	5	0.6	85	1.2	30	350	400
Children	1-3y	12.9	12.5	15	500	90	8	3.3	90	0.7	1.1	7	0.9	120	1.2	30	390	600
	4-6y	18.3	16.0	20	550	125	11	4.5	90	0.9	1.3	9	1.2	135	2.2	35	510	
	7-9y	25.3	23.0	26	650	175	15	5.9	90	1.1	1.6	11	1.5	170	2.2	45	630	
Boys	10-12y	34.9	32.0	33	850	240	16	8.5	100	1.5	2.1	15	2.0	220	2.2	55	770	600
Girls	10-12y	36.4	33.0	30	850	250	28	8.5	100	1.4	1.9	14	1.9	225	2.2	50	790	600
Boys	13-15y	50.5	45.0	43	1000	345	22	14.3	140	1.9	2.7	19	2.6	285	2.2	70	930	600
Girls	13-15y	49.6	43.0	36	1000	340	30	12.8	140	1.6	2.2	16	2.2	245	2.2	65	890	600
Boys	16-18y	64.4	55.0	50	1050	440	26	17.6	140	2.2	3.1	22	3.0	340	2.2	85	1000	600
Girls	16-18y	55.7	46.0	38	1050	380	32	14.2	140	1.7	2.3	17	2.3	270	2.2	70	860	600

*Adequate Intake (AI)

Note: For adequate intake of Biotin and Pantothenic acid, refer to the text on summary of recommendations

5G. RECOMMENDATIONS FOR DIETARY FAT INTAKE IN INDIANS—ICMR-NIN, 2020

Age/Gender/ physiological groups	Physical activity	Minimum level of Total fat (% E)	Minimum level* of Fat from foods other than visible fats % E	Visible fat	
				%E	g/day
Adult Men	Sedentary	20	10	10	25
	Moderate				30
	Heavy				40
Adult Women	Sedentary	20	10	10	20
	Moderate				25
	Heavy				30
	Pregnant women	20	10	10	30
	Lactating women				30
Infants	0-6 m	40-60	Human milk		
	6-24 m	35	10[c]	25	25
Children	3-6y	25	10	15	25
	7-9y				30
Boys	10-12y				35
	13-15y				45
	16-18y				50
Girls	10-12y				35
	13-15y				40
	16-18y				35

*If higher than 10%E, visible fat requirement proportionately reduces

5H. DAILY NUTRIENT RECOMMENDATIONS FOR THE ELDERLY IN INDIA-ICMR-NIN, 2020

Nutrients		Energy (Kcal)	Dietary Fibre	Protein (g)	Vit-A (µg)	Thiamin B_1 (mg)	Riboflavin B_2 (mg)	Niacin (mg)	Vit-C (mg)	Vit-B_6 (mg)	Folate (µg)	Vit-B_{12} (mg)	Vit-D (IU)	Calcium (mg)	Magnesium (mg)	Iron (mg)	Zinc (mg)	Iodine (µg)
Men ≥60 yrs	EAR	1700	–	43.0	460	1.2	1.6	12	65	1.6	250	2.0	400	1000	370	11	14	95
	RDA	–	30	54.0	1000	1.4	2.0	14	80	1.9	300	2.2	800	1200	440	19	17	140
Woman ≥60 yrs	EAR	1500	–	36.3	390	1.1	1.6	9	55	1.6	180	2.0	400	1000	310	11	11	95
	RDA	–	25	46.0	840	1.4	1.9	11	65	1.9	200	2.2	800	1200	370	19	13.2	140

5I. AMDR BY AGE AND PHYSIOLOGICAL GROUPS–ICMR-NIN, 2020

Acceptable Macronutrient Distribution Range (AMDR) by Age and Physiological Groups as Percent of Energy (%E)

Age group Nutrients	1-2 years	3-18 years	Adults	Pregnant and lactating women
Protein (PE ratio)*	5-15	5-15	5-15	5-15
Total Fat	30-40	25-35	15-35	20-35
n-6 PUFA#	4-10	4-10	4-10	4-10
n-3-PUFA	0.5-1	0.5-1	0.5-1	0.5-1
Carbohydrate	40-60	45-65	45-65	45-65

*Depends on protein quality and total energy intake

#n-6 to n-3 ratio should be between 5-10:1

Note: For good health, adults should consume minimum of 100 to 130g of carbohydrates and atleast 20g fats (food sources)

Summary of Recommended Intakes for Other Minerals and Trace Elements in Adults

S No.	Minerals/Trace Element	Recommended intake (per day)
1	Phosphorous	1000 mg
2	Sodium	2000 mg
3	Potassium	3500 mg
4	Copper	1.7 mg
5	Manganese	4 mg
6	Chromium	50 μg
7	Selenium	40 μg

5J. BALANCED DIET FOR MODERATE ACTIVE MAN–ICMR-NIN, 2020

Food Composition	Amount (g/day)	Nutrient	Vegetarian diet	Non-vegetarian diet	EAR	RDA
Cereals and Millets	360	Energy (Kcal)	2690	2650	2710	–
		Protein (g)	87.5	81.7	43	54
Pulses (Legumes)/ flesh foods[1]	120	Visible fat (g)	35	35	30	30
Green leafy vegetables	100	Calcium	1084	1054	800	1000
Other Vegetables	200	Iron (mg)	33.3	31.1	11	19.0
Roots and Tubers (excluding potatoes)	100	Zinc (mg)	16.3	15.9	14.1	17
Fruits	150	Magnesium (mg)	968	891	370	440
Milk	300	Vitamin A (μg)*	1802	1796	460	1000
Fats and Oils	30	β carotene	9842	9779	2760	6000
Oil seeds and Nuts (gingely seeds and Pea nuts)	30	Thiamine (mg)	2.0	1.9	1.5	1.8
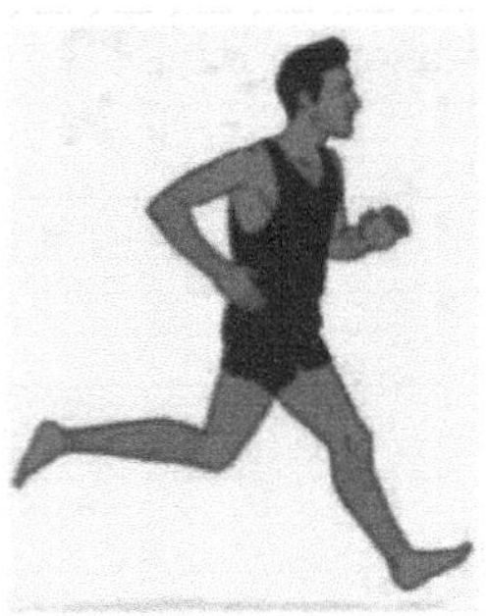		Riboflavin (mg)	1.9	1.9	2.1	2.5
		Niacin (mg)	19	20.0	15	18
		Vitamin B_6 (mg)	2.4	2.4	2.1	2.4
		Vitamin C (mg)	209	209	65	80
		Total Folates (μg)	559	491	250	300
		Vitamin B_{12} (μg)	1.5	2.4	2.0	2.2

Note: Total protein from the above diet=88g, Digestible protein = 71g, PDCAAS=84%.

[1]Pulses can be replaced with animal foods (egg, meat, fish and chicken) for non-vegetarians.

*Retinol derived from β carotene from diet was also added to the total Vitamin A.

For cereals and millets, it is recommended to consume 50% as whole grains.

5K. BALANCED DIET FOR SEDENTARY MAN–ICMR-NIN, 2020

Foods Composition	Amount (g/day)	Nutrient	Vegetarian diet	Non-vegetarian diet	EAR	RDA
Cereals and Millets	275	Energy (kcal)	2130	2084	2110	–
		Protein (g)	67.2	69.1	43	54
Pulses (Legumes)/flesh foods[1]	80	Visible fat (g)	25	25	25	25
Green leafy vegetables	100	Calcium (mg)	968	958	800	1000
Other Vegetables	200	Iron (mg)	27.4	26.3	11.0	19.0
Roots and Tubers (excluding potatoes)	100	Zinc (mg)	13.5	13.2	14.1	17.0
Fruits	150	Magnesium (mg)	798	762	370	440
Milk	300	Vitamin A (μg)*	1768	1765	460	1000
Fats and Oils	25	B-carotene (μg)	9638	9605	2760	6000
Oils seeds and Nuts (gingely seeds and Pea nuts)	30	Thiamine (mg)	1.7	1.6	1.2	1.4
Spices	10	Riboflavin	1.6	1.6	1.6	2.0
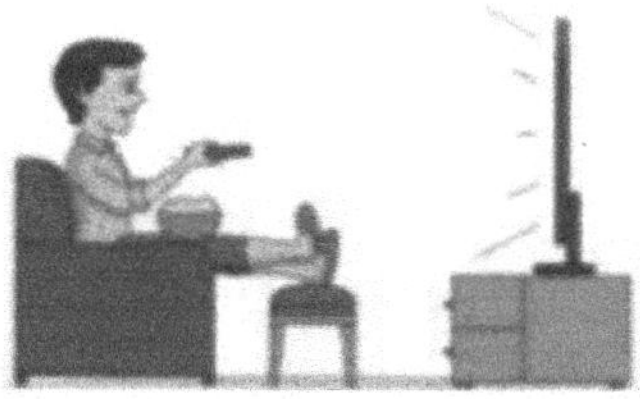		Niacin (mg)	15.6	16.0	12	14
		Vitamin B_6 (mg)	2.0	2.0	1.6	1.9
		Vitamin C (mg)			65	80
		Total Folates (μg)	483	450	250	300
		Vitamin B_{12} (μg)	1.5	2.0	2.0	2.2

Note: Total protein from the above diet = 71g, Digestible protein = 58g, PDCAAS=85%

[1]Pulses can be replaced with animal foods (egg, meat, fish and chicken) for non-vegetarians.

*Retinol derived from β carotene from diet was also added to the total Vitamin A

For cereals and millets, it is recommended to consume 50% as whole grains

5L. BALANCED DIET FOR MODERATE ACTIVE WOMAN–ICMR-NIN, 2020

Food Composition	Amount (g/day)	Nutrient	Vegetarian diet	Non-vegetarian diet	EAR	RDA
Cereals and Millets	300	Energy (kcal)	2135	2084	2130	–
		Protein (g)	74.2	73.3	36.0	46.0
Pulses (Legumes)/flesh foods[1]	90	Visible fat (g)	20	20	25	20
Green leafy vegetables	100	Calcium (mg)	999	989	800	1000
Other Vegetables	200	Iron (mg)	29.0	27.9	15.0	29.0
Roots and Tubers (excluding potatoes)	100	Zinc (mg)	14.0	13.6	11.0	13.2
Fruits	150	Magnesium (mg)	841	806	310	370
Milk	300	Vitamin A (μg)*	1804	1741	390	840
Fats and Oils	20	B-carotene (μg)	9489	9457	–	–
Oil seeds and Nuts (gingely seeds and Pea nuts)	30	Thiamine (mg)	1.75	1.70	1.4	1.7
Spices	10	Riboflavin	1.65	1.64	2.0	2.4
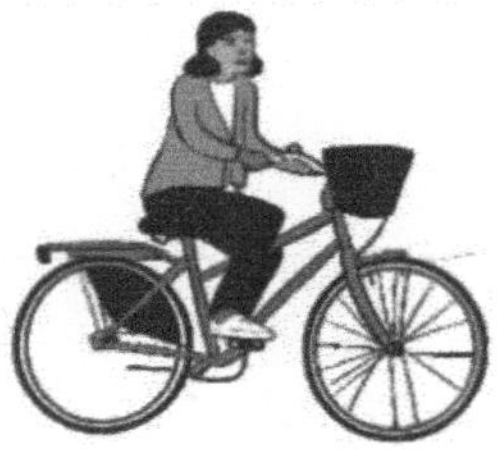		Niacin (mg)	16.3	16.8	12	14
		Vitamin B_6 (mg)	1.96	1.97	1.6	1.9
		Vitamin C (mg)	187	187	55	65
		Total Folates (μg)	191	459	180	220
		Vitamin B_{12} (μg)	1.5	2.0	2	2.2

Note: Total protein from the above diet = 76g, Digestible protein =62g, PDCAAS = 85%

[1]Pulses can be replaced with animal foods (egg, meat, fish and chicken) for non-vegetarians.

*Retinol derived from β carotene from diet was also added to the total Vitamin A.

For cereals and millets, it is recommended to consume 50% as whole grains.

5M. BALANCED DIET FOR SEDENTARY WOMAN–ICMR-NIN, 2020

Food Composition	Amount (g/day)	Nutrient	Vegetarian diet	Non-vegetarian diet	EAR	RDA
Cereals and Millets	200	Energy (kcal)	1690	1650	1660	–
		Protein (g)	58.2	57.4	36.0	46.0
Pulses (Legumes)[1]	60	Visible fat (g)	15	15	20	20
Green leafy vegetables	100	Calcium (mg)	905	895	800	1000
Other Vegetables	200	Iron (mg)	23.8	22.8	15.0	29.0
Roots and Tubers (excluding potatoes)	100	Zinc (mg)	11.0	10.5	11.0	13.2
Fruits	150	Magnesium (mg)	684	649	310	370
Milk	300	Vitamin A (μg)*	1730	1727	390	840
Fats and Oils	15	β-carotene (μg)	9412	9380	–	–
Oil seeds and Nuts (gingely seeds and Pea nuts)	30	Thiamine (mg)	1.36	1.30	1.1	1.4
Spices	10	Riboflavin	1.5	1.48	1.6	1.9
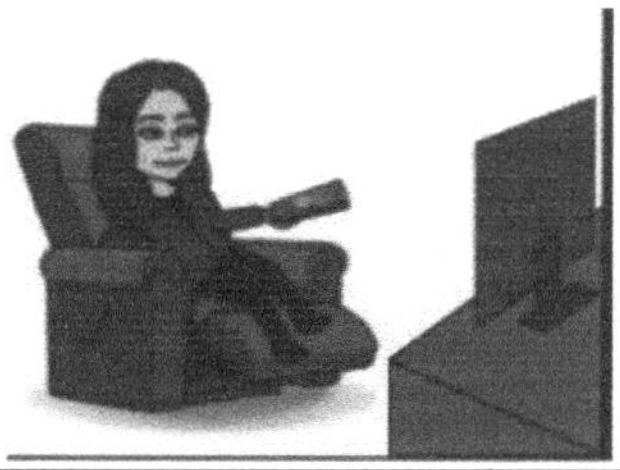		Niacin (mg)	13.0	13.5	9.0	11
		Vitamin B_6 (mg)	1.7	1.7	1.6	1.9
		Vitamin C (mg)	187	187	55	65
		Total Folates (μg)	426	395	180	220
		Vitamin B_{12} (μg)	1.5	2.0	2	2.2

Note: Total protein from the above diet = 60g, Digestible protein =50g, PDCAAS=87%

[1]Pulses can be replaced with animal foods (egg, meat, fish and chicken) for non-vegetarians.

*Retinol derived from β carotene from diet was also added to the total Vitamin A.

For cereals and millets, it is recommended to consume 50% as whole grains.

5N. BALANCED DIET FOR PREGNANT WOMAN–ICMR-NIN, 2020

Food Composition	Amount (g/day)	Nutrient	Vegetarian diet	Non-vegetarian diet	EAR	RDA
Cereals and Millets	325	Energy (kcal)	2060	2040	2480	–
		Protein (g)	71.7	71.6	54	68
Pulses (Legumes)[1]	90	Visible fat (g)	15	15	30	30
Green leafy vegetables	100	Calcium (mg)	980	970	800	1000
Other Vegetables	200	Iron (mg)	27.2	26.0	21	27
Roots and Tubers (excluding potatoes)	100	Zinc (mg)	13.1	12.8	12.0	14.5
Fruits	150	Magnesium (mg)	786	747	370	440
Milk	400	Vitamin A (μg)*	1821	1818	406	900
Fats and Oils	25	β-carotene (μg)	9634	9597	–	–
Oil seeds and Nuts (gingely seeds and Pea nuts)	40	Thiamine (mg)	1.64	1.60	1.6	2.0
Spices	10	Riboflavin	1.8	1.84	2.3	2.7
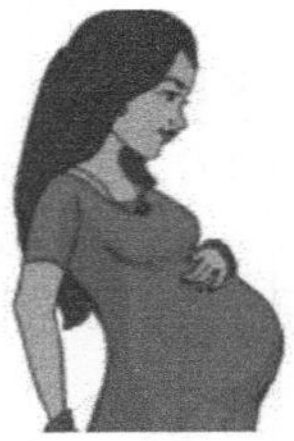		Niacin (mg)	16.0	16.7	14	16
		Vitamin B_6 (mg)	2.0	2.0	1.9	2.3
		Vitamin C (mg)	210	210	65	80
		Total Folates (μg)	484	447	480	570
		Vitamin B_{12} (μg)	2.0	2.4	2.2	2.5

Note: Total protein from the above diet = 78.8g, Digestible protein = 70g, PDCAAS = 88%

[1]Pulses can be replaced with animal foods (egg, meat, fish and chicken) for non-vegetarians.

*Retinol derived from β carotene from diet was also added to the total Vitamin A.

For cereals and millets, it is recommended to consume 50% as whole grains.

5O. KEY NUTRIENTS IN DIFFERENT FOOD GROUPS–ICMR-NIN, 2020

(All values are for 100 g edible portion)

Micro-nutrients	Cereals[a]	Pulses[b]	Leafy Vegetables[c]	Other vegetables	Roots and Tubers[d]	Fruits[e]	Milk (Buffalo)[f]	Milk (Cow)[f]	Egg	Chicken	Mutton	Beef	Fish	Liver (Sheep, Goat, Lamb)
Iron (mg)	3.00	5	8.5	2.12	0.6	0.56	0.2	0.2	1.82	1.5	1.3	2.2	0.6	6.3
Zinc (mg)	2.16	2.1	0.2	0.3	0.3	0.11	0.4	0.3	1.2	1.7	3	4.6	0.6	3.6
Vitamin A (µg)	2.43	8.6	259.1	22.4	70.0	32.36	49.8	58.3	198	21.4	9	15.5	5.6	6690
Riboflavin (mg)	0.15	0.14	0.1	0.07	0.0	0.01	0.13	0.11	0.2	0.09	0.16	0.12	0.03	0.36
Dietary folate (µg)	24.03	127.7	16.7	24.4	31.3	17.61	8.6	7	49.3	9.3	6.4	8.1	15.4	92
Vitamin B_{12} (µg)	Nil	Nil	Nil	Nil	Nil	Nil	1.5	1.5	1.8	NA	2.8	1.7	1.4	91.9

[a] Mean values of nutrients from commonly consumed cereals (67% weightages) such as rice and wheat were taken and 33% weightage was also given to millets such as Bajra, Jowar, Maiz and Ragi

[b] Mean values of nutrients from Lentils, Tur dhal, Bengal gram, Black gram, Cowpea, Green gram, Peas, Rajmah, Red gram and Soyabean were considered

[c] Carotenoid conversion to retinol equivalents

[d] Mean values of nutrients from Beetroot, Carrot, Colocasia, Onion, Radish, Tapioca and Yam were considered

[e] Mean values of nutrients from Amla, Apple, Banana, Cherries, Grapes, Guava, Jack fruit, Lemon, Lichi, Mango, Melon, Orange, Papaya, Pine apple, Pomegranate, Sapota, Custard apple, Strawberry were considered.

[f] Good source of bioavailable calcium

NA=Not available ; NR=Not reported

- Low absorption of non heme iron can be improved by consuming more vitamin C rich foods (Amla, Lemon, Oranges, Guava, etc.) in raw form as much as possible
- Meat, poultry and liver contains high bio-available heme iron and also increases absorption (meat factor) of non-heme iron (including fish)

5P. BALANCED DIET FOR ADULTS–SEDENTARY/ MODERATE/HEAVY ACTIVITY (NO. OF PORTIONS)

	Type of work						
	g/portion	Sedentary		Moderate		Heavy	
		Man	Woman	Man	Woman	Man	Woman
		No. of portions					
Cereals and millets	30	12.5	9	15	11	20	16
Pulses	30	2.5	2	3	2.5	4	3
Milk and milk products	100 ml	3	3	3	3	3	3
Roots and tubers	100	2	2	2	2	2	2
Green leafy vegetables	100	1	1	1	1	1	1
Other vegetables	100	2	2	2	2	2	2
Fruits	100	1	1	1	1	1	1
Sugar	5	4	4	6	6	11	9
Fat	5	5	4	6	5	8	6

To calculate the days requirement of above mentioned food groups for an individual, multiply grams per portion with number of portions.

5Q. BALANCED DIET FOR INFANTS, CHILDREN AND ADOLESCENTS (NO. OF PORTIONS)

Food groups	g/portion	Infants 6-12 months	1-3	4-6	7-9	Years					
						10-12		13-15		16-18	
						Girls	Boys	Girls	Boys	Girls	Boys
Cereals and millets	30	0.5	2	4	6	8	10	11	14	11	15
Pulses	30	0.25	1	1.0	2	2	2	2	2.5	2.5	3
Milk (ml) and milk products	100	4[a]	5	5	5	5	5	5	5	5	5
Roots and tubers	100	0.5	0.5	1	1	1	1	1	1.5	2	2
Green leafy vegetables	100	0.25	0.5	0.5	1	1	1	1	1	1	1
Other vegetables	100	0.25	0.5	1	1	2	2	2	2	2	2
Fruits	100	1	1	1	1	1	1	1	1	1	1
Sugar	5	2	3	4	4	6	6	5	4	5	6
Fat/oil (visible)	5	4	5	5	6	7	7	8	9	7	10

[a] Quantity indicates top milk. For breastfed infants, 200 ml top milk is required.

One portion of pulse may be exchanged with one portion (50 g) of egg/meat/chicken/fish.

For infants introduce egg/meat/chicken/fish around 9 months.

(Source: Dietary Guidelines for Indians–A Manual. 2nd ed. Hyderabad: NIN, ICMR; 2011)

5R. SAMPLE MEAL PLAN FOR ADULT MAN (SEDENTARY)

Meal Time	Food Group	Raw	Cooked Recipe	Servings Amounts
Breakfast	Milk	100 ml	Milk	1/2 Cup
	Sugar	15 g	Tea or Coffee	2 Cups 1 Cup
	Cereals	70 g	Breakfast Item	
	Pulses	20g		
Lunch	Cereals	120 g	Rice	2 Cups
			Pulkas	2 Nos.
	Pulses	20 g	Dhal	1/2 Cup
	Vegetables	150 g	Veg. curry	3/4 Cup
	Vegetables	50 g	Veg. salad	7-8 Slices
	Milk	100 ml	Curd	1/2 Cup
Tea	Cereals			
	Milk	50 ml	Tea	1 Cup
	Sugar			
Dinner	Cereals	120 g	Rice	2 Cups
			Pulkas	2 Nos.
	Pulses	20 g	Dhal	1/2 Cup
	Vegetables	150 g	Veg. curry	3/4 Cup
	Milk (Curd)	50 ml		
	Vegetables	50 g		
	Fruit	100 g	Seasonal	1 Medium

1 Cup = 200 ml

Note: For Non-Vegetarians–Substitute one pulse portion with one portion of egg/meat/chicken/fish

Use 25g visible fat and <5g salt during preparation of meal per day.

Breakfast Items: Idli – 4 Nos. / Dosa – 3 Nos. / Upma – 1-1/2 Cup / Bread – 4 Slices/ Porridge – 2 Cups / Corn flakes with milk – 2 Cups

Snacks: Poha – 1 Cup / Toast – 2 Slices

Dhokla – 4 Nos.

5S. SAMPLE MEAL PLAN FOR ADULT WOMAN (SEDENTARY)

Meal Time	Food Group	Raw	Cooked Recipe	Servings
Breakfast	Milk	100 ml	Milk or	1/2 Cup
	Sugar	10 g	Tea or	2 Cups
			Coffee	1 Cup
	Cereals	50 g	Breakfast Item	
	Pulses	20 g		
Lunch	Cereals	100 g	Rice	1 Cup
			Phulkas	2 Nos.
	Pulses	20 g	Dhal	1/2 Cup
	Vegetables	100 g	Veg. curry	1/2 Cup
	Vegetables	50 g	Veg. salad	7-8 Slices
	Milk	100 ml	Curd	1/2 Cup
Tea	Cereals	50 g	Snack	
	Milk	50 ml	Tea	1 Cup
	Sugar	10 g		
Dinner	Cereals	100 g	Rice	1 Cup
			Phulkas	2 Nos.
	Pulses	20 g	Dhal	1/2 Cup
	Vegetables	100 g	Veg. curry	1/2 Cup
	Milk (Curd)	50 ml		
	Vegetables	50 g		
	Fruit	100 g	Seasonal	1 Medium

1 Cup = 200 ml

Note: For Non-Vegetarians – Substitute one pulse portion with one portion of egg/meat/chicken/fish
Use 20 g visible fat and < 5g salt during preparation of meal per day.

Breakfast Items: Idli – 3 Nos. / Dosa – 2 Nos. / Upma – 1 Cup / Bread – 3 Slices / Porridge -1-1/2 Cups / Corn flakes with milk – 1-1/2 Cup.

Snacks: Poha – 1 Cup/Toast – 2 Slices
Dhokla – 4 Nos.

(Source: Dietary Guidelines for Indians – A Manual. 2nd Edition Hyderabad: NIN, ICMR; 2011)

5T. NUTRITIVE VALUE OF RAW FOODSTUFFS

Annexure – I

Foodstuff	Energy (kcal)	Carbohydrates (gm)	Protein (gm)	Fats (gm)	Calcium (mg)	Iron (mg)
1.	2.	3.	4.	5.	6.	7.
Cereals:						
Bajra	361	67.5	11.6	5.0	42	8.0
Jowar	349	72.6	10.4	1.9	25	4.1
Maize	125	24.6	4.7	0.9	09	1.1
Ragi	328	72.0	7.3	1.3	344	3.9
Rice (hand pounded)	346	76.7	7.5	1.0	10	3.2
Rice (milled)	345	78.2	6.8	0.5	10	0.7
Rice (parboiled)	346	79.0	6.4	0.4	09	1.0
Wheat	346	71.2	11.8	1.5	41	5.3
Wheat flour (refined)	348	73.9	11.0	0.9	23	2.7
Pulses:						
Bengal gram, whole	360	60.9	17.1	5.3	202	4.6
Bengal gram dal	372	59.8	20.8	5.6	56	5.3
Bengal gram roasted	369	58.1	22.5	5.2	58	9.5
Black gram dal	347	59.6	24.0	1.4	154	3.8
Green gram dal	348	59.9	24.5	1.2	75	3.9
Khesari dal	345	56.6	28.2	1.6	90	6.3
Lentil	343	59.0	25.1	0.7	69	7.6
Peas, dry	315	56.5	19.7	1.1	75	7.0
Red gram dal	335	57.6	22.3	1.7	73	2.7
Soyabean	432	20.9	43.2	19.5	240	10.4
Leafy Vegetables:						
Amaranth	45	6.1	4.0	0.5	397	3.5
Ambat chukka	15	1.4	1.6	0.3	363	0.8
Bathua leaves	30	2.9	3.7	0.4	150	4.2
Bengal gram leaves	97	14.1	7.0	1.4	340	23.8
Cabbage	27	4.6	1.8	0.1	39	0.8
Cauliflower leaves	66	7.6	5.9	1.3	626	40.0
Coriander leaves	44	6.3	3.3	0.6	184	1.4
Curry leaves	108	18.7	6.1	1.0	830	0.9
Drumstick leaves	92	12.5	6.7	1.7	440	0.8
Fenugreek leaves	49	6.0	4.4	0.9	395	1.9
Gogu	56	9.9	1.7	1.1	172	2.3
Mint	48	5.8	4.8	0.6	200	15.6
Mustard leaves	34	3.2	4.0	0.6	155	16.3
Radish leaves	28	2.4	3.8	0.4	265	–
Spinach	26	2.9	2.0	0.7	73	1.1
Tamarind leaves	115	18.2	5.8	2.1	101	0.3

Contd.

Contd.

Grapes (blue variety)	58	13.1	0.6	0.4	20	0.5
Guava, country	51	11.2	0.9	0.3	10	0.3
Jack fruit	88	19.8	1.9	0.1	20	0.6
Lemon (citrus)	57	11.1	1.0	0.9	70	0.3
Lichi	61	13.6	1.1	0.2	35	0.7
Lime	59	10.9	1.5	1.0	20	0.3
Lime sweet (masumbi)	43	9.3	0.8	0.3	30	0.7
Mango, ripe	74	16.9	0.6	0.4	16	1.3
Melon (water)	16	3.3	0.2	0.2	12	7.9
Orange	48	10.9	0.7	0.2	20	0.3
Papaya, ripe	32	7.2	0.6	0.1	13	0.5
Pineapple	46	10.8	0.4	0.1	9	2.4
Pomegranate	65	14.5	1.6	0.1	70	1.8
Raisins	308	74.6	1.8	0.3	80	7.7
Sapota	98	21.4	0.7	1.1	27	1.3
Seethaphal	104	23.5	1.6	0.4	47	4.3
Tomato, ripe	20	3.6	0.9	0.2	20	0.6
Wood apple	134	18.1	7.1	3.7	110	0.5
Milk and Milk Products:						
Cheese	348	6.3	24.1	25.1	790	2.1
Curd	60	3.0	3.1	4.0	149	0.2
Milk, buffalo	117	5.0	4.3	6.5	210	0.2
Milk, cow	67	4.4	3.2	4.1	120	0.2
Milk, goat	72	4.6	3.3	4.5	170	0.3
Milk, human	65	7.4	1.1	3.4	28	–
Other Fresh Foods:						
Beef muscle	144	–	22.6	2.6	10	0.8
Egg duck	181	0.8	13.5	13.7	70	2.5
Egg hen	173	–	13.3	13.3	60	2.1
Goat meat, muscle	118	–	22.4	3.6	12	–
Liver, goat	107	–	20.0	3.0	17	–
Liver, sheep	150	1.3	19.3	7.5	10	6.3
Mutton	194	–	18.5	13.3	150	2.5
Pork, muscle	114	–	18.7	4.4	30	2.2
Miscellaneous Foodstuffs:						
Betel leaves	44	6.1	3.1	0.8	230	10.6
Bread (white)	245	51.9	7.8	0.7	11	1.1
Jaggery	383	95.0	0.4	0.1	80	2.6
Oil or ghee	900	–	–	100.0	–	–
Sago	351	87.1	0.2	0.2	10	1.3
Sugar	398	99.4	0.1	–	12	0.2

(Source: Nutritive Value of Foodstuffs – Gopalan C, Ramashashtri BV, Balasubramanium SC–Nutritive Value of Indian Foods. Revised 1st edition, Hyderabad: NIN, ICMR; 2010)

ANNEXURE-6

Anthropometry

6A. WEIGHT-FOR-AGE GIRLS [BIRTH TO 5 YEARS (Z-SCORES)]

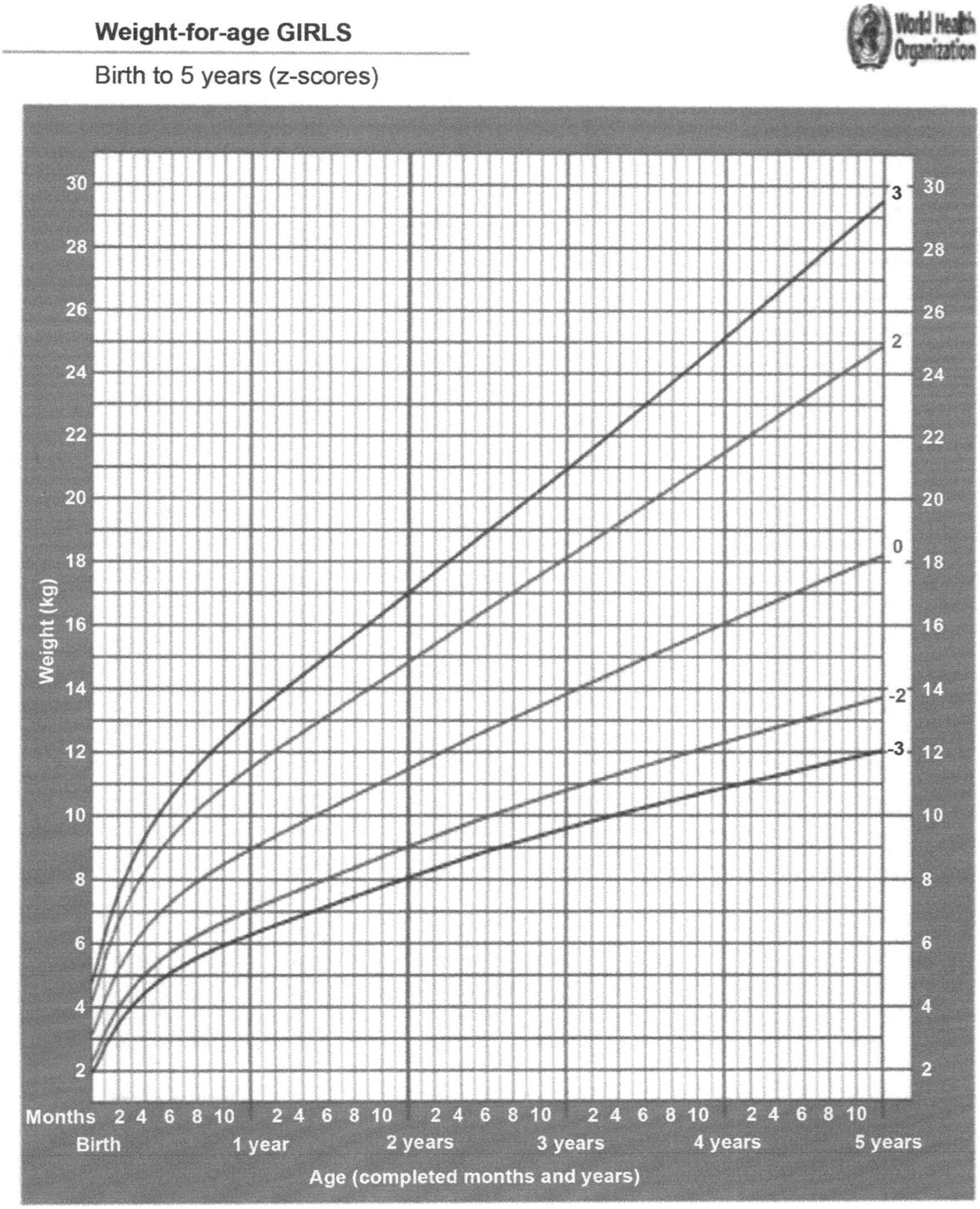

(Ref: WHO Child Growth Standards, 2007)

6B. WEIGHT-FOR-AGE BOYS [BIRTH TO 5 YEARS(Z-SCORES)]

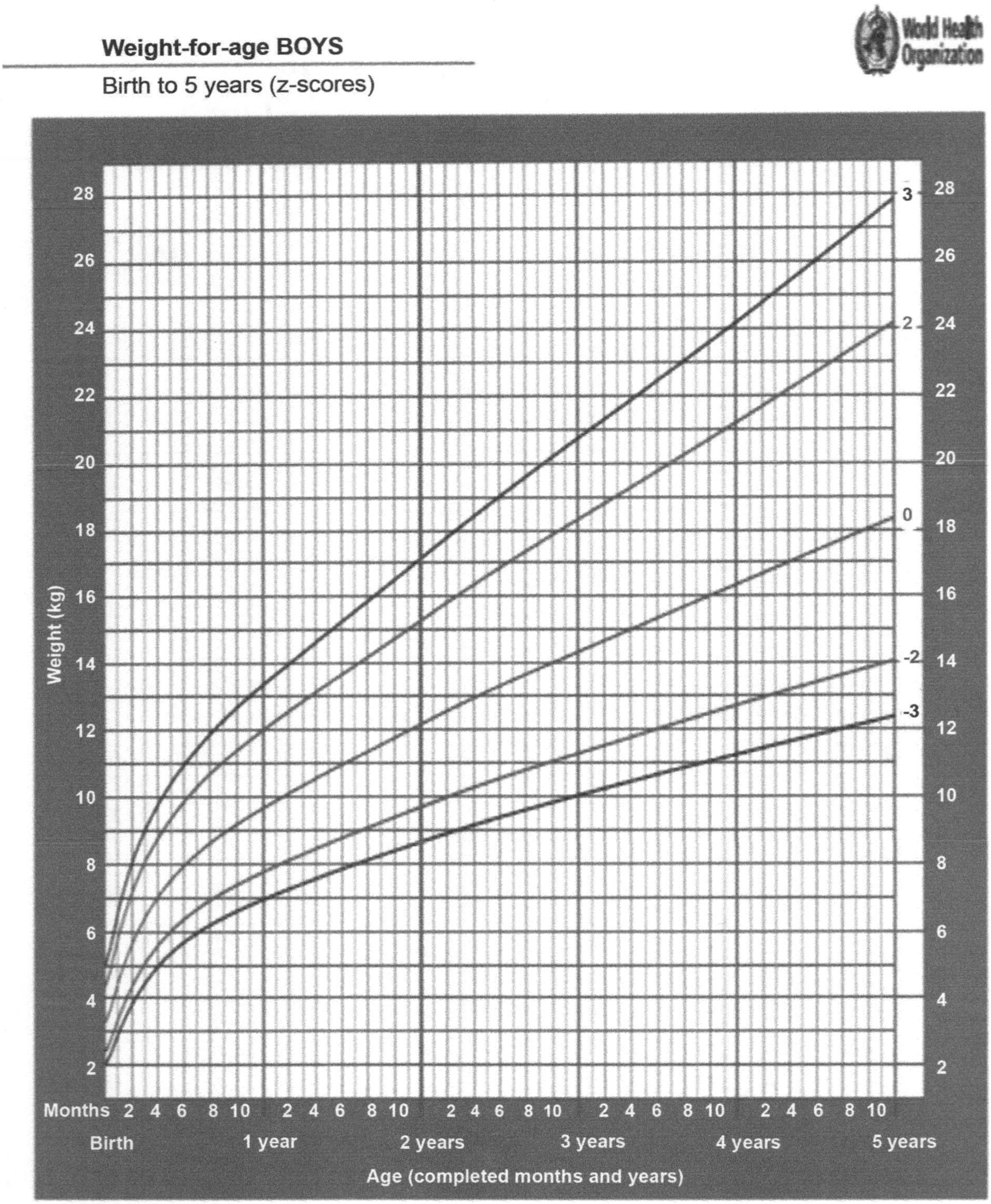

(Ref: WHO Child Growth Standards, 2007)

6C. BMI-FOR-AGE GIRLS [5 YEARS TO 19 YEARS (Z-SCORES)]

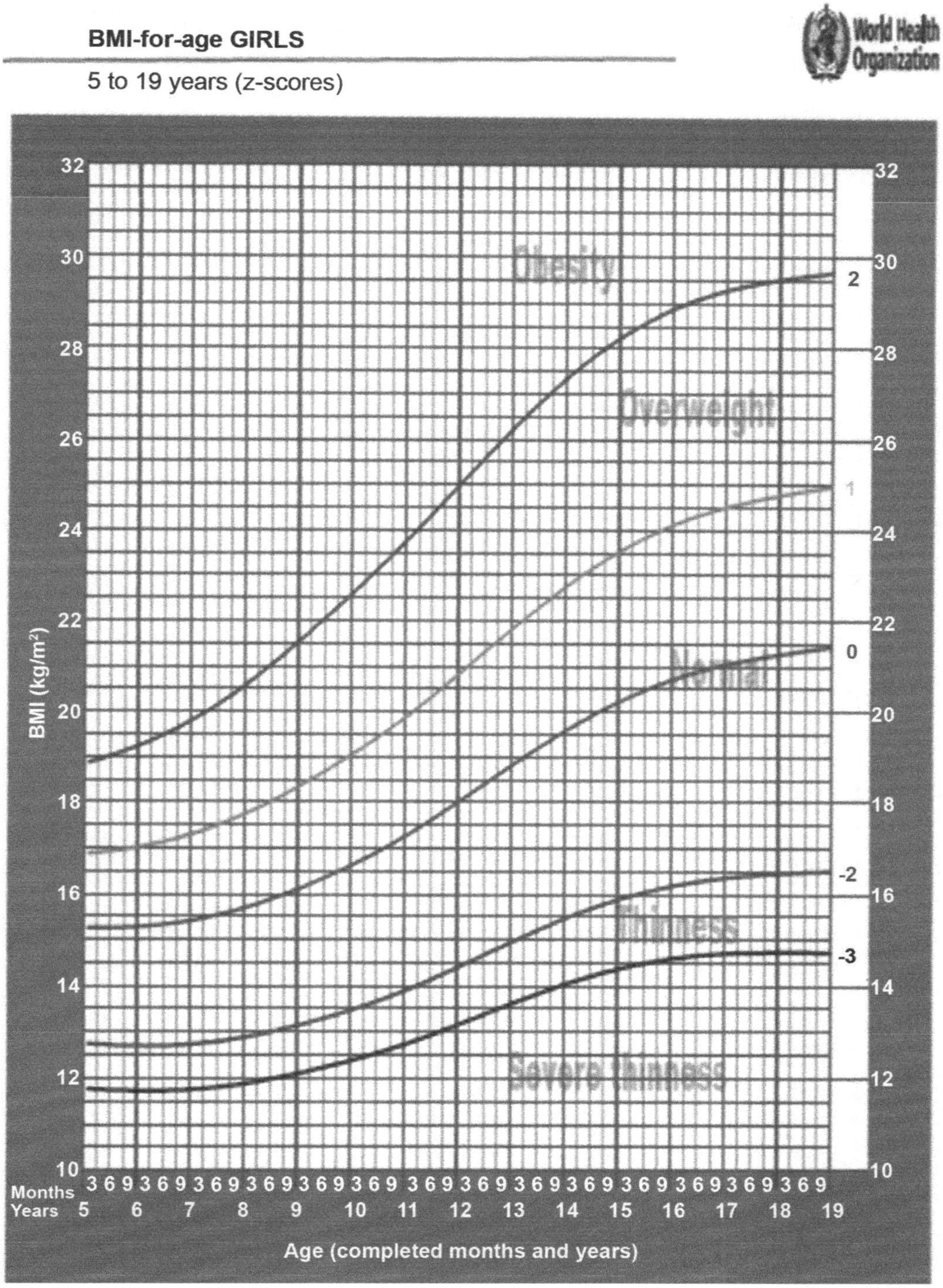

(Ref: 2007 WHO Reference)

6D.BMI-FOR-AGE BOYS [5 YEARS TO 19 YEARS (Z-SCORES)]

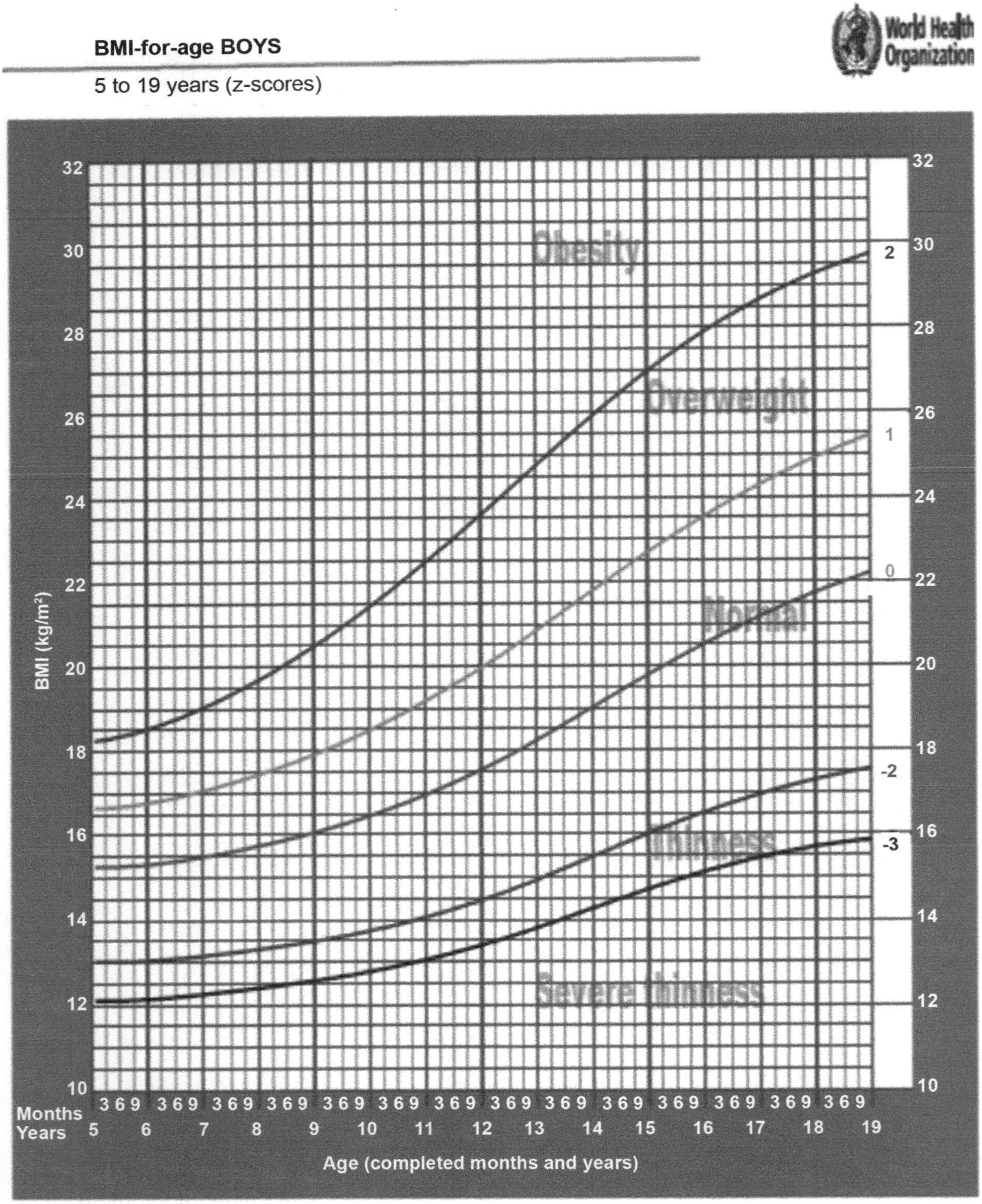

(Ref: 2007 WHO Reference)

ANNEXURE-7

Developmental Milestones

Age	Development Milestone			
	Physical development	Mental development	Social/ Emotional development	Communication/ Language development
From birth to 2 months	Cannot support head from birth till 1 month. Sleeps 20 hours a day till a month. Around 2 months, able to hold head. Begins to push while lying on your tummy at 2 months. Makes easy movements with hands and legs.	Starts paying attention to faces. Acknowledges you from a distance. Follows things through eyes. Cries if gets bored with an activity.	Starts smiling in response to your voice. Brings hands to mouth to calm self for a short while.	Starts cooing and purling cognizes sounds and tries to turn head towards it.
By the age of 4 months	Keeps head steady Senses color, visuals and oral exploration. Controls eyes' movements. Lifts head when lying over your stomach. May roll from tummy to back Can hold a toy and shake it.	Expresses mood (happy or sad) Starts using hands and eyes together like seeing andreaching for toys. Watches faces with focus. Acknowledges affection.	Smiles impulsively or may laugh. Cries if no one plays with her/him. Copies some acts like smile and frown.	Cries if angry, hungry or tired. Starts babbling with expressions. Begins speaking vowels.
By the age of 6 months	Rolls from front to back and back to front.	Starts looking around for things	Knows when sees a stranger.	Starts responding when hears own name.
	Supports self and starts sitting with round back. Carries weight on legs when stands and may bounce. Pushes backward before going ahead.	Shows curiosity about things and tries to get them. Passes things from one hand to another.	Loves playing, especially with parentsand other babies. Grasps things with palm on purpose. Reacts to your emotions, usually remains happy joys being cuddled.	Speaks vowels together like "ah", "eh", "oh" etc. Begins speaking consonants like "m", "b" etc. Shows emotions by making sounds.

Contd.

Contd.

By the age of 9 months	Stands with support. Starts crawling. May get into sitting position by self and sits without support with straight back.	Seeks the things you hide. Plays peek-a-boo. Starts picking things with thumb and index finger. Puts things in her/ his mouth.	Emotional attachment to mother. Clings to familiar people. Afraid of strangers. Chooses some favorite toys.	Starts making sounds like "mamama" or "bababa" etc. Starts waving and understands that it is connected to "bye-bye". Points at things with finger. Understands "no"
By the age of 12 months	Starts sitting and standing without any help. May take few steps without holding anything as support. Walks while holding furniture or sidesteps around furniture.	Likes to mess up by shaking, banging and throwing things away. Copies gestures like clapping or dancing. Follows directions like "pick up your toy".	Feels shy and nervous in front of strangers. Gives and takes objects. Makes sounds and repeats actions in order to get attention. May ask you to do somethings like holding out both hands to get picked up. Cries when any of the parents leave the house.	Uses gestures like shaking head to say "no". Says "mama" or "dada" or "uh-oh". Tries to repeat words you say.

Source: www.nhp.gov.in

Viva Voce

Q1. Difference between family and household.

Ans. Family: Family is a group of individuals related to each other biologically or by law (marriage or adoption), living together, sharing common income and eating from a common kitchen.

Household: one or more people who live in a single residence (house, apartment etc.) but are unrelated.

Families can be part of a larger household, and households can include members of several unrelated families who do not reside together.

Q2. Define nuclear, joint and three generation family.

Ans. Nuclear Family: The family comprises the husband, wife, and their children (as long as the children are dependent and unmarried).

Joint Family: it comprises blood related persons and their wives and children from three or more generations living in a single home, with a common kitchen and commonly held property (movable or immovable) and headed by the eldest member.

Three generation family/Extended family: is an extension of the nuclear family, in which the couple along with their children and dependent parents live together.

Q3. Enumerate advantages and disadvantages of nuclear and joint family.

Ans.

	Nuclear Family	Joint Family
Advantages	Economic Independence	Division of labor
	Women empowerment	Preservation of social values
	Privacy is maintained	Due to joint property ownership members share a common purse and this helps in accommodating unemployed member if any.
		Care of children, old people and handicapped is better as someone is always available to look after.
Disadvantages	Fragile Unity	Status of women is compromised.
	Social value erosion	Lack of freedom
	Undue stress of child rearing and old persons care on the couple	Conflicts are common

Q4. What are vulnerable groups in a family?

Ans. In family there are certain groups of human beings which either by nature or because of deep rooted customs is week and vulnerable such as women, children, disabled persons, aged etc. Others comprise of pregnant women, postnatal mothers, infants, persons suffering from illnesses etc.

Q5. What are vital events?

Ans. It refers to the **live birth, death, fetal death, marriage, divorce and adoption, etc**.

Q6. What is dependency ratio?

Ans. The proportion of persons above 65 years of age and children below 15 years of age are considered to be dependent on economically productive age group (15-64 years). As dependency ratio increases, there is increased strain on the productive part of the population to support the upbringing and pensions of the economically dependent. In India, as per 2020 data dependency ratio is 48.7 which means roughly 49 dependents for every 100 productive people.

Q7. Who is considered a literate as per the census definition

Ans. As per the census (1991, 2001, 2011,2021) definition in India, any person who can read and write, with understanding, in any one language of India and who is more than 7 years of age is considered as literate. According to census 2021, literacy rate in India is 74.04% with male (82.14%) literacy rate significantly higher than female (65.46%).

Q8. What are the various scales used to classify socioeconomic status in urban and rural areas of India?

Ans.

Socio-economic status scale for urban area	Socio-economic status scale for rural area
Modified Kuppuswamy scale	Modified Udai Pareek
Modified B G Prasad	Modified B G Prasad
Kulshreshtha	Radhukar
Srivastava	Shirpurkar
Jalota	

Q9. Enumerate the diseases associated with upper and lower socio-economic status.

Ans. Diseases prevalent among high SES: due to behavioral risk factors (like alcoholism, smoking, sedentary lifestyle, faulty dietary habits, stress etc.) more prevalent among elite strata of the society, this SES is commonly affected by non-communicable disease including mental illnesses.

Diseases prevalent among low SES: Socioeconomic deprivation appears to predispose to a wide range of health issues, from disease to access to provision of and outcomes of health care. Health conditions that may happen due to low SES are malnutrition, anemia, drug abuse, food and water borne diseases due to poor food and water hygiene, Malaria, HIV/AIDS, Tuberculosis, and diseases due to parasites.

Q10. How much is the per capita income in India at present?

Ans. Per capita income, also known as income per person, is the mean income of the people in an economic unit such as a country, state or city. To know per capita income, the total income of a unit is divided by the population of that unit.

According to the data released by the National Statistical Office (NSO), Ministry of Statistics and Programme Implementation, the 'Per Capita Income' during 2019-20 is reported as ₹ 94,566. Among all states/UT, the state per capita income of Goa is highest in the country followed by Delhi and Sikkim whereas Bihar has the lowest NSDP per capita

Q11. Define poverty line. What are the criteria used for deciding cutoff for poverty line in India.

Ans. Poverty line is the amount of money needed for a person to meet his basic needs. As per report of the Rangrajan Committee (2014), the 'Monthly per capita consumption expenditure' (MPCE) of Rs 972 in rural and Rs 1407 in urban areas is set for poverty line and it is based on the minimum income required for meeting the nutritional requirement of 2400 kcal/person/day in rural and 2100kcal/person/day in urban areas.

Hence Below Poverty Line (BPL) is defined as below:

Criteria	Rural India	Urban India
Per capita calorie intake(kcal/person/day)	<2400	<2100
Per capita income	< Rs.32/day	< Rs.47/day

Q12. Name any five schemes run by Government of India (GoI) for below poverty line strata.

Ans. Schemes run by GoI for BPL strata are:

I. **RSBY (Rashtriya Swasthiya Bima Yojana)** has been launched by Ministry of Labor and Employment, **Government** of **India** to provide **health** insurance coverage for Below Poverty Line (**BPL**) families. The objective of RSBY is to provide protection to **BPL** households from financial liabilities arising out of health shocks that involve hospitalization.

II. **National Maternity Benefit Scheme:** In this scheme the pregnant women from poor family who are below poverty line are given financial assistance for pre- and post- pregnancy care. Every pregnant woman will get Rs. 500 per pregnancy and for first two delivery women is eligible for the benefits of scheme.

III. **Indira Gandhi National Old-Age Pension Scheme (IGNOAPS):** Person (male or female) should be aged 60 years or more and below poverty line (BPL). The amount of old age pension is Rs. 600-1000 per month from the Central Government depending on the state share of the pension.

IV. **National Family Benefit Scheme (NFBS)-** In case of death of the primary bread earner of families living below the poverty line, the bereaved families are assisted with a financial assistance of Rs. 20,000. However, the deceased person must be in the age group of 18 to 64 years.

V. **Antyodaya Anna Yojana (AAY):** It is a **Government of India sponsored scheme.** AAY involved identification of poorest of the poor families amongst BPL and providing them food grains at a highly subsidized rate. The identified families (rural/semi-urban/urban) for this AAY Scheme are provided with the Green Color AAY Ration card.

Other schemes: Annapurna Scheme, Indira Awas Yojana, National Rural Employment Guarantee Act (NREGA), Minimum Needs Program.

Q13. Enumerate diseases associated with overcrowding.

Ans. Effects on quality of life due to crowding may be due to increased physical contact, lack of sleep, lack of privacy and poor hygiene practices. Overcrowding is one of the major factors in the transmission of diseases with outbreak potential such as acute respiratory infections, meningitis, typhus, cholera, scabies, etc. Outbreaks of disease are more frequent and more severe in such condition.

Q14. What are the breeding sites and diseases transmitted by culex, anopheles and aedes mosquitoes?

Ans.

Mosquito	Breeding Sites	Diseases Transmitted
Anopheles	Clean water (pools, slow running stream, rice fields etc.)	• Malaria; filaria (not in India) • Bite during night (mainly indoor)
Culex	Dirty and Polluted water (open drains, cesspools, leaking septic tanks etc.)	• Japanese encephalitis, Bancroftian filariasis, West Nile fever, Epidemic viral arthritis. • Bite during night
Aedes aegypti	Artificial collections of water in and around human dwellings (tyres, flowerpots, coolers, broken pots etc.)	• Dengue, Chikungunya, Rift valley fever, yellow fever • Bite during daytime

Q15. What is the breeding site for housefly and discuss diseases transmitted by it?

Ans. Housefly breeds on organic matter like human excreta, manure, garbage, decaying fruits and vegetables. It transmits diseases by mechanical transmission through feet and legs, vomit drops and defecation. Diseases transmitted by housefly includes cholera, diarrhea, dysentery, typhoid, paratyphoid, amoebiasis, anthrax, trachoma.

Q16. What is safe, wholesome/potable water?

Ans. Criteria for safe and wholesome/potable water are:

- Water should be free from pathogenic agents, harmful chemical substances, radiological hazards, odor and color.
- It should be pleasant to taste and usable for domestic purposes.
- It should fulfil the criteria defined by national standards for drinking water quality.

Q17. Enumerate the household methods for disinfection of water.

Ans. Household methods for disinfection of water are:

Boiling, chlorination (sodium hypochlorite, calcium hypochlorite), reverse osmosis, filtration using ceramic filters.

Q18. What are diseases associated with cattle and pet.

Ans. Cattles and pets can transmit zoonotic diseases like anthrax, brucellosis, salmonellosis, rabies, plague, scrub typhus, Japanese encephalitis, leptospirosis, taeniasis.

Q19. What are social institutions? Give suitable examples.

Ans. Social institutions are complex set of social norms, beliefs, values and role relationship that arise in response to the needs of society. Social institutions exist to satisfy social needs. These social institutions are responsible to constrain and control, punish and reward members of the society. We find informal and formal social institutions in societies. Institutions such as family and religion are examples of informal social institutions while law, economics and (formal) education are formal social institutions.

Q20. Name the diseases to which social stigma are attached?

Ans. Diseases with social stigma are COVID-19, tuberculosis, leprosy, HIV/AIDS, STDs etc.

Q21. What are customs, mores and folkways?

Ans. Custom is often referred to as a folkway. But there is a difference between the two that the folkways are of more general and wider character than the customs.

Folkways are behaviors that are learned and shared by a social group that are not morally significant, but they can be important for social acceptance. Thus, for example-shaking hands, eating four meals etc. are folkways rather than of customs.

Customs are traditional and widely accepted way of behaving or doing something that is specific to a particular society, place, or time. Customs are related to the survival and growth of the group.

They are not made obligatory by the group. They are sanctioned informally.

Mores are social norms that are widely observed within a particular society or culture. Mores determine what is considered morally acceptable or unacceptable within any given culture.

Q22. What is acculturation?

Ans. **Acculturation** is mixing of people of two cultures that affects the lifestyle of both the groups. It usually happens due to trade and commerce, industrialization, propagation of religion, education or conquest.

Q23. Give examples of tradition, custom, habit and belief related to health.

Ans. **Tradition:** piercing ear and nose, application of kajal into eyes

Custom: pre-lacteal feeding, walking barefoot to temple

Habit: nail biting, eating junk foods

Belief: papaya is an abortifacient, leprosy is due to past sin

Q24. What is social diagnosis and social therapy?

Ans. **Social diagnosis** is the identification of social causes which are responsible for diseases, e.g. 'poor economic conditions, low literacy and overcrowding'.

Social therapy is the use of social interventions targeted at social causes of diseases for prevention of diseases and promotion of health, e.g., creating awareness for acceptance of family planning services, awareness to remove social stigma associated with diseases like HIV/AIDS etc.

Q25. What are food taboos, food fads and food fallacy

Ans. **Food taboos:** Non consumption of certain foods due to religious, cultural, social or other reasons, e.g., Hindus don't eat beef, orthodox Brahimins do not eat onion and garlic etc.

Food fads: Extreme likes or dislikes for a particular food usually for a short period, e.g., consuming only fruits etc.

Food fallacies: Wrong belief about food as per the modern scientific knowledge, e.g., orange and curd cause cold, peas and beans cause constipation etc.

Q26. What is the difference between clinical diagnosis and community diagnosis?

Ans.

Procedures	Clinical Diagnosis	Community Diagnosis
Assessment	Patient	Family formal and informal leaders, other community members
To detect problems	Examine patients	Observations in community, topographical features, leadership patterns, conflicting power groups
Investigations	Lab tests	Data collection- primary and secondary sources
Preliminary diagnosis	Doctor's initial evaluation	Data processing and analysis
Explain diagnosis	To patient	Data presentation to community
Start treatment	Medications, surgery etc.	Action Plan
Behavior changes	May/May not be required	Must require and results in lasting improvement in community health status
Controlling authority	Doctor	Community
Follow up	Assess progress, confirm diagnosis followed by treatment	Monitor, evaluate and plan new health actions

Q27. What is the significance of conducting community survey?

Ans. A community survey helps to discover attitudes, opinions, experiences, and needs of the target community. It further provides an opportunity to collect community feedback on various social products, schemes and policies. Depending on the feedback, policy makers try to align the product or service with the needs and expectations of the community.

Q28. What is Community Diagnosis?

Ans. Community diagnosis is a comprehensive assessment of health status of the community in relation to its social, physical and biological environment.

Q29. What is the importance of community diagnosis in health planning and management?

Ans. Community diagnosis helps policy makers in the following ways:

- To find the common problems or diseases, which are troublesome to the community and are easily preventable.
- To find the actual problems of the community people which might not have perceived by them as problems.
- To access the group of underprivileged people who are unable to use the available facilities due to poverty, prevailing discriminations and other reasons.
- To impart knowledge and change people's attitude towards prevailing problems. Community diagnosis by defining existing problems, determining available resources and setting priorities for planning, implementing and evaluating health action, by and for the community thus helps in health planning and management.

Q30. What dietary advice and treatment will you give to a three-year child suffering from vit. A deficiency?

Ans. Dietary advice- Rich sources of vitamin A such as green leafy vegetables, deep yellow/orange fruits, eggs, milk and meat should be included in the diet. As far as possible fortified ghee, butter, hydrogenated vegetable oil should be consumed. Periodic massive doses as per UIP should be administered to the child till he attains 5 years of age.

In case of diagnosed xerophthalmia, along with dietary advice, the following regime should be followed:

2,00,000IU (110mg) of retinol palmitate (oil miscible vitamin A) is administered orally for 2 days. In cases of persistent vomiting/diarrhoea, water miscible vitamin A 1,00,000 IU is administered as IM injection, followed by 2,00,000IU 1-4 weeks later.

Q31. What dietary advice will you give to a patient of Diabetes Mellitus?

Ans. The ideal diet for people with diabetes lays emphasis on having a healthy and balanced meal. All varieties of cereals, dhal/whole grams, vegetables, fruits should be incorporated in the daily menu. A thali/plate should preferably include a cereal, dhal or lean meat, vegetables and milk products. Amount of oil used in food preparations should be minimal and a combination of different varieties of oil is better. It is necessary to include one fresh fruit (orange, sweet lime, apple, papaya) daily as a snack. Avoid banana, mango, watermelon, sapota, custard apple. Avoid plain sugar and refined carbohydrates, have food at regular intervals consisting of 3 main meals and 1-2 snacks in-between to control blood sugar levels. (http:/nhp.gov.in)

Q32. What dietary advice will you give to a pregnant mother?

Ans. Advice:

- Eat one extra meal a day, to ensure adequacy of all nutrients.
- Prefer high fibre cereals and legumes-include sprouts.
- Take milk and dairy products– these are rich in calcium, proteins and vitamins.
- Eat fresh seasonal fruits and vegetables as these provide vitamins and iron.
- Cereals, pulses and whole grains are good source of proteins.
- A handful (45 gm) of nuts and atleast two cups of daal provide daily requirement of proteins in vegetarians.
- Green leafy vegetables are rich source of iron and folic acid.
- For non-vegetarians, meat, egg, chicken or fish are good sources of protein, vitamins and iron.
- Don't take fad diets.
- Take iron and folate supplements regularly.

Q33. What dietary modifications should be advised for geriatric people?

Ans. Except for a marginal reduction in energy requirement the need for the other nutrients remains almost the same. For each year above 30 years, it is a rule of thumb to subtract 10 calories/year for men and 7 calories/year for women. Accordingly, the estimated energy requirements based on BMR and physical activity levels (PAL), for the sedentary elderly man and woman weighing 65 kg and 55 kg are 1700kcal and 1500kcal respectively.

Principles of diet for elderly: simple but nutritious food, green leafy vegetables, plenty of fruits, inclusion of whole cereals, frequent small meals, plenty of fluids, avoiding fasting, avoiding fried foods, consuming low salt and sugar, easy to cook foods.

Foods to be preferred: Dalia, Khichdi, Upma, Kheer, Poha, Fruit juices, Vegetable soups, Meat stew.

Q34. How many calories are provided by breastmilk.

Ans. Average 413kcal (6-8 months), 379 kcal (9-11 months), 346 kcal (12-13 months) in an average breastfed infant. (WHO, UNICEF,1998)

Q35. What do you understand by IYCF? List the major practices in IYCF.

Ans. IYCF stands for infant and young child practices, a set of national guidelines, related to nutrition of newborns and children up to the age of 2 years to achieve the optimum nutrition.

Major practices in IYCF- 1. Initiation of breastfeeding within 1 hour of birth. 2. Exclusive breastfeeding for first 6 months. 3.Appropriate complementary feeding after 6 months. 4. Continued breastfeeding for 2 years or beyond.

Q36. Is there any national health programme for elderly in India? What is its main objective?

Ans. National Programme for Health Care of the Elderly (NPHCE).

Objective: To provide preventive, curative and rehabilitative services to the elderly persons at various levels of healthcare delivery system.

Q37. What is vegan diet. Which nutrient may be deficient in vegans?

Ans. A diet that does not include any animal product such as nonvegetarian food, milk or milk products is a vegan diet. Vitamin B12 is usually deficient in vegans.

Q38. Name foods items rich in iron and calcium.

Ans. Iron : Bengal gram, amaranth, dark green leafy vegetables, jaggery, cauliflower leaves, radish leaves, whole grains, dry fruits, nuts, meat.

Calcium : Millets and pulses including ragi, rajmah, Bengal gram, Leafy vegetables, Nuts and oil seeds, Animal products including fish, milk and its products, egg.

Q39. What is the difference between the terms target couple and eligible couple. What is the relevance of estimating these couples in a community?

Ans. Target couples are those married couple having two or three children and where wife is in the reproductive age group, whereas eligible couple is any currently married couple where wife is in reproductive age group. Thus, target couples are a part of eligible couple but they are given priority for family welfare services.

Estimation of such couples in the community is utilized for organizing the family welfare services.

Q40. How many minimum visits should be made at ANC clinic?

Ans. Minimum Four visits should be made: First- within 12 weeks

Second- 14-26 weeks Third- 28-34 weeks Fourth- 36weeks-term

Q41. Enumerate high risk pregnancy criteria.

Ans. Past Obstetric history of C-Section, still birth, abortion, congenital malformation, obstructed labour, grand multipara.

Associated risk factors in present pregnancy: Young primi (<20years), elderly primi (>35years), short stature(<140cm), Hb<7gm%, PIH, pre-eclampsia, eclampsia, gestational diabetes mellitus, multiple pregnancy, malpresentation, placenta previa.

Q42. What are the common complications during post-natal period?

Ans. Excessive bleeding, puerperal pelvic infection, mastitis, breast abscesses, thromboembolism.

Q43. What are the components of essential newborn care?

Ans.

1. Immediate and thorough drying of the baby
2 Early skin to skin contact between mother and the newborn
3. Properly timed cord clamping
4. Non-separation of the mother and baby for early breastfeeding initiation

Q44. Differentiate between SAM and MAM:

Ans.

Severe Acute Malnutrition (SAM)	Moderate Acute Malnutrition (MAM)
Child's weight for his/her/height/length lies below -3SDof WHO growth standards or MUAC is <11.5cm or bilateral oedema of feet is present or visible severe wasting is present.	Child's weight for his/her/height/length lies between -3SD and -2SD of WHO growth standards or MUAC is between 12.5cm and 11.5cm and there is no oedema of feet is present. Moreover, the child is alert and clinically well.
A child having SAM with complications must be hospitalized.	A child with MAM can be managed in OPD setting having provision for supplementary feeding.

Q45. What are common health problems in adolescents?

Ans.

1. Injuries including road traffic injuries, drowning, violence and self-harm.
2. Mental health problems mainly depression
3. Alcohol and other substance abuse
4. HIV/AIDS and other RTIs due to unsafe sexual practices
5. Early pregnancy and childbirth
6. Micronutrient deficiencies

Preventive checkup of other family members

Enter the relevant information in the format given below for all family members (One page per family member) Add additional pages if required

Date of Examination	Name	Age/ Sex	Significant Findings on History	Significant Findings on Examination	Height	Weight	BMI	Blood Pressure	Hemoglobin	Diagnosis	Action Taken	Follow up

Preventive checkup of other family members

Enter the relevant information in the format given below for all family members (One page per family member) Add additional pages if required

Date of Examination	Name	Age/ Sex	Significant Findings on History	Significant Findings on Examination	Height	Weight	BMI	Blood Pressure	Hemoglobin	Diagnosis	Action Taken	Follow up

Preventive checkup of other family members

Enter the relevant information in the format given below for all family members (One page per family member) Add additional pages if required

Date of Examination	Name	Age/ Sex	Significant Findings on History	Significant Findings on Examination	Height	Weight	BMI	Blood Pressure	Hemoglobin	Diagnosis	Action Taken	Follow up

Preventive checkup of other family members

Enter the relevant information in the format given below for all family members (One page per family member) Add additional pages if required

Date of Examination	Name	Age/ Sex	Significant Findings on History	Significant Findings on Examination	Height	Weight	BMI	Blood Pressure	Hemoglobin	Diagnosis	Action Taken	Follow up

STUDENT'S NOTES

Supervisor's Signature

Section III

Clinicosocial Cases

Section III: Clinicosocial Cases

	Topic	Competency	Signature of Supervisor with Date	Grade
1.	List of Clinicosocial Cases	-		
2.	Clinicosocial Case Format	-		
3.	Specimen Clinicosocial Case for Communicable Diseases- Tuberculosis	CM 1.9- Demonstrate the role of effective Communication skills in health in a simulated environment. CM 1.10- Demonstrate the important aspects of the doctor patient relationship in a simulated environment. CM 8.1- Describe and discuss the epidemiological and control measures including the use of essential laboratory tests at the primary care. Level for communicable diseases CM 8.3- Enumerate and describe disease specific National Health Programs including their prevention and treatment of a case. PE 34.3- Discuss the various regimens for management of Tuberculosis as per National Guidelines. CT1.15 Prescribe an appropriate antituberculosis regimen based on the location of disease, smear positivity and negativity and comorbidities based on current national guidelines including directly observed tuberculosis therapy (DOTS)		
4.	Specimen Clinicosocial Case for Non-Communicable Diseases – Diabetes	CM 1.9, CM 1.10, CM 8.2- Describe and discuss the epidemiological and control measures including the use of essential laboratory tests at the primary care level for non-communicable diseases (diabetes, Hypertension, Stroke, obesity and cancer etc.)		

5.	Specimen Case Scenarios for Case Based Learning	-		
A.	Adolescent with Anaemia	CM 1.9, CM 1.10, IM 9.15- Describe the national programs for anaemia prevention PE 9.6- Assess and classify the nutrition status of infants, children and adolescents and recognize deviations PE 29.5- Discuss the National anaemia Control program		
B.	Under-5 with Acute Respiratory Infections	CM 1.9, CM 1.10, CM 10.5- Describe Universal Immunization Program; Integrated Management of Neonatal and Childhood Illness (IMNCI) and other existing Programs.		
C.	Under-5 with Diarrhoea	CM 1.9, CM 1.10, CM 10.5, PE 10.4- Identify children with under nutrition as per IMNCI criteria and plan		
D.	Post-Menopausal Woman with Hypertension	CM 1.9, CM 1.10 CM 12.2- Describe health problems of aged population CM 12.3- Describe the prevention of health problems of aged population CM 8.2- Describe and discuss the epidemiological and control measures including the use of essential laboratory tests at the primary care level for Non Communicable diseases (Diabetes, Hypertension, Stroke, obesity and cancer etc.)		
E.	Clinicosocial Case Scenario–Adult with Tuberculosis	CM 1.9,1.10, 8.1, 8.3, PE 34.3, 34.4 CT1.15 Prescribe an appropriate antituberculosis regimen based on the location of disease, smear positivity and negativity and comorbidities based on current national guidelines including directly observed tuberculosis therapy (DOTS)		
F.	Short Cases	CM 1.9, 1.10		

CHAPTER 1

List of Clinicosocial Cases

1. Acute diarrhea in an under-five child
2. Acute respiratory infection (ARI) in an under-five child
3. Malnutrition (Undernutrition) in an under-five child
4. Iron-deficiency anemia
5. Diabetes mellitus
6. Hypertension
7. Tuberculosis
8. COPD
9. Cerebral palsy
10. Mental retardation
11. Polio
12. Fever with rash
13. Malaria
14. Dengue
15. Rabies/Dog bite

Other suggested cases that have already been covered in Section II:

1. Antenatal woman
2. Post-natal woman
3. Eligible couple
4. Geriatric

CHAPTER 2

Clinicosocial Case Format

- Factors related to the individual

a. **Socio-demographic profile**

- Name
- Age
- Marital status
- Occupation
- Socioeconomic status

Address

Gender

Education

Family Composition

b. **History**

- Chief complaints in chronological order
- History of present illness
- History of past medical/ surgical illness
- Family history
- In females menstrual and obstetric history
- Immunization history and Developmental milestone among children
- Personal history including habits and addiction
- Clinical examination
  - Anthropometry
  - General
  - Systemic

c. **Health seeking behaviour**

- KAP regarding disease/prevention
- Attitude towards healthcare system
- Healthcare services
  - Availability
  - Accessibility

- Affordability
- Utilization

d. Environmental history

- Physical environment
  - Housing- general, area, overcrowding, ventilation, lighting, other comforts, Water supply, Waste disposal
- Biological environment
- Psycho- Emotive factors in the family
  - Interaction bondages
    - Between family members
    - With index case
    - Impact of the disease on family
  - Family support system
    - Understanding of the problem
    - Readiness to provide support
    - Care provider within the family
  - Factors in the workplace
    - General description (including School if applicable)
    - Attitude and support (emotional, physical, financial) on part of
      - Employer/Superiors
      - Colleagues
      - Subordinates
  - Factors in the immediate community
    - Cohesiveness within
    - Interaction with family members and index case
    - Availability of support system
      - Healthcare
      - School/Special school
      - NGOs/Voluntary bodies
      - Public health bodies
  - Factors in the community at large
    - General attitude
    - Towards disease

    - Towards disease prevention and rehabilitation
    - Availability of treatment facility
    - Availability of rehabilitation facility

- Summarize

  What is the social pathology in the present family?

  (The major weakness e.g., "Alcoholism", "poor purchasing power", "adverse attitude towards girl child")

- Summarize

  What is social diagnosis.

  (e.g., "Gross physical handicap", "with poor rehabilitation facility", "with broken family" , "adversely predisposed family")

- (SWOT analysis)
  - Strength
  - Weakness
  - Opportunity
  - Threats
- What is the plan of management?
  - Medical
  - Lifestyle
  - Disability limitation
  - Vocational rehabilitation
  - Emotional rehabilitation
  - Physical and financial support
  - Plan of management for family members

*Detailed relevant history needs to be elicited for each clinicosocial case.

Chapter 3

Specimen Clinicosocial Case for Communicable Diseases-Tuberculosis

Date:________________

Identification details

Name:

Age:

Gender:

Education:

Occupation (try to rule out high risk groups like people employed in mining works, tobacco industry, stone crushing, carpet weaving etc.):

SES:

History of present illness (in chronological order):

Complaints	Onset(sudden/gradual)	Duration	Describe symptoms

Treatment History

Is the person a diagnosed case of TB: Y/N; If yes

Where TB was diagnosed: When TB was diagnosed:

What are the drugs patient is consuming? Duration of treatment: ________________________

____

____

Has he/she discontinued the treatment: Y/N; If yes, specify reasons ________________________

Any history of immunosuppressants drug intake: Y/N

Past History

Any history of Tuberculosis, Diabetes mellitus, Hypertension, Asthma or COPD in the past.

Personal History (to rule out risk factors for TB)

Food habits: Vegetarian/Non-vegetarian/Mixed

Bowel habits: Bladder habits:

Sleep: Time of sleep, duration of sleep, onset, latency, disturbed sleep.

Smoking: Y/N; Sharing hukka: Y/N; Smokeless tobacco: Y/N Alcohol: Y/N

Physical activity:

Dietary History

Number of meals consumed daily

Dislike for food items if any:

Dietary Assessment (24 hour Recall Method)

Assess the nutritional requirement

Name	Calorie requirement (Kcal/day)	Protein Requirement (g/day)	Fat Requirement (Visible) (g/day)	Dietary Fiber requirement (g/day)	Any special needs

Daily diet consumption by the individual (24 hour Recall Method) - In terms of cooked food

S. No.	Name	Meal	Name of food items	Quantity (ml/g/ number)	Calories (Kcal)	Protein (g)	Fat (g)	Dietary Fiber (g)
1.		Break Fast Mid-morning snack Lunch Evening tea/snack Dinner Post-dinner snack						

- Excess/Deficit of calorie intake if any:
- Excess/Deficit of protein intake if any:

Psychosocial History:

Detailed environmental history as stated in previous section.

Knowledge, attitude and practices towards illness

Knowledge	Attitude	Practices
Cause of TB:	Towards recovery:	Cough hygiene etiquettes:
Transmission:		Sputum disposal:
Management:		Availing services under NTEP:
		Compliance to treatment:
		Supplementary nutrition:

Physical examination

Investigations

Clinical Diagnosis including category of the patient:

Advice

To patient:

To family members:

Supervisor's Signature

CHAPTER 4

Specimen Clinicosocial Case for Non-Communicable Diseases—Diabetes

Date:____________

Identification details

Name:

Age:

Gender:

Address

Education:

Occupation:

Income:

SES:

History of present illness

A. Symptoms in chronological order

Complaints	Onset (sudden/gradual)	Duration	Describe symptoms

B. Treatment History if any

System of medicine utilized for management of diabetes: Allopathy/AAYUSH/Other

Drug history:

Duration of taking drugs:

C. Complications if any

Macrovascular

History of chest pain/palpitation/dyspnea on exertion(cardiovascular): Y/N

History of weakness in limbs/reduced reflexes(cerebrovascular): Y/N

Microvascular

History of blurring of vision/sudden loss of vision/ floaters/(retinopathy): Y/N

History of reduced urine output/Oedema of face or legs (nephropathy): Y/N

History of numbness/tingling/foot ulcers(neuropathy): Y/N

Past history

History of previous illness/hospitalization for similar complaints: Y/N

Hypertension / any coronary artery disease / TIA / stroke / COPD / seizure disorder/ intake of any other chronic medication / blood transfusion / trauma: Y/N

Personal history

Food habits: Vegetarian/Non-vegetarian/Mixed

Bowel habits: Bladder:

Sleep: time of sleep, duration of sleep, onset, latency, disturbed sleep.

Smoking: Y/N; Sharing hukka: Y/N; Smokeless tobacco: Y/N Alcohol: Y/N

Physical activity: sedentary lifestyle/active

Hygiene:

Yoga/meditation/sports/Music/Other recreational activities

Dietary history

No. of meals everyday:

Intake of fresh fruits and salads: Y/N

Dietary assessment (24 hour Recall Method) Assess the nutritional requirement

Name	Calorie requirement (Kcal/day)	Protein Requirement (g/day)	Fat Requirement (Visible) (g/day)	Dietary Fiber Requirement (g/day)	Any special needs

Daily diet consumption by the individual (24 hour Recall Method) - In terms of cooked food

S. No.	Name	Meal	Name of food items	Quantity (ml/g/ number)	Calories (Kcal)	Protein (g)	Fat (g)	Dietary Fiber (g)
1.		Break Fast Mid morning snack Lunch Evening tea/ snack Dinner Post-dinner snack						

Daily calorie intake: ; Excess/Deficit:

Daily protein intake: ; Excess/Deficit :

Daily fat intake: ; Excess/Deficit :

Daily salt consumption:

Family History:

Psychosocial History:

Detailed environmental history as stated in previous section.

Physical Examination

General examination:

Systemic examination:

Lab investigations:

Clinicosocial diagnosis

Advice given:

Supervisor's Signature

Chapter 5

Specimen Case Scenarios for Case Based Learning

A. Adolescent with Anaemia

Date:_____________

Sociodemographic details:

Rani, 16-year-old girl, school dropout, Hindu by religion, residing in Prem Nagar, Faridabad, belonging to a 8 membered three generation family. Her father, Mr. Mahesh, head of the family, 42 years old, is educated till 8th class. He is a machine operator in a factory and earns Rs.8000/- per month. Mrs. Sarita (wife of Mr. Mahesh) 36 years old, works as a domestic helper and earns Rs. 2000 per month and is educated till 5th class. Mr. Mahesh has three daughters and one son, 16 years old Rani, 14 years old Tina, 13 years old Meena and 7 years old Amit. His parents are illiterate and his mother manages the daily household work of the house.

Informant: self, mother was present at the time of history taking and examination.

Presenting complaints: The girl complaints of fatigue, headache, generalized weakness, shortness of breath and difficulty in concentrating since last 1 month.

History of present illness: The girl developed shortness of breath and fatigue which was gradual in onset and progressive in nature. The shortness of breath was aggravated on doing physical work like washing clothes, climbing stairs, walking for 200 metres and used to get relieved on taking rest. She had 2 episodes of fainting in last 15 days.

The girl also complained of heavy menstrual bleeding for past 6 months. Headache is generalized, gets precipitated on watching TV or knitting for longer durations and gets relieved on taking rest without any medication. There's no radiation of headache to neck or shoulders. She is not using spectacles/ lenses at present. However, she has never visited an eye specialist in recent past.

Past history: There is no h/o similar episodes/complaints in the past but having history of repeated episodes of worm infestation.

Family history: No h/o similar complaints in the family. There is no h/o DM, HTN, TB, thalassemia, repeated blood transfusions to parents/ siblings

Menstrual history: Menarche was attained at 12 years of age. Cycles are irregular since 6 months and are of 22 days, lasts for 5-8 days. She uses 6-8 pads per day. H/o passage of blood clots is present and is associated with dysmenorrhea.

Personal history: She is vegetarian by diet. She is having habit of eating chalk in the school. She has normal bladder and bowel habits. Her sleep cycle is normal. There's no reported addiction of tobacco (in any form), alcohol, or any other substance of abuse.

Psychosocial History: Home- lives with family. Situation at home is not good as there is financial crisis, father has debts and there is less earning due to lockdown now. They have difficulty in getting food and other basic amenities.

Education / Employment – not studying currently, school dropout. Parents think that she will help her mother as house maid and earn some money. She is not working at present.

Activity – She sleeps for 6 hours and most of the time she indulges with mobile and internet activities. There's no physical activity.

Drugs – Never used Tobacco / Alcohol / other substances.

Sexuality – Sexually inactive.

Safety – Feels safe at home and neighborhood.

Suicide – Able to cope with her situation, never thought of ending her life, doesn't have suicidal ideation, doesn't feel helpless, hopeless or worthless.

Dietary history: Based on 24-hour recall:

Breakfast: 1 bread slice, 1 glass milk with 1 tsf sugar Lunch: 1 roti, 1 katori aloo Shimla mirch sabzi Snacks: 2 glucose biscuits, 1 cup tea with 1 tsf sugar Dinner: 1 Katori boiled rice, 1 katori dal

Environmental history: The family resides in a kaccha-pucca house with one living room and attached washroom. It has two windows and one door, one ceiling fan and one tube light. Water is stored in uncovered containers taken from a common tap outside the house on specific timing. Refuse is collected in uncovered container and is kept just outside the door and discarded into public bin on daily basis. Sanitary latrine is present in the house. Kitchen is not separate.

Sociocultural history: Socio cultural practices followed by the family are that arranged marriage is done with age of marriage for girls and boys to be 18 and 21 years respectively. The family prefers vegetarian diet and do not support the practice of alcohol and tobacco intake.

Examination: Girl appeared pale and lethargic but was oriented to time, place and person. Weight was 42 kg, Height- 156 cm, BMI-17.3Kg/m2

Vitals: Pulse- 92/min, RR -14/min, Afebrile

General Examination: Pallor is Present. Hands and feet were cold to touch. Icterus, Clubbing, Cyanosis, lymphadenopathy and edema were absent. Tenderness in legs was present.

Systemic Examination: ***Respiratory system:*** No visible abnormality on inspection. On auscultation equal breath sounds heard bilaterally, no wheeze, rhonchi or crepitations heard. ***Cardiovascular system:*** S1 S2 heard, no added sounds heard. ***Abdominal:*** Soft, non-tender, No palpable mass. ***CNS:*** No Abnormality Detected.

LONG CASE-QUESTIONS

1. **Write the clinicosocial diagnosis of Index case.**
2. **Enumerate factors responsible for the present problem of the index case.**
3. **Mention the Socio-economic class of the family according to modified Kuppuswamy scale. Justify.**
4. **Comment on physical environment and mention risks to health of index case.**
5. **Calculate and comment on the diet of index case. What suggestions will you given to the Index case regarding diet (specific proportions for calories, protein and iron intake)**
6. **Discuss the relevant health programmes and services available to improve the health of index case.**

STUDENT'S NOTES

Supervisor's Signature

B. Under-5 with Acute Respiratory Infections

Date:__________

Socio-Demographic details:

Informant is mother and case is Rahul, 2 year and 10 months old boy, Hindu by religion, residing in urban area of Delhi in a 5 membered family which include, his father, mother, elder sister (8 years) and brother (5 years). His father Naresh, head of family, is 30 years old, 12th pass, carpenter by occupation and earning about Rs.20000/month. Mrs. Megha, wife of head of family, aged 27 years is educated till 10th class and is a homemaker. The family has been residing in a rented house for the past 9 years.

Presenting Complaints: According to mother, Rahul has been suffering from fever and cough for past 6 days and difficulty in breathing for last 2 days.

History of present illness: The child was apparently normal 6 days ago when he developed cough which was productive in nature, white in color, progressive and associated with fever which was coming on and off, high grade and was getting relieved on medications. He also had difficulty in breathing for last 2 days and was unable to sleep.

Past History: When asked, the mother said that the child has had frequent episodes of cough and fever in the last one year, which was accompanied by in drawing of chest.

Birth History: Rahul was a full term normal vaginal delivery at a government hospital in Delhi. Antenatal, intranatal and postnatal periods were uneventful. Baby cried immediately after birth; birth weight was 2.5kg. Breastfeeding started/ was initiated within an hour of birth and no evidence of congenital anomalies. Colostrum was given and prelacteal feed in the form of honey was given to the child. He received birth dose of BCG, OPV, Hep B and Vit K. His birth order is 3.

Immunization: Immunization card is present with mother. Besides birth doses of BCG, OPV and Hep B, he has received 3 doses of OPV, Pentavalent, Rotavirus on time. 2 doses of measles and IPV were also given timely. The child has received vitamin A only twice and not taken any other vaccine after that.

Family history: No significant family history.

Feeding history: Breast feeding initiated within an hour of birth and supplemented with cow milk given by bottle. Nothing else was given till 6 months of age. After 6 months, complementary foods were started with boiled and mashed pulses and then further included mashed potatoes, mashed apple, mashed rice and banana. He is registered with Anganwadi centre. Child normally takes 2 biscuits and cup of milk (1 tsf sugar) in morning, half katori rice with dal in afternoon, 1 banana in evening and mashed potato (half katori) and a cup of milk (1 tsf sugar) in night. But since few days his diet has decreased. In the day the child sleeps for 2 hours but at night he sometimes gets restless and cries.

Environmental history: The family lives in a two rooms pucca rented house. The room has 1 CFL of 15 watts. There is no exhaust fan or windows. Kitchen is not separate. The mother cooks in the corner of one room on a table and LPG is used as cooking fuel. Toilet is shared between two families who are staying on rent adjacent to each other. Mosquitoes, flies and cockroaches were present at the time of visit. Surroundings were unhygienic with puddles of water. Waste is disposed in an uncovered dustbin and emptied into a common dustbin on the street. Surrounding drains are uncovered. Water supply is from Delhi Jal Board and stored in buckets for daily use. Same water is used for drinking and stored in a mud pot which is covered by a plate, but no method of water purification is used before drinking. Hygiene practices are poor. Due to scarcity of water, family does not bathe daily.

Examination: Anthropometry: Height: 90 cm, Weight: 12 kgs, Head circumference: 47 cm, Chest circumference: 50cm, Mid upper arm circumference: 14 cm.

General Physical Examination: Child is irritable, but conscious and well-oriented. He is thin built, hair have normal luster, normal facies, eyes sunken, lips and teeth normal, tongue pale, skin is dry, nails appear normal. He is lethargic, pale, dyspneic, weak cry, not icteric, not cyanosed, no clubbing, no lymphadenopathy, no generalized edema. Vital signs: Temperature: 101degree F Heart rate:123/ min Respiratory rate:54/ min

Systemic Examination: Respiratory system– Respiratory rate 54/min. No visible abnormality on inspection. On auscultation equal breath sounds heard bilaterally. Cardiovascular System – No visible abnormality on inspection. Heart rate 123/minute. S1, S2 heard with no abnormal sound heard. Abdominal – No abnormality detected on inspection, palpation, percussion or auscultation. Genitourinary – No abnormality visible in hernial orifice and external genitalia. CNS – Child is lethargic. No abnormality detected.

Developmental Milestones: He started walking without support at 1 year of age, running at 18 months, he can ride tricycle and walk upstairs and downstairs. He can tell his name, age, and sing few words of nursery rhymes.

LONG CASE-QUESTIONS

1. **Write the clinicosocial diagnosis for this case.**
2. **Classify the illness as per IMNCI guidelines.**
3. **Calculate the total calorie intake from the dietary history provided. Find the deficit/excess of the various nutrients and comment on them with respect to their RDA.**
4. **Assess the biological environment of the family.**
5. **What advice would you give for this case at the individual, family and community level?**
6. **Plot the given anthropometric measurements on appropriate growth chart.**
7. **Comment on the immunization status of the child.**

STUDENT'S NOTES

Supervisor's Signature

C. Under-5 with Diarrhoea

Date:____________

Socio-Demographic details:

Informant is mother and case is Ashraf, a 4 year old male child, Muslim by religion, residing in an urban area of Hisar. The child belongs to a 3 membered family. His father, Islam, head of family, is a vegetable vendor, is 8th pass, earns Rs 17,000 per month and mother, Mariam is illiterate and works as a maid at two houses and earns Rs 6000 per month.

Presenting complaints: According to mother, child complained of pain in abdomen and loose stools for past 2 days and fever for last 1 day.

History of Presenting Complaints: The child was apparently well two days back when he woke up early morning and had an acute onset of loose stools, watery in consistency, foul smelling, not associated with blood or mucous. He has had 10-12 episodes of loose stools associated with pain in abdomen and nausea in the past two days. One day back, he developed fever. Fever was 100°F, on and off, high grade and got relieved on medications. He was given Syrup Paracetamol by his mother. He is unable to eat or drink because of nausea.

Past History: The mother informed that the child had frequent episodes of loose stools almost every two to three months but not every episode was accompanied with fever. The child also gets cold and cough very frequently.

Birth History of child: His mother did not attend any ANC visit, no supplements and no TT vaccine received during pregnancy. The child was born at home and delivery was conducted by a dai. Baby cried immediately after birth, no congenital abnormality was detected, birth weight of the child was 2200 grams. Breastfeeding was initiated 6 hours after delivery.

Immunization History: Immunization History – Immunization card was available with the mother. Child has been immunized with all vaccines up to one year. Afterwards no vaccine has been given as the mother could not find time to take the child to vaccination.

Feeding History: Breast feeding was initiated after 6hous. Colostrum was given, prelacteal feed was given in the form of honey. After 2 days artificial feeding was initiated due to inadequate breast milk secretion. The child was then started on diluted (1:1) packaged toned milk. The mother additionally started giving mashed vegetables, rice water and dal water after 6 months. Milk was fed by bottle which was washed with soap-water before every use. Bottle feeding continued till 3 years of age.

The child does not go to anganwadi as the mother finds it difficult to drop and pick up the child due to her work timings. The child stays hungry frequently but does not agree to eat homemade food. He prefers junk food. Presently the child is given packaged mother dairy milk. His usual diet is: Breakfast- 1 glass of milk (200ml) + 1tsf sugar + 1 slice of bread

Lunch- 1 chapatti + half katori daal

Evening- 1 cup of tea + 1 tsf sugar + 2 Parle G biscuit

Dinner- half katori daal + Half katori rice

But in last 24 hours he consumed half katori khichdi twice a day and 1 banana.

The mother during the day leaves the child at neighbor's house and goes for her work. The mother also gives history of pica for her child.

Environmental history: The family lives in a one room, pucca, rented house. Kitchen is not separate. The mother cooks in the corner of one room on a table and LPG is used as cooking fuel. There was no refrigerator for storage of perishable food stuffs however non-perishable food were being stored in covered containers. The room was ill lighted and ill ventilated. Water supply is from Municipal Corporation, stored in uncovered buckets for daily use and drawn out with the help of any glass. Toilet is shared between five families staying adjacent to each other on rent on the same floor. Surroundings were found to be unhygienic. Mosquitoes, flies and cockroaches were all present at the time of visit. Waste is disposed in an uncovered dustbin. Surrounding drains were uncovered. Hygiene practices were found to be poor.

Examination: Anthropometry: Height- 93 cm, Weight- 12 kgs, Mid upper arm circumference: 12.0 cm.

General Physical Examination: The child appears thin built, hairs have normal luster, normal facies, eyes sunken, lips dry, tongue pale, normal teeth, skin is dry nails appear normal. He is irritable, conscious, well oriented, pale, thirsty but due to nausea not able to drink properly, weak cry, skin pinch goes back slowly, not icteric, not cyanosed, no clubbing, no lymphadenopathy, nogeneralized edema. Vital signs: Temperature: 100-degree F, Heart rate: 123/ min, Respiratory rate: 30/ min.

Systemic Examination: *Respiratory system* – Respiratory rate 30/min. No visible abnormality, equal movement of chest seen on breathing. On auscultation bilateral equal breath sounds heard. *Cardiovascular System* – No visible abnormality on inspection. Heart rate 123/minute. S1, S2 heard with no abnormal sound heard. *Abdominal* – Abdomen is tender and bloated. On skin pinch, tenting was found to be of grade 2. (skin pinch went back slowly). *Genitourinary* – No abnormality visible in hernial orifice and external genitalia. *CNS* – Child is irritable. No abnormality was detected.

LONG CASE-QUESTIONS

1. **Write the clinicosocial diagnosis for the given case.**
2. **What are the risk factors that could have contributed to diarrhea in this case?**
3. **In the above scenario, classify diarrhea as per IMNCI. Which category does the child fall into and how will the case be managed at primary health care level?**
4. **Conduct dietary assessment and give suitable recommendations for index case.**
5. **What advice would you give to the mother regarding prevention and management of diarrhea?**
6. **Discuss the immunization schedule for a 4-year-old unimmunized child.**

STUDENT'S NOTES

Supervisor's Signature

D. Post-Menopausal Woman with Hypertension

Date:__________

Socio-Demographic details:

Mrs. Ratia, 54 years old female is a housewife, educated up to 8th standard and is a resident of urban area, Nangal. She lives in a 4 membered Hindu family. Her family comprises of her husband and two children, a son who is 30 years old and a daughter who is 18 years old. Her husband Raghu, head of the family, is a graduate, working as a government servant and having monthly income of Rs. 40,000. Mr. Piyush, son of head of the family is a teacher in a private school and getting monthly salary of Rs. 20,000. Ms. Priyanka, daughter of head of the family is a student presently.

Presenting Complaints: The patient presented with headache for the last one day.

History of Presenting Complaints: Mrs. Ratia is a known case of Hypertension since 2 years. She was diagnosed with this condition when she started having frequent episodes of headache. Headache was severe and generalized in nature and not associated with fever. There was no radiation to neck, shoulders or jaw. There were no precipitating or relieving factors. She got her blood pressure examined at the Mohalla clinic where her blood pressure was found to be consistently high on repeated measurements.

When her disease was diagnosed 2 years back, she tried to control it by making dietary modifications and somewhat reduced salt intake but was unable to do so in the following 3 months during which she still had raised blood pressure of 180/90 mm of Hg and thus was prescribed Tab Amlodipine 10mg OD by a physician. She has been taking the same off and on. She has not visited the physician for follow up visits. She takes the medicine if she gets headache but frequently misses the tablet when she feels okay. Headache gets relieved on taking the medication.

Past History: The patient is aware of the disease she suffers from and is non-compliant with her medication as well as lifestyle modification advice.

Apart from hypertension, she does not suffer from any other significant medical problem like dyslipidemia, Coronary artery disease, diabetes, COPD and/or tuberculosis. She has never had prolonged hospitalization, major accident, blood transfusion and has never taken any chronic medication.

Family History: No family history of hypertension, diabetes, coronary artery disease or COPD.

Personal History: She is non- smoker, non-alcoholic, with no other substance abuse. She sleeps for 8 hours at night and 1 hour during the day. She is aware that physical activity is important but considers it done in her routine household works like cooking and dusting. She takes bath daily and maintains personal hygiene.

Menstrual history: She attained menarche at the age of 15 years, her cycles were regular, flow was normal, not associated with dysmenorrhea. 5 years back she attained menopause She has not had any episode of peri-menopausal or post-menopausal bleed.

Dietary History: The patient is vegetarian and takes 4 meals per day. She is well aware of the fact that high salt foods are a risk factor for hypertension and needs to be avoided.

By 24- hour recall method, her dietary intake was found to be:

Breakfast- 1 cup of tea (50ml toned milk) + 2 slices of white bread fried in ghee and sprinkle with salt and pepper

Lunch- 1 katori aloo baigan sabji + 2 paratha + 1 katori raita + pickle

Evening- 2 samosa+ pudina chatni with 1 cup of tea.

Dinner- 1 cup green gram daal + 2 cup polished rice +Papad + pickle

Environmental history: The family stays in a 3 room, self-owned pucca house on the first floor with a separate kitchen, bathroom and toilet. The stairs leading to the first floor don't have railings or guards. The rooms were well ventilated but cross-ventilation was absent. Natural and artificial light were both found to be inadequate. There was one ceiling fan in each room. Kitchen was standing type, with marble flooring, well ventilated and ill lighted. Source of drinking water is from Municipal Corporation; RO was being used for water purification. For waste disposal, the waste was stored in an uncovered dustbin and emptied in the MCD collection van every day. There were flies and mosquitoes present at the time of visit. The drains were uncovered. Puddles and stray dog were present in the peri-domestic area.

General Physical Examination: Weight- 80kgs, Height- 156 cm, BMI- 32.9kg/m2, Pulse rate-82/min, BP- 180/90 mm of Hg, Temperature- afebrile to touch.

No pallor, Icterus, clubbing, cyanosis, raised JVP, edema or lymphadenopathy present.

Systemic Examination: Patient was well built, conscious, cooperative and well oriented to time, place and person. R*espiratory system:* RR is 18/min. No visible chest deformity, Trachea centrally placed, Symmetrical chest expansion, Normal vesicular breadth sounds heard. *Cardiovascular system:* S1 S2 heard, no murmurs or added sound heard. *Abdominal:* Soft, non-tender/ no organomegaly, bowel sounds present. *CNS*: No neurological deficit present.

Long Case-Questions

1. **Write the clinico social diagnosis for this case.**
2. **Identify the potential hazards for the above case?**
3. **Which scale will you use for assessing socio-economic class? Why? Mention its two disadvantages.**
4. **What screening tests would you like to advise for this case**
5. **Assess diet of index case and mention dietary interventions required**
6. **What lifestyle related advice would you give to the index case**
7. **Name one intervention for each applicable levels of prevention for the case**

STUDENT'S NOTES

Supervisor's Signature

E. Clinicosocial Case Scenario–Adult with Tuberculosis

Date:___________

Socio-demographic details:

Mr. Lekhraj Gujjar, 30 years old male, married, residing in Patel Nagar, Faridabad, Hindu by religion, belongs to a 5 membered three generation family.

Name	Age (years)	Sex	Marital Status	Relationship to the head of family	Education	Occupation	Income per month
Veerpal Gujjar	59	M	Widower	Father	Illiterate	Unemployed	–
Lekhraj Gujjar	30	M	Married	Head of family	Higher Secondary	Machine Operator in a Factory	20000/per month
Sheetal Gujjar	26	F	Married	Wife	Illiterate	Housewife	–
Mukesh	6	M	Unmarried	Daughter	1st standard	Student	–
Muskan	3	F	Unmarried	Son	–	Unemployed	–

Presenting complaints: Fever and cough for last 1 month

History of presenting illness: The index case was apparently well 1 month ago when he developed mild fever without any periodicity, resolved on medication, and was associated with cough. The cough was productive, with whitish sputum, which did not resolve with medication. The frequency of cough and volume of sputum gradually increased. The fever was also accompanied by night sweats and a decrease in appetite. Fever was not associated with chills or rigor, rash, difficulty in breathing, chest pain, pain in throat, rhinorrhea, hemoptysis, diarrhea, lower abdominal pain, burning micturition, pain abdomen, bony pains or pain in any other part of the body, myalgia, weakness or loss of weight.

Treatment History: Patient has taken homeopathic medicine and steam the inhalation for fever and cough.

Past History: There is no previous history of jaundice, malaria, tuberculosis, diabetes, hypertension or other infectious diseases.

Family History: His father is a hypertensive on treatment for the last 8 years. His father was diagnosed with Tuberculosis 6 years back and was started on antitubercular drugs. As a side effect, he developed itching and altered color of urine leading to discontinuation of the treatment after 3 months.

Personal History: Non-vegetarian with reduced appetite, smokes cigarettes about 1/2-1 pack each day for the last 10 years, non-alcoholic, no history of substance abuse. Bowel and bladder habits are normal. He has been having disturbed sleep with frequent awakening with night sweats.

Dietary History:

Diet as recalled from last 24 hours	Items
Morning	1 glass tea with milk and 1 tsf sugar
	2 Roti with 1 katori sabji (seasonal)
	1 boiled egg
Mid-Morning snack	1 tea
Lunch	1/2 katori rice, 1 katori sabji, 2 Roti
Evening snack	1 glass tea with milk and 1 tsf sugar, 2 biscuits
Dinner	1/2 katori rice, 1 katori daal, 2 katori Sabji

Environmental History: They reside in an owned, 2 room pucca house. Lighting and ventilation were inadequate in the house. The kitchen was separate, and LPG was used as a cooking fuel and there was no smoke outlet. The water supply is from Municipal Corporation and is intermittent. The drinking water is stored in plastic bottles. Waste disposal is done in a closed bin in the house which is collected outside the house by the MCD every day. There is one bathroom in the house. The drainage in the house is covered but mosquitoes and flies were in the house at the time of visit. There were collections of water and uncovered waste was being dumped outside and around the area.

General Physical Examination: Height- 170.9 cm, Weight- 65 kg, BMI- 22.49 kg/m2, Temperature- 99.50F, Pulse- 108/min, BP- 126/86 mm Hg.

Pallor was present. Clubbing, icterus, cyanosis, edema, lymphadenopathy were not present. JVP was not raised.

Systemic Examination: Patient is conscious, co-operative and well oriented to time, place and person. *Respiratory system:* No visible chest deformity, trachea centrally placed, symmetrical chest expansion, normal vesicular breadth sounds heard, mild crepitations heard on bilateral lower lung fields. *Cardiovascular system:* S1 S2 heard, no murmurs or added sounds heard. *Abdominal:* Soft, non-tender/ no organomegaly, bowel sounds present. *CNS:* No neurological deficit present.

Lab Investigations:

Blood Glucose- 96 mg/dl (Fasting) 135 mg/dl (PP)

Hb-12 mg%

LONG CASE-QUESTIONS

1. **What is the clinico social diagnosis for the case?**
2. **What is the socioeconomic status of the family?**
3. **From the given diet, calculate total calorie intake, and deficit and intake of relevant parameters. Formulate a suitable diet.**
4. **What other investigations would you order based on your clinical differential diagnosis?**
5. **What is the latest diagnostic algorithm and treatment protocol for managing such a case?**
6. **What advice would you give at each of the following levels: individual, family and community?**

STUDENT'S NOTES

Supervisor's Signature

F. Short Cases

Reena is 8 months old and weighs 5 kg. Her temperature is 38.5 °C. She was brought to the OPD by her grandmother as the mother is a maid and gone for work. She had been having fever and cough for 3 days and runny nose for last 5 days. She is able to drink, not vomiting, not having convulsions and was not lethargic or unconscious. On examination her breathing rate was 56 breaths per minute. Chest indrawing and stridor were not present. There was no rash. The child had received BCG, Hep B (0), OPV (0,1,2), Pentavalent (1,2), IPV (1) vaccinations till date. The child was breast fed till 6 months and now half katori khichdi and half banana are given twice a day in addition to breast-milk. The child belongs to 8 membered joint family belonging to lower socio-economic class, residing in one-room kutcha make-shift house with poor lighting and ventilation. There is no independent water supply in the house and family keeps water in uncovered buckets outside the house. There is no toilet within the house and family goes to adjacent railway tracks for defaecation. There are 2 elder siblings of the patient who are 2 and 4 years old with unknown vaccination status.

1. Assess nutritional status of the child and plot measurement on growth chart.
2. Discuss the physical environment and risks associated.
3. What medical management will you advise for this case as per IMNCI guidelines.
4. Discuss immunisation for this child.
5. Discuss family level interventions for health improvement.

Anshika, 18 months old female child, weighing 8 kg, is brought to the OPD by her mother with loose stools, decreased appetite for last three days. The child also had two-three episodes of vomiting, and general listlessness for one day. The child is not having fever or convulsions but does not respond to commands. On history examination, the skin pinch goes back very slowly and eyes seem sunken. The child was born with birth weight of 2200 g at home. Breastfeeding was started after 3 days of birth but due to inadequate milk production, she was given diluted cow milk with bottle. Mother started solid foods after 8 months and currently child takes two chapattis, a few biscuits, half katori dal and 200 ml toned milk in a day. The child lives in a one-room pucca, well-ventilated but poorly lit house in a resettlement colony in West Delhi with mother father and one elder brother. Father is a rickshaw puller and mother is a housewife. Both parents are illiterate. Total family income is Rs 7000 per month. Family uses a public toilet shared by 10 families. The child goes out barefoot in the street. Handwashing and bathing habits of the family are not satisfactory. The child has received all due vaccination till 9 months of age.

1. Assess nutritional status of the child and plot measurement on growth chart.
2. Calculate socio-ecomomic class using appropriate scale.
3. Discuss the physical environment that could have impacted the health of the case.
4. What medical management will you advise for this case as per IMNCI guidelines.
5. Discuss immunisation for this child.
6. Discuss family level interventions for health improvement.

Seema, 19-year-old lady, is 5 months into her pregnancy, presented in the antenatal OPD with complaints of fatigue, breathlessness during exertion. She had conceived once earlier 10 months ago but had a spontaneous abortion. She conceived spontaneously 3 months after the abortion. Since conception, she has had two antenatal visits to a private doctor and was advised IFA tablets after her Hb level was found to be 10 gm/dl but she has not been able to take them due to nausea. On examination, she weighed 40 kg and was 140 cm tall. She has moderate pallor and per abdomen examination was normal. Her diet consists of six chapattis, three katori dal, two katori sabzi and a glass of milk as assessed by 24-hour recall method. She resides in a two-room pucca house, with separate kitchen and toilet, in Tilak Nagar area, with her husband who is 12th pass, works as salesman and earns Rs 15000 per month. The outside of the house in unclean, with open drains and garbage dumps nearby. The husband's company provides ESI benefits. She has one household help for washing and cleaning. She is not aware of any health services nearby for emergencies.

1. Calculate and comment on diet and nutritional status of the case (Calorie and protein intake, BMI).
2. What dietary advise will you give for this case?
3. Discuss further medical management of the case in terms of anemia, antenatal check-up and planning for delivery.
4. Discuss contraception advise for the case post delivery.
5. Comment on physical environment and risks associated.

Hari Kishan Singh, a 62-year-old male came for routine check-up six months after he was started on Tablet Metformin 500 mg BD for diabetes. He weighs 85 kg and is 165 cm tall. He complains of frequent episodes of dizziness and also fainted twice in last 15 days after which his blood sugar was found to be low. He is a chronic smoker and smokes one packet bidi per day. He consumes alcohol thrice a week – around four beer / two large pegs on an average each time. He is a supervisor in a private packaging firm and spends most of the time sitting in the office. He has started going for evening walk occasionally for last one month. He eats three meals in a day and consumes 2700 kcal and 70 g protein per day as calculated by dietary assessment. He does not consume sweets or sugary foods since his diagnosis. He is complaint with his medication. He earns Rs 35000/- per month and resides in a two BHK house, with adequate lighting and ventilation, with his wife. His two sons are married and live in another city.

1. Comment on socio-economic status of the family using appropriate scale.
2. Calculate BMI and comment.
3. Comment on diet and Discuss dietary management of the case.
4. What other lifestyle interventions are required for this case.
5. Discuss screening tests recommended for this case.

Sapna, sixteen-year-old girl, came to the OPD with her mother with complaints of dysmenorrhea and menorrhagia for last three months. She also complains of breathlessness and easy fatiguablity for the last two months. She weighs 38 kg and her height is 150 cm. On examination, moderate pallor seen in palpebral conjunctiva and tongue. No other significant clinical finding. She takes

a diet of four chapattis, one katori dal, one katori sabzi, 3 cups tea and two bread slices per day. Milk and fruit intake only occasionally – 1-2 times per week. Menarche was at 13 years and she uses cloth during her periods. She is a school dropout after class 5 as she had to take care of three younger siblings and does household chores when her parents go for work. The family lives in a one room house with no separate kitchen. The toilet used is a public facility shared by around 12-15 families in the community. Surroundings have open drains, stagnant water in ditches and garbage dump around 200 m away from the house. Waste is thrown outside in the street daily. Mother knows about anganwadi but does not let the children go there alone as she is apprehensive for their safety. Father is daily wage labourer and mother works as a maid. Total family income is Rs 8000/- per month and family has a BPL card.

1. Comment on type of family and socio-economic status.
2. Comment on nutritional status based on anthropometry and diet.
3. Discuss social factors related to clinical profile of the case.
4. Discuss specific programme interventions related to menstrual hygiene and prevention of RTI/STI.
5. Comment on physical environment and mention associated risk factor.

Anjana, 26-year-old lady, who had home delivered a baby boy one weeks ago, was visited by an ASHA worker post delivery during home-visit. The delivery was conducted by a trained dai at home. No history of fever, pain abdomen or in the legs, excessive per vaginal bleeding. Mother and baby were confined to a separate room since the delivery as they believe 13 days are unclean after child-birth. Breast feeding was started 4 hours after delivery after the ritual of giving pre-lacteal feed of honey was done. She is able to breast feed the baby and on-demand feeding is being done with some amount of clean boiled water being given 2-3 times to the baby. Mother is being given a semi-solid diet consisting of 2 cup khichdi with one spoon ghee thrice a day and two glasses of milk everyday. Antenatal period was uneventful. She had received four antenatal check-ups and took IFA tablets given at the health centre. She has two older daughters, 3 and 2 years old respectively, and were also delivered at home. On examination, she had moderate pallor. She stays in a two room house with her husband, mother and father-in-law and two daughters. Husband is 12th pass, works as a helper in a transport company and travels frequently. Family income is Rs 20,000/- per month.

1. Discuss type and socio-economic class of the family.
2. What contraceptive advice will you give to this lady?
3. Comment on socio-cultural practices related to child feeding and advise to be given.
4. Calculate and comment on adequacy of dietary intake.
5. What are supportive programme services available for improvement of nutritional status in this case?

Volume 2

Practical Manual & Logbook in Community Medicine

(Based on Latest CBME)

(Includes Family Adoption Programme)

Revised and Updated

Authors

Dr. Priya Arora
Professor, Community Medicine
Army College of Medical Sciences
New Delhi

Dr. Pooja Goyal
Professor & Head, Community Medicine
ESIC Medical College and Hospital
Faridabad, Haryana

Dr. Shveta Lukhmana
Associate Professor, Community Medicine
VMMC and Safdarjung Hospital
New Delhi

Dr. Abhishek Singh
Associate Professor, Community Medicine
SHKM Government Medical College
Mewat, Haryana

Foreword By

- **Col. (Dr) Puja Dudeja**
- **Dr. Abhishek V. Raut**
- **Dr. Prasanna Mithra P.**
- **Dr. Avijit Roy**

Peepee Publishers and Distributors Private Limited®

Practical Manual & Logbook in Community Medicine (Based on Latest CBME)

Published by
Pawaninder P. Vij and Anupam Vij

Peepee Publishers and Distributors (P) Ltd.
Head Office: 160, Shakti Vihar, Pitam Pura, Delhi-110 034 (India)

Correspondence Address:

7/31, First Floor, Ansari Road, Daryaganj
New Delhi-110 002 (India)

Ph: 41512412, 9811156083

e-mail: peepee160@yahoo.co.in

e-mail: peepee160@gmail.com

www.peepeepub.com

join us on facebook.com/pp.publishers

LM-03

First Edition: 2022

Revised and Updated: 2025

ISBN: 978-81-9651-878-3

Contents

Volume 2

Section IV: Epidemiology and Biostatistics

Section V: Visits to Institutions of Public Health Importance

Section VI: Spots

Section IV

Epidemiology and Biostatistics

Section IV: Epidemiology and Biostatistics

	Topic	Competency	Signature of Supervisor with Date	Grade
A. APPLIED EPIDEMIOLOGY AND BIOSTATISTICS				
1.	Epidemiology: Historical Perspective	CM 7.1 Define Epidemiology and describe and enumerate the principles, concepts and uses		
2. A.	Indicators: Measuring Mortality and Morbidity	CM 1.7 Enumerate and describe health indicators CM 7.4 Define, calculate and interpret morbidity and mortality indicators based on given set of data		
B.	Maternal and Child Health	OG 1.1 Define and discuss birth rate, maternal mortality and morbidity OG 1.2 Define and discuss perinatal mortality and morbidity including perinatal and neonatal mortality and morbidity audit		
3.	Measurement of Risk	CM 7.5 Enumerate, define, describe and discuss epidemiological study designs		
4.	Association and Causation	CM 7.8 Describe the principles of association, causation and biases in epidemiological studies CM 6.3 Describe, discuss and demonstrate the application of elementary statistical methods including test of significance in various study designs		
5.	Screening: Concept, Criteria and Uses	CM 7.6 Enumerate and evaluate the need of screening tests		
6.	Epidemic Investigation	CM 7.7 Describe and demonstrate the steps in the Investigation of an epidemic of communicable disease and describe the principles of control measures CM 8.4 Describe the principles and enumerate the measures to control a disease epidemic CM 20.2 Describe various issues during outbreaks and their prevention		

7.	Presentation of data	CM 6.2 Describe and discuss the principles and demonstrate the methods of collection, classification, analysis, interpretation and presentation of statistical data		
8.	Measures of Central Tendency and Dispersion	CM 6.4 Enumerate, discuss and demonstrate common sampling techniques, simple statistical methods, frequency distribution, measures of central tendency and dispersion		
9.	A. Sampling: Methods and Application B. Standard Error	CM 6.4 Enumerate, discuss and demonstrate common sampling techniques, simple statistical methods, frequency distribution, measures of central tendency and dispersion		
10.	Public Health Planning: Logistic Management	CM 8.5 Describe and discuss the principles of planning, implementing and evaluating control measures for disease at community level bearing in mind the public health importance of the disease CM 16.1 Define and describe the concept of health planning		
	Annexures			
		B. RESEARCH METHODOLOGY		
11.	Introduction to research methodology and Report Writing	CM 6.1 Formulate a research question for a study		
12.	Conducting a research study (project)	CM 6.2 Describe and discuss the principles and demonstrate the methods of collection, classification, analysis, interpretation and presentation of statistical data CM 6.3 Describe, discuss and demonstrate the application of elementary statistical methods including test of significance in various study designs		
	Hints and Answers to Exercises			

A. Applied Epidemiology and Biostatistics

Chapter 1

Epidemiology: Historical Perspective

Date:____________

Specific learning objectives: At the end of the session, Phase III (Part-1) student will be able to:

1. Discuss historical perspective of epidemiology.
2. Define epidemiology.

Epidemiology:

Epidemiology has been defined by John M Last in 1988 as "The study of the distribution and determinants of health-related states or events in specified populations and the application of this study to the control of health problems".

Epidemiology is the study of how disease is distributed in populations and the factors that influence or determine this distribution.

Epidemiological Approach

1. Asking Questions
2. Making Comparisons

Let us learn how epidemiologic observations have led to effective prevention of diseases in human populations.

Sir John Snow (1813-1858) and Cholera:

One of the most prominent communicable diseases in 18th Century was cholera. It was thought that cholera was transmitted by a miasma, or cloud, that clung low on the surface of the earth.

During 1848-49 epidemic, Snow began examining the victims and found that their initial symptoms were always related to the gastrointestinal tract. Snow reasoned that, if cholera was spread by bad air, it should cause pulmonary symptoms, but since the symptoms were gastrointestinal, perhaps it was transmitted by water or food consumption. He also went house-to-house to map the location of cases of cholera. This kind of map is now known as a spot map and is commonly used for investigation of epidemics.

Distribution of Cholera Cases in the Golden Square Area of London, August-September, 1848

In 1850's London residents obtained water in their homes by signing up with one of the many water supply companies supplying home water. The water intakes for the water supply companies were from a much-polluted part of the Thames River. Sometime between 1849 and 1854, one of the companies, the Lambeth Company, moved its source to a comparatively upstream point of the Thames where the water was relatively free from the sewage of London.

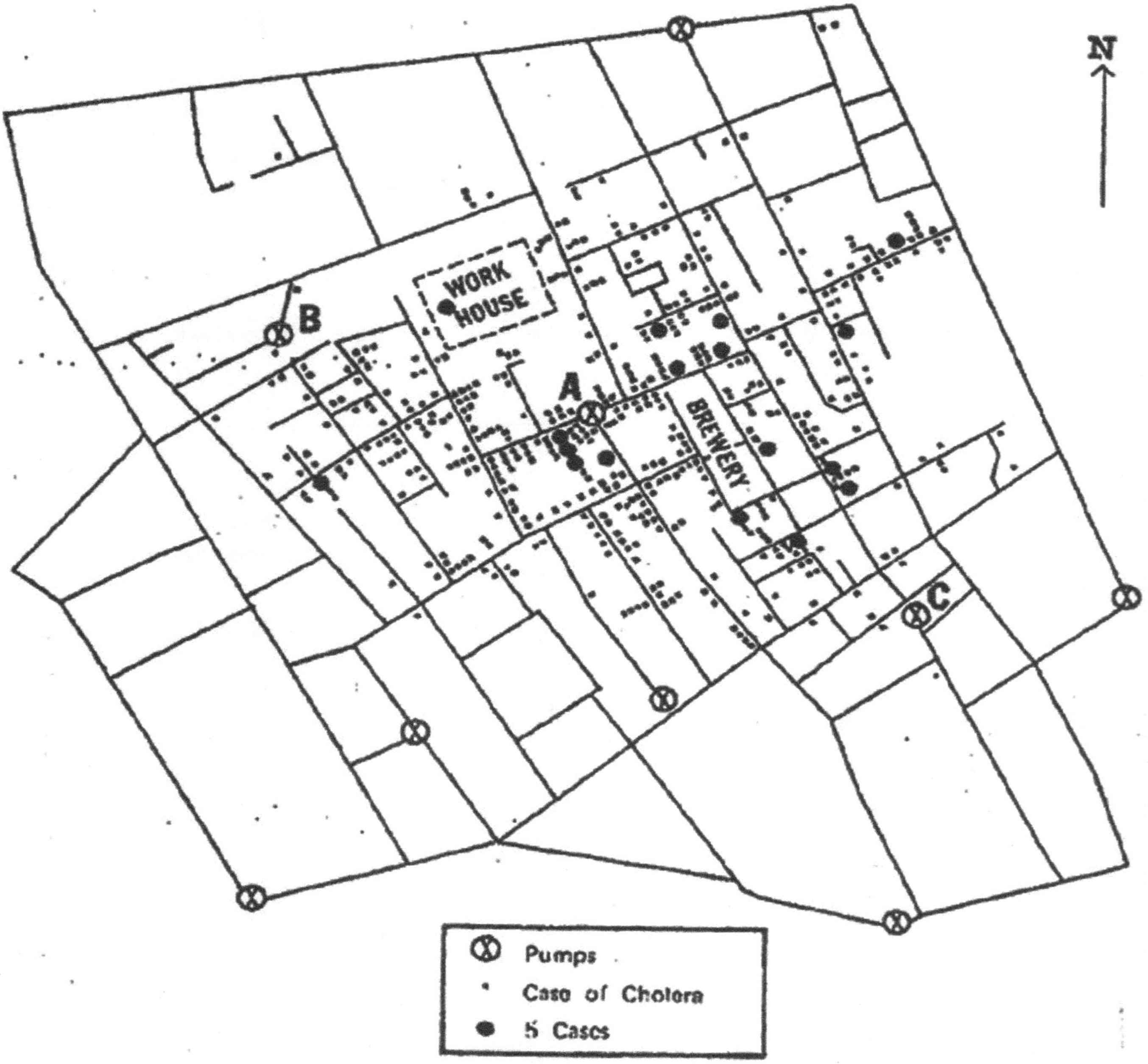

Again in 1854, when another epidemic of cholera occurred among residents of London, Snow investigated the death in the area and observed that water was supplied by two companies in an interpenetrating manner in the area. The house son the same street received water from one or the other company. A casual look into the deaths in the area provided him no clue. Then he found more about the total number of houses supplied by each company, calculated death rates per 10,000 population, for first seven weeks during the a work house in that area had its own private well, and there were only 5 deaths among its 535 inmates, also a brewery on Broad Street like wise never used the water from the Broad Street Pump, Its workers drank beer and it had no cases among its 70 workers. He put his observations as follows:

John Snow's observations of 1854:

Water supply source	Population Covered	Deaths Reported	Deaths per 10,000 population
Southwark and Vauxhall	40,046	1263	315
Lambeth Company	26,107	98	37
Rest of London	2,56,423	1422	56

Data adapted from Snow J: On the mode of communication of cholera. In Snow on Cholera: A Reprint of Two Papers by John Snow, M.D. New York, The Commonwealth Fund, 1936.

He failed to convince the authorities of his observation that water was the source. It was discovered later that broad street public well had been dug only three feet from an old cesspit that had begun to leak fecal bacteria. A baby who had contracted cholera from another source had its nappies (diapers) washed into this cesspit.

He removed the handle of broad Street pump, making it non usable, where incidence of cholera was highest. Subsequently the number of new cases decreased in the region impressively.

EXERCISE 1.1

(a) Based on the above mentioned case study, describe the distribution of cases of cholera in terms of time, place and person.

(b) How did his observations help in control of new cases?

STUDENT'S NOTES

STUDENT'S NOTES

STUDENT'S NOTES

Supervisor's Signature

CHAPTER 2

A. Indicators: Measuring Mortality and Morbidity

Date:____________

Specific learning objectives: At the end of the session, Phase III (Part-1) student will be able to:

1. Define various events of disease measurement -Birth, Sickness, Disability and Death.
2. Explain the difference between numerator and denominator, and their importance in population measurements.
3. Define, distinguish, calculate and interpret ratios, proportions and rates used in epidemiology.
4. Quantify and measure severity of disease in population, by appropriate indices.

Morbidity: It has been defined as "any departure, subjective or objective from a state of physiological or psychological well-being". It usually refers to people who are ill or the period/duration / spells of illnesses experienced by them.

Since epidemiological measurements purport to measure the distribution and determinants of disease, quantification of the health events / disease is a prerequisite for this.

The fundamental epidemiologic measure is the frequency with which events of interest, usually disease or death, occur in the population. Frequency is a simple count of affected individuals that is essential for determining the allocation of health care resources in a particular community. Frequency can be measured in different ways and it can be related to different denominators, depending upon the purpose of the research and the availability of data.

There are three tools for epidemiology to measure the disease frequency.

These are:

(a) Rate

(b) Ratio

(c) Proportion

RATE: It measures the occurrence of some particular event (development of disease or occurrence of death) in population during a given time-period. It indicates the change in an event that takes place in a population over a period of time. It is generally expressed as per thousand of population; but any suitable multiplier may be used. Rates tell us how fast a disease is occurring in a population.

$$\text{e.g., Crude death rate} = \frac{\text{Number of deaths (defined place and time period)}}{\text{Mid-year population (defined place and time period)}} \times 1000$$

RATIO: It expresses a relation in size between two random quantities. The numerator is not a component of the denominator. Ratio is the result of dividing one quantity by another. It is expressed as X: y or X/y.

For example:

1. A city of 3,000,000 persons has 375 doctors. Calculate the ratio of doctors per person.

   $375/3,000,000 \times 10^n = 0.000125$ doctors per person

   To make it easier to understand, you can use $10^n = 10^4 = 10,000$. Then the ratio becomes:

   $0.000125 \times 10,000 = 1.25$ doctors per 10,000 persons

   You could also divide each value by 1.25, and express this ratio as 1 doctor for every 8,000 persons.

2. The sex ratio of CHD patients (Male: Female) is 80:20 or 4:1. For every female CHD patient, there are 4 male CHD patients.

   The ratio also indicates another very important measure-the "odds". Here, given that CHD has occurred, the "odds" of being a male in such a disease are 4 times as compared to being a female.

   PROPORTION: It is type of ratio in which the numerator is included in the denominator. It may be expressed as a percentage. Proportions tell us what fraction of the population is affected.

   The Proportion indicates an important measure in research methodology - The Probability.

For example:

No of wasted under-five children at a certain time = 50

Total no of children at the same time = 100

$$\text{Prevalence} = \frac{50}{100} \times 100 = 50\%$$

Hence, we can draw a conclusion that the probability (or chance) that no. of children that would suffer from wasting is 0.5 or 50%.

Disease frequency: To measure frequency of disease, we commonly use-

(i) Incidence

(ii) Prevalence

INCIDENCE: This rate provides the number of new cases of a disease developed in the POPULATION AT RISK during a specified time interval. Incidence is a measure of events—the disease is identified in a person who develops the disease during a specified period and did not have the disease previously. Because the incidence is a measure of events (i.e., from being non-diseased to being diseased), incidence is a measure of risk.

$$\text{Incidence} = \frac{\text{Number of new cases of a particular disease in a specified time period}}{\text{Total population at risk during that period}} \times 1000$$

It has two sub-categories:

(A) **CUMULATIVE INCIDENCE:** (Syn. Incidence Proportion, attack rate, risk)

Number of new cases of a disease during a given period of time divided by total population at risk. It provides an estimate of the probability or risk that an individual will develop a disease during a specified period of time. It assumes that the entire "population at risk" at the beginning of the study period has been followed up for a specified interval of time for the development of the outcome under investigation. Hence the definition of CI is exactly the same as used to define incidence. CI is a proportion because the persons in the numerator, those who develop disease during the specified period, are included in the denominator (the entire population).

$$CI = \frac{\text{Number of people who develop the outcome / disease during the specific time period of follow up}}{\text{Total no. of people who were at risk of developing the outcome / disease at the start of the follow up}} \times 10^n$$

EXAMPLE

In a study of patients with Cancer, 50 of the 179 patients of cancer died during the 10-year follow- up period. Calculate the risk of death for these patients.

Numerator = 50 deaths among Cancer patients

Denominator = 179 patients of Cancer, $10^n = 10^2 = 100$

Risk = (50/179) × 100 = 27.9%

(B) **INCIDENCE DENSITY** (Syn Incidence Rate): During the course of disease measurement, some participants may not be followed up for the entire duration of observation because of death from any other cause or simply loss to follow up. An alternative and more valid method would be to include all individuals irrespective of time at which they entered and were lost to follow-up, considering them for only the period for which information was obtained about them. This is INCIDENCE DENSITY.

$$\text{Incidence Density} = \frac{\text{Number of New-cases of disease during a given period of time}}{\text{Total person-time of observation}} \times 1000$$

The denominator consists of the sum of the units of time that each individual was at risk and was observed. This is called person-time and is often expressed in terms of person-months or person years of exposure.

EXAMPLES*

1. The diabetes follow-up study included 218 diabetic women and 3,823 nondiabetic women. By the end of the study, 72 of the diabetic women and 511 of the nondiabetic women had died. The diabetic women were observed for a total of 1,862 person years; the nondiabetic women were observed for a total of 36,653 person years. Calculate the incidence rates of death for the diabetic and non-diabetic women.

   For diabetic women, numerator = 72 and denominator = 1,862

   Person-time rate = 72/1,862

   = 0.0386 deaths per person-year

   = 38.6 deaths per 1,000 person-years

For nondiabetic women, numerator = 511 and denominator = 36,653

Person-time rate = 511/36,653 = 0.0139 deaths per person-year

= 13.9 deaths per 1,000 person-years

2. In 2003, 44,232 new cases of acquired immunodeficiency syndrome (AIDS) were reported in the United States. The estimated mid-year population of the U.S. in 2003 was approximately 290,809,777. Calculate the incidence rate of AIDS expressed as per 100,000 population for the year 2003.

Numerator = 44,232 new cases of AIDS

Denominator = 290,809,777 estimated mid-year population

Incidence rate = (44,232/290,809,777) × 100,000

= 15.21 new cases of AIDS per 100,000 population

*** Source: https://www.cdc.gov/csels/dsepd/ss1978/lesson3/section2.html**

PREVALENCE: It is the total number of individuals who have an attribute or disease at a particular time (or during a particular period) divided by the population at risk of having the attribute, or disease at this point in time or midway through the period, i.e., what proportion of the population is affected by the disease at/ during that time.

$$\text{Prevalence Rate} = \frac{\text{No. of existing cases of disease (both old and new) at a specific time}}{\text{Total population}} \times 100$$

PREVALENCE HAS TWO SUB-CATEGORIES

POINT PREVALENCE: Prevalence of a disease at any particular point of time. It is the proportion of persons with a particular disease or attribute on a particular date or at a particular time.

$$\text{Point Prevalence} = \frac{\text{No. of new and old cases at a given point of time}}{\text{Total population at a given point of time}} \times 100$$

EXAMPLE

There are 100 children in a class, while screening for dental caries at a particular point of time it was found that 10 of them have dental caries.

Point Prevalence = 10/100 ×100

= 10%

10 percent of the children of class have dental caries or the point prevalence of dental caries in this particular class is 10 percent.

PERIOD PREVALENCE: Prevalence measured over a particular interval of time. It is the proportion of persons with a particular disease or attribute at any time during the interval. This is especially useful for short term ailments like acute diarrhea / respiratory infections.

$$\text{Period Prevalence} = \frac{\text{No. of new and old cases in a specified time period}}{\text{Total population for the same time period}} \times 100$$

EXAMPLE

In a study included 150 participants and followed for a period of 1 year, following sequence of events happen – at the beginning, 30 had disease of interest and another 10 new cases developed during the year.

Period Prevalence = 30+10/150 * 100

= 0.26 * 100

= 26%

RELATIONSHIP BETWEEN INCIDENCE AND PREVALENCE P = I × D

Where P = Prevalence

I = Incidence

Other commonly used measures of disease frequency are:

- Attack Rate
- Secondary Attack Rate
- Proportional Morbidity Rate
- Morbidity Ratio

EXERCISE 2.1

Define various measures of disease frequency.

EXERCISE 2.2

For each of the fractions shown below, indicate whether it is a ratio, a proportion, a rate, or none of the three.

1. $\frac{\text{Number of men in State A who died from CHD in 2020}}{\text{Number of men in State A who died in 2020}}$

2. $\frac{\text{Number of men in State A who died from CHD in 2020}}{\text{Estimated number of men living in State A on July 1, 2020}}$

3. $\frac{\text{Number of men in State A who died from CHD in 2020}}{\text{Number of men in State A who died from cancer in 2020}}$

4. $\frac{\text{Number of women in State A who died from Breast Cancer in 2020}}{\text{Number of women in State A who died from cancer (all types) in 2020}}$

5. $\frac{\text{Number of men in State A who died from lung cancer in 2020}}{\text{Estimated revenue (in Rupees) in State A from cigarette sales in 2020}}$

EXERCISE 2.3

(a) During a six - hour work shift at a paint factory, 20 employees visited the factory medical officer with complaints of nausea, vomiting, headaches and dizziness. If 800 persons worked in the factory, what is the attack rate of the disease?

(b) In 2020, 10,266,674 new cases of COVID-19 were reported in India. The estimated mid-year population of India in 2020 was approximately 1,380,004,385. Calculate the incidence rate of COVID-19 in India in 2020.

EXERCISE 2.4

For a given year, the prevalence of disease X in a certain geographic area is 0.004 (400 per 100,000) and the incidence is 0.0008 (80 per 100,000). What is the average duration (in years) of this disease?

EXERCISE 2.5

There was an outbreak of Hepatitis A in a locality. Secondary cases within 30 days of onset were also reported. The findings of a community survey for the cases and sanitation facilities are summarized in the following table.

	HOUSEHOLDS WITHOUT ACCESS TO SANITARY LATRINE			HOUSEHOLDS WITH SANITARY LATRINE		
Age (in years)	**No. of contacts Exposed to Primary cases**	**No.of Secondary cases**	**Attack Rate**	**No. of contacts exposed to primary cases**	**No. of Secondary cases**	**Attack Rate**
0-4	143	42		123	7	
5-14	206	27		216	9	
15+	321	37		381	12	
Total	670	106		720	28	

Q. 2.5.1 Calculate the secondary attack rate in each category.

Q. 2.5.2 What inference do you draw from this result?

EXERCISE 2.6

4 individuals in a household of 15 developed Measles within two weeks after one member came from a trip outside town with measles rashes. 2 other members had already had Measles during childhood.

Q. 2.6.1 Define Primary and Secondary Case. Identify the same in the given example.

Q. 2.6.2 Calculate Secondary Attack Rate.

EXERCISE 2.7

Given table illustrates the occurrence of Hepatitis B in a group of persons with high-risk behavior. 15 Injectable drug users were tested prior to the onset of study and five who tested positive were excluded from the study. Rest 10 were followed up for a period of six years starting in January 2014. All were tested in the month of January every year. The table below summarizes the findings these ten subjects. A bracketed plus sign (+) indicates when a subject was found to be positive for Hepatitis B; a question mark (?) indicates when a subject became lost to follow-up. The dashed lines indicate continued follow-up.

Subject	**Follow up**						
	2014	**2015**	**2016**	**2017**	**2018**	**2019**	**Disease free duration (yrs.)**
1	----------	(+)					1
2	----------	?					1
3	---------	----------	(+)				2
4	---------	?					1
5	---------	----------	----------	?			3
6	---------	---------	---------	----------	?		4
7	---------	---------	---------	---------	---------	---------	6
8	----------	---------	---------	---------	---------	?	5
9	---------	(+)					1
10	---------	(+)					1

Q. 2.7.1 Calculate the incidence density of Hepatitis B in the group.

EXERCISE 2.8

An epidemiological study was conducted in which a cohort of 20 persons was studied to record the occurrence of disease X. Fig 2 represents 10 new cases of the disease X over the observation period in a population of 20 persons. Rest of the persons remained free from disease throughout the follow-up period. Each horizontal line represents one person. The circle indicates the date of onset of illness. The solid line represents the duration of illness. Marked circle represents death and cross represents recovery.

Q. 2.8.1 Calculate the period prevalence of the disease X in the cohort during 2020.

Q. 2.8.2 Calculate cumulative incidence of the disease X in the population for the year 2020.

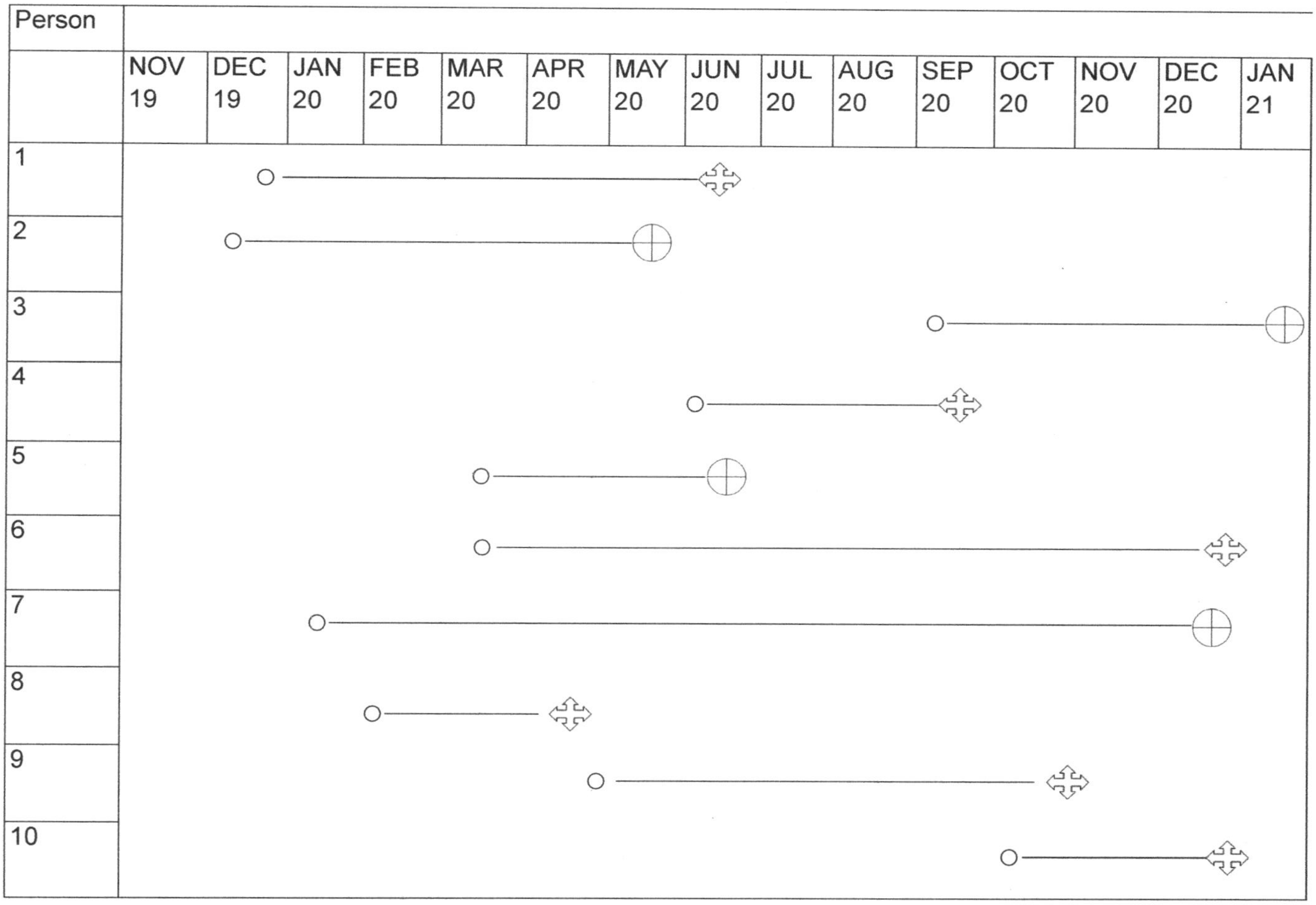

EXERCISE 2.9

In a medical college hostel, there were 392 students residing in six different blocks. A total of 20 students developed COVID 19. All cases occurred in Block I and II which had a common dining hall. During the course of investigation, it was found that 186 students were residing in Block I and II.

On Thursday evening, Mr. A, who had come back on Monday after visiting his local guardian, complained of sore throat, fever and loss of taste. His nasopharyngeal swab was sent for testing and he was told to stay in his room till the results of the test were available. Mr. A had come in contact with 27 persons during this time. Mr. B, Mr. C and Mr. D, complained of pain in the throat and fever on following Sunday afternoon and were tested and diagnosed as COVID-19. All students who had come in contact with these positive cases were told to stay in their rooms and report in case of any symptoms. The contacts were tested on 7th day of exposure to positive cases. Rest of the cases occurred after 14 days of onset of illness in Mr. A.

Q. 2.9.1. What do you understand by (a) Quarantine (b) Isolation (c) Contact Tracing?

Q. 2.9.2. What is a primary case? Identify the primary case in this.

Q. 2.9.3. Identify secondary cases.

MEASURES OF MORTALITY

Mortality rate is a measure of the frequency of deaths in a defined population over a certain period of time. The denominator used to calculate overall mortality is the average number of the population over a period of time or the mid-year population.

Various types of mortality rates and defined for various purposes. There are three types of mortality rates:-

- Crude Rates
- Specific Rates
- Standardized Rates.

CRUDE DEATH RATE is defined as the number of deaths (from all causes) per 1000 estimated mid- year population in one year in a given place. Thus, crude death rate is an estimate of the portion of a population that dies due to any cause during a specified period.

$$\text{Crude Death Rate} = \frac{\text{Number of deaths during the year}}{\text{Mid-year Population}} \times 1000$$

This does not take into consideration factors such as age, sex, cause etc.

SPECIFIC RATES: They are used to refine the crude death rate. They use a subset of the population with specific characteristics as denominator. Some of them are:

1. **Age specific death rate: e.g.**

$$\text{Specific death rate in age group 15-20 years} = \frac{\text{Number of deaths of persons aged 15-20 during a calendar year}}{\text{Mid-year population of persons aged 15-20}} \times 1000$$

2. **Cause or disease specific death rate:** e.g.

$$\text{Specific death rate due to Tuberculosis} = \frac{\text{Number of deaths from tuberculosis during a calendar year}}{\text{Mid-year population}} \times 1000$$

3. **Case fatality rate:** Determines what percentage of people who have a certain disease die within a certain time after their disease was diagnosed. It is a measure of killing- power of the disease. The case-fatality rate is a proportion, not a true rate. As a result, some epidemiologists prefer the term case-fatality ratio.

$$\text{Case Fatality Rate} = \frac{\text{Total number of deaths due to a particular disease during a specified time period}}{\text{Total number of cases due to the same disease}} \times 100$$

4. **Proportional mortality rate:** It expresses the number of deaths due to a particular cause (or in a specific age group) out of all deaths. Thus we have:

(a) Proportional mortality from a specific disease- This indicates the degree to which that specific cause of death contributes to total mortality. e.g.

$$\text{Proportional mortality for Tuberculosis} = \frac{\text{Deaths due to TB in a population in a given year}}{\text{Total deaths in the same population in the same year}} \times 100$$

(b) Age specific proportional mortality
e.g Under 5 proportional mortality rate

$$= \frac{\text{No. of deaths under 5 years of age in the given year}}{\text{Total no. of deaths of all age groups in that year}} \times 100$$

5. **Survival rate:** It is the proportion of survivors in a group of patients studied and followed over a period. It is a method of describing prognosis in certain disease conditions. The survival period is usually recorded from the date of diagnosis or start of the treatment.

$$\text{Survival rate} = \frac{\text{Total number of patients alive after 5 years}}{\text{Total number of patients diagnosed or treated}} \times 100$$

EXERCISE 2.10

In 2020, 600 cases and 90 deaths due to Hepatitis A occurred in town X with a population of 99,000. Prior to 2020, the town had never reported any case of Hepatitis A. The details of cases and deaths are as follows:

AGE (YEARS)	POPULATION	CASES	DEATHS
0-14	18,000	175	10
15-44	42,000	225	50
45+	39,000	200	30
	99,000	600	90

1. Calculate crude deaths rate for Hepatitis A in town X ?
2. Assuming that there was no case of the disease in town X prior to 1998, what was the incidence of Hepatitis A?
3. What is the age specific death rate and case fatality rate for residents in the three age-groups
4. What is the case fatality rate for Hepatitis A in town?

EXERCISE 2.11

For disease X, which causes death in most patients within a short duration after diagnosis, which of the following will be true:

(a) Incidence rates and mortality rates will be similar
(b) Mortality rates will be higher than incidence rates
(c) Incidence rates will be higher than mortality rates
(d) Incidence rates will not be related to mortality rates

EXERCISE 2.12

When mortality rate is a good reflection of the incidence rate?

(a) Low case fatality, long duration
(b) High case fatality, long duration
(c) High case fatality, short duration
(d) Low case fatality, short duration

EXERCISE 2.13

What is the effect on prevalence of a disease due to the following?

(a) Increase in incidence

(b) Decrease in mortality

EXERCISE 2.14

In calculation of incidence rate of a disease, which of the following is taken as denominator?

(a) Number of persons exposed to disease

(b) Total Population of the area

(c) Person-time

STANDARDISED RATES

Mortality rates can be used to compare the rates in one area with the rates in another area, or to compare rates over time. But these Rates are comparable only if the populations upon which they are based are comparable. To eliminate the distortion caused by different underlying age distributions in different populations, statistical techniques are used to adjust or standardize the rates among the populations to be compared.

Age adjustment or age standardisation removes the confounding effect of different age structures and yields a single standardised or adjusted rate be which the mortality experience can be compared directly. The adjustment can be made for age, sex, race, parity etc.

Standardisation can be carried out by two methods:

- Direct standardization
- Indirect standardization

Direct Method:

$$\text{Standardised death rate} = \frac{\text{Expected no. of total deaths}}{\text{Total standard population}} \times 1000$$

Indirect Method:

Standardised death Rate = Crude death rate × Index death rate

$$\text{Where, index death rate} = \frac{\text{Observed deaths}}{\text{Expected deaths}}$$

The direct method is feasible only if the actual specific rates in the subgroups of the observed population are available.

STANDARDISED MORTALITY RATIO (SMR)

It is a ratio of total number of deaths that occur in the study group to the number of deaths that would have been expected to occur if that study group had experienced the death rates of a standard population (or other reference population)

$$\text{SMR} = \frac{\text{Observed deaths}}{\text{Expected deaths}} \times 100$$

STUDENT'S NOTES

STUDENT'S NOTES

STUDENT'S NOTES

STUDENT'S NOTES

STUDENT'S NOTES

STUDENT'S NOTES

STUDENT'S NOTES

STUDENT'S NOTES

Supervisor's Signature

B. Indicators: Maternal and Child Health

Date:__________

Specific learning objectives: At the end of the session, Phase III (Part-1) student will be able to:

1. Define the indicators of maternal and child health.
2. Calculate and interpret various MCH indicators.
3. Learn about causes of maternal and child mortality.

The various indicators of MCH are:

1. **Maternal Mortality Ratio (MMR) =**

Maternal Death- The death of a woman while pregnant or within 42 days of termination of pregnancy irrespective of the duration and site of pregnancy, from any cause related to or aggravated by the pregnancy or its management but not from accidental or incidental causes.

$$\text{MMR} = \frac{\text{Total no. of female deaths due to complications of pregnancy, child birth or within 42 days of delivery from Puerperal Causes in an area during a given year}}{\text{Total no of live births in the same area and same year}} \times 1000$$

Late Maternal Death - Death of a woman from direct or indirect obstetric causes more than 42 days but less than one year after termination of pregnancy.

Other statistical measures of maternal mortality

- Maternal mortality rate – Number of maternal deaths in a given period per 100,000 women of reproductive age-group
- Adult lifetime risk of maternal death – the probability of dying due to a maternal cause during a woman's reproductive life-span
- Proportion of maternal deaths of women of reproductive age – the number of maternal deaths in a given time period divided by the total number of deaths, among women aged 15-49 years

2. **Still Birth Rate**

$$\text{SBR} = \frac{\text{Fetal death weighing over 1000 g at birth during the year}}{\text{Total (live + still) births weighing over 1000 g at birth during the year}} \times 1000$$

3. **Perinatal Mortality Rate***

$$= \frac{\text{Late fetal deaths (Weighing} \geq 1000\text{ g) + Early neonatal deaths (First week) in one year}}{\text{Live births in the same year (weighing 1000 g or more)}} \times 1000$$

* If birth weight not available – use gestational age of 28 weeks

When both not available, use crown-heel length of 35 cm

4. **Neonatal Mortality Rate**

$$\text{NMR} = \frac{\text{Number of deaths of children under 28 days of age in a year}}{\text{Total live births in the same year}} \times 1000$$

5. **Post Neonatal Mortality Rate**

$$\text{PNMR} = \frac{\text{No. of deaths of children between 28 days and one year of age in a given year}}{\text{Total live births in the same year}} \times 1000$$

6. **Infant Mortality Rate**

$$\text{IMR} = \frac{\text{No. of deaths of children less than 1 year of age in a year}}{\text{No. of live births in the same year}} \times 1000$$

7. **1-4 Year Mortality Rate** =

$$\frac{\text{No. of deaths of children aged 1-4 years in a year}}{\text{Total no. of children aged 1-4 years at the middle of the year}} \times 1000$$

8. **Under 5 Mortality Rate:** The probability of a newborn dying before completion of five years of age. It is calculated by the life table approach.

9. **Child Survival Rate**

$$\frac{\text{1000-Under 5 mortality rate}}{10}$$

10. **Crude Birth Rate** = $\frac{\text{No. of live births during the year}}{\text{Estimated mid-year population}} \times 1000$

11. **General Fertility Rate** = $\frac{\text{No. of live births in an area during the year}}{\text{Mid-year female population aged 15-44 years in the same area and year}} \times 1000$

12. **General marital fertility rate (GMFR):** It is the number of live births per 1000 married women in the reproductive age group (15-44 years) in a given year.

13. **Age Specific Fertility Rate:** It is the number of live births in a year to 1000 women in any specified age group. The age-specific fertility rates throw light on the fertility pattern. They are also sensitive indicators of family planning achievement.

$$\text{AFSR} = \frac{\text{Number of live births in a particular age group}}{\text{Mid-year female population of the same age-group}} \times 1000$$

14. **Age-specific Marital Fertility Rate (ASMFR):** It is the number of live births in a year to 1000 married women in any specified age group.

15. **Total Fertility Rate:** It is the average no of children a woman would have it she were to pass through her reproductive years bearing children at the same rate as the woman now in each age group. It is computed by summing the age-specific fertility rates for all ages. This measure gives the approximate magnitude of "completed family size".

16. **Total Marital Fertility Rate: Average no of children that would be born to a married woman if** she experiences the current fertility pattern throughout her reproductive span.

17. **Gross Reproduction Rate:** Average number of girls that would be born to a woman if she experiences the current fertility pattern throughout her reproductive span (15-44 or 49) assuming no mortality.

18. **Net Reproduction Rate:** It is defined as the number of daughters a new born girl will bear during her lifetime assuming fixed age specific fertility and mortality rates. NRR is a demographic indicator. NRR of 1 is equivalent to attaining approximately the 2-child norm.

19. **Pregnancy Rate:** It is the ratio of number of pregnancies in a year to married women in the ages 15-44 or 49 years.

20. **Abortion Rate:** The number of all types of abortions; expressed as per 1000 women of childbearing age.

EXAMPLE

Given that in a town in a year

Total number of live births – 19635, No. of Infant deaths – 1130, No. of deaths within first week –603, Infant deaths during first 28 days – 875, foetal deaths weighing > 1000 g – 150

Infant Mortality Rate = (1130/19635) × 1000= 57.5 per 1000 live births

Neonatal Mortality Rate = (875/19635) ×1000 = 44.6 per 1000 live births

Post Neonatal Mortality Rate = (1130-875)/(19635) × 1000 = 13.0 per 1000 live births

Perinatal Mortality Rate= (603+150)/ (19635+150) × 1000 = 38.1 per 1000 births

EXERCISE 2B.1: The quarterly report (Jan-March 2021) from a primary Health centre Ujjwa catering to 60,000 population reflects

Births: 200

Infant deaths: 10

Deaths of infants in first week of life: 4

Still births: 2

Calculate the relevant rates, compare with National average and the MCH targets. Comment.

EXERCISE 2B.2: In a town with a population of 100,000 there were 5000 births and 240 infant deaths in the year 2020. Out of these 160 infants died in the first 28 days of life and 100 of them died in the 1st week of life. There were 110 still births in the same year. Calculate Infant mortality rate, post neonatal mortality rate, perinatal and neonatal mortality rate.

EXERCISE 2B.3: In Rampur in Uttar Pradesh, the mid year population in 2020 was 250,000. The deaths in 2020 were 2000 and there were 5000 births. There were 150 infants deaths of which 100 died in the first 28 days of life and 60 of them died in the first week of life. There were 100 still births. Calculate : Crude Birth Rate, Infant Mortality Rate, Neonatal Mortality Rate, Perinatal Mortality Rate, Post-neonatal Mortality Rate.

EXERCISE 2B.4: Draw a pie chart depicting major causes of maternal mortality in India.

EXERCISE 2B.5: Define

- Maternal Mortality Rate
- Adult lifetime risk of Maternal death
- Proportion of maternal deaths of woman of reproductive age group
- Direct and indirect obstetric death

EXERCISE 2B.6: List the major causes of neonatal and infant mortality in India.

EXERCISE 2B.7: Find out about current TFR and NRR in India and the national targets for these indicators.

STUDENT'S NOTES

STUDENT'S NOTES

STUDENT'S NOTES

STUDENT'S NOTES

STUDENT'S NOTES

Supervisor's Signature

CHAPTER 3

Measurement of Risk

Date:______________

Specific learning objectives: At the end of the session, Phase III (Part-1) student will be able to:

1. Know about various types of epidemiological studies.
2. To measure and interpret relative risk, attributable risk of exposure to a factor on the occurrence of disease.
3. Construct an appropriate study design for an epidemiological study.

A. EPIDEMIOLOGICAL METHODS

Observational Descriptive

Analytical

- Case - Control
- Cross - sectional
- Cohort

Ecological

Experimental/Intervention

- Randomized Controlled Trials (RCT)
- Field Trials
- Community Trials
- Clinical Trials

These study methods are not water tight compartments; they complement one another Observational studies allow nature to take its own course. The investigator measures but does not intervenes. Descriptive study describes the occurrence of a disease in a population. Analytical study analyses relationship between health status and other variables. Experimental or intervention studies involve an active attempt to change a disease determinant or the progress of a disease.

ANALYTICAL EPIDEMIOLOGY

CASE CONTROL STUDY (Syn: case comparison study, case compeer study, case history study, case referent study, retrospective study) The observational epidemiologic study of persons with the disease (or other outcome variable) of interest and a suitable control (comparison, reference) group of persons without the disease. The relationship of an attribute to the disease is examined by comparing the diseased and non-diseased with regard to how frequently the attribute is present or, if quantitative, the levels of the attribute, in each of the groups. In short, the past history of exposure to a suspected RISK FACTOR is compared between "cases" and "controls," persons who resemble the cases in such respects as age and sex but do not have the disease or condition of interest. It helps us to calculate Odds Ratio

ODDS RATIO (OR)

It compares the odds that a particular characteristic or exposure will be present in individuals who have a particular disease

Summarized in a 2 x 2 table -

Table : To calculate odds of having an exposure amongst diseased individuals

	Cases	Controls	TOTAL
Exposed	a	b	a+b
Non-exposed	c	d	c+d

N=a+b+c+d

$$\text{ODDS RATIO} = \frac{\text{Odds that a case was exposed}}{\text{Odds that a control was exposed}} \quad \frac{a/b}{c/d} = \frac{(ad)}{(bc)}$$

The OR gives a reliable estimate of the Relative Risk as it gives as a reasonably accurate idea of the RR. However, for this there are two assumptions which should be met with:

(a) The outcome, i.e. the disease of interest should be a "rare disease".

(b) The "controls" i.e. the comparison group should be "representative" of the same total population from which the cases are selected.

COHORT STUDY (Syn: concurrent, follow-up, incidence, longitudinal, prospective study): The analytic method of epidemiologic study in which subsets of a defined population can be identified who are, have been, or in the future may be exposed or not exposed, or exposed in different degrees, to a factor or factors hypothesized to influence the probability of occurrence of a given disease or other outcome. The main feature of cohort study is observation of large numbers over a long period (commonly years) with comparison of incidence rates in groups that differ in exposure levels. The alternative terms for a cohort study, i.e., follow-up, longitudinal, and prospective study, describe an essential feature of the method, which is observation of the population for a sufficient number of person-years to generate reliable incidence or mortality rates in the population subsets. This generally implies study of a large population, study for a prolonged period (years), or both. **These study designs help us to calculate the following.**

1. **RELATIVE RISK (Syn Risk Ratio, Incidence Risk Ratio)**

It is the ratio of incidence of the outcome among exposed individuals to the incidence among non-exposed individuals.

The data to be used in calculating RR are first summarised in a 2 × 2 table

$$\text{RR} = \frac{\text{Incidence of disease in exposed group}}{\text{Incidence of disease in non-exposed group}} \quad \frac{a/(a+b)}{c/(c+d)}$$

Table : To calculate RR of contracting a disease given exposure to a risk factor			
Cohort	**Diseased**	**Non-diseased**	**TOTAL**
Exposed to putative aetiologic factor	a	b	a+b
Non-exposed to putative aetiologic factor	c	d	c+d

N= a+b+c+d

Relative Risk is a direct measure (or index) of the "strength" of the association between suspected cause and effect. A relative risk of one indicates no association; relative risk greater than one suggests "positive" association between exposure and the disease under study. If RR is less than one, the exposure is a protective factor (negative association).

A. Attributable Risk (AR):

Difference in risk of disease between an exposed group and non-exposed group.

$$AR = \frac{\text{Incidence Rate of disease among exposed minus Incidence Rate of disease among non-exposed}}{\text{Incidence rate of disease among exposed}} \times 100$$

Attributable risk indicates, among the exposed, to what extent the disease under study can be attributed to the exposure / risk factor under consideration. If we use a multiplier (like say 1000), we can obtain the expected number of individuals (out of 1000) who will not get the disease if the risk factor is eliminated among the exposed.

Risk Difference i.e. the difference in absolute risk (I_E-I_{NE}) between the two groups is used as an indicator of comparison of effectiveness of different treatment modalities or interventions in an experimental set up. The reciprocal of RD is known as Number Needed to Treat (NNT). It gives the number of patients who would need to be given a new treatment for having one more additional person cured as compared to the conventional treatment.

Population Attributable Risk Percentage (PAR %) (Syn. Etiologic Fraction in Total Population) (EFTP)

It is the incidence of the disease in the total population minus the incidence of disease among those who were not exposed to the suspected causal factor. It provides an estimate of the amount by which the disease could be reduced in that population if the suspected factor was eliminated.

CROSS-SECTIONAL STUDY (Syn: disease frequency survey, prevalence study): A study that examines the relationship between diseases (or other health-related characteristics) and other variables of interest as they exist in a defined population at one particular time. The presence or absence of disease and the presence or absence of the other variables (or, if they are quantitative, their level) are determined in each member of the study population or in a representative sample at one particular time. The relationship between a variable and the disease can be examined (1) in terms of the prevalence of disease in different population subgroups defined according to the presence or absence (or level) of the variables and (2) in terms of the presence or absence (or level) of the variables in the diseased versus the non-diseased. Note that disease prevalence rather than incidence is normally recorded in a cross- sectional study. The temporal sequence of cause and effect cannot necessarily be determined in a cross-sectional study.

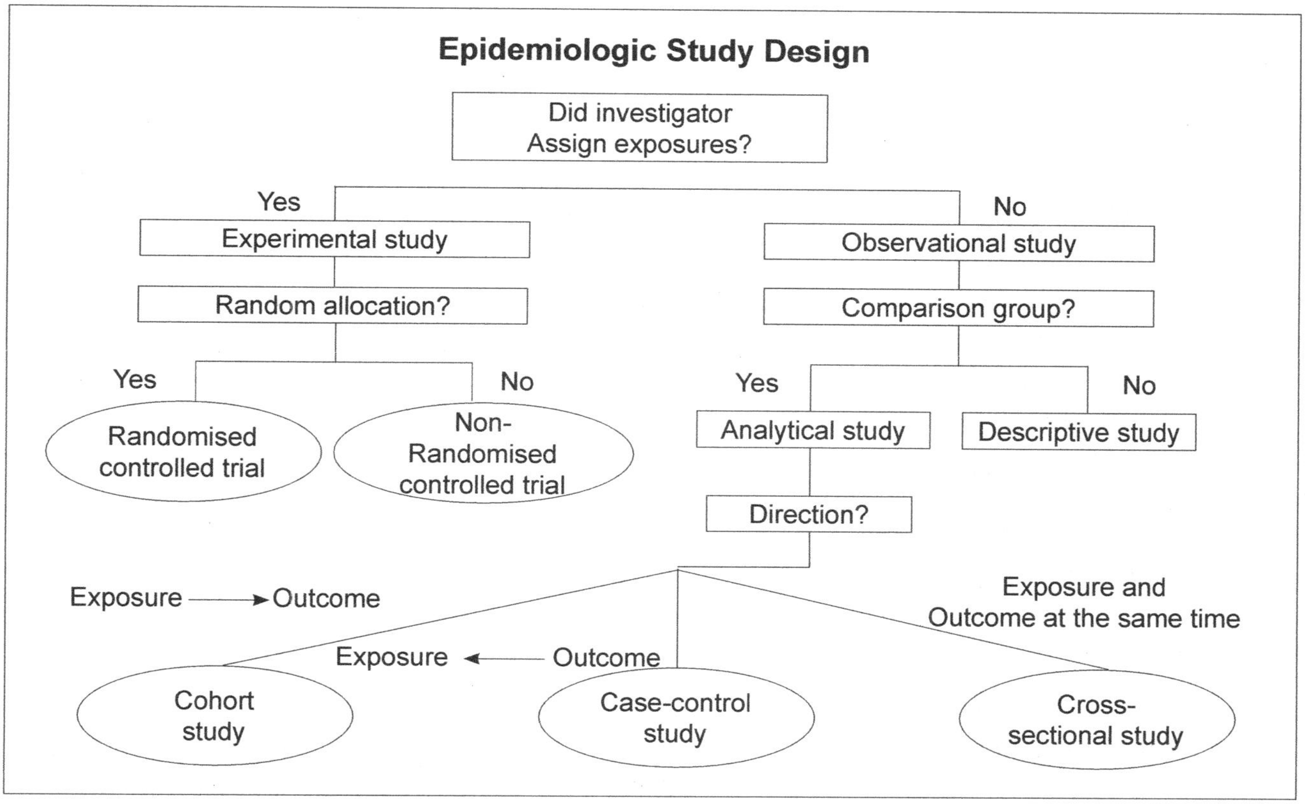

EXERCISE 3.1

3.1.1 Compare and contrast case control and cohort study:

3.1.2 Case control and cohort are examples of ________________________ epidemiological method.

3.1.3 What do the above three studies yield or establish viz - incidence (absolute risk), prevalence or odds ratio.

3.1.4 In a hospital-based study 200 babies born between Jan. 2020 to Dec 2020 were observed for a period of one year, to assess morbidity and mortality due to pneumonia. What is the study design, give reason for your answer.

3.1.5 A Study began in Bangalore in 1995 and a group of 5000 adults were asked about consumption of fresh fruits and vegetables. The occurrence of cancer in this group was studied between 2001 and 2005. What is the study design?

3.1.6 The physical examination records of the entire incoming fresher class of 1994 at the University of Delhi were examined in 2005 to see if their recorded height and weight at the time of admission was related to their chance of developing CHD by 2016. What is the study design?

3.1.7 In a small pilot study, 20 women with breast cancer and 20 women with no apparent disease were contacted and asked whether they had ever used oral contraceptives. Each woman with cancer was matched by age, race, weight, and parity to a woman without disease. What is the study design?

3.1.8 At the age of 6 weeks, all the children enrolled in a well baby clinic were randomly given one of two types of a new vaccine against rotavirus infection. ASHA worker visited the homes of these children two weeks later and asked whether the children had experienced any of a list of side-effects.

3.1.9 Identify the study design for each of the following:

3.1.9.1 Study of past morbidity and mortality trends estimate disease occurrence in the future.

3.1.9.2 Obtaining histories from a group of known patients and comparing with the non-diseased group to determine the relative frequency of exposure.

3.1.9.3 Study of incidence of lung cancer in men who have quit smoking.

3.1.9.4 A representative sample of middle-aged sedentary adults were selected from four census wards in Delhi, and each person was examined for coronary artery disease (CAD). All persons without disease were randomly assigned to either a two-year program of regular cycling or a two-year yoga program. Both groups were observed semiannually for incidence of CAD.

3.1.10 Which of the following is an advantage of cohort study? Give reason for your answer:

- Multiple exposures can be studied.
- Multiple outcomes can be studied.

EXAMPLE

Following table gives information for a follow up study where a group of 10000 tobacco chewers were followed up for a period of 10 years for the occurrence of oral cancer. 20,000 non-chewers were also followed up for the same period. Both groups were periodically screened for oral cancer with same frequency.

Tobacco Chewing	Develop Oral Cancer	Do not Develop Oral Cancer	Total
Yes (Exposed)	50	9950	10000
No (Non- Exposed)	10	19990	20000
	60	29940	30000

(a) What is the study design? Justify.

Since it is a follow-up study that starts with assessment of exposure and measures the occurrence of disease during the follow-up period; it is a cohort study.

(b) Calculate Relative Risk and Attributable Risk for the study.

Relative Risk = Incidence among exposed / Incidence among Non Exposed

$$= \frac{50/10000}{10/20000}$$

= 10 ; Means tobacco chewers are 10 times more at risk of developing oral cancer

$$\text{Attributable Risk} = \frac{\text{Incidence rate among exposed} - \text{Incidence rate among Non exposed}}{\text{Incidence rate among Exposed}} \times 100$$

$$= \frac{50/10000 - 10/20000}{50/10000} \times 100$$

= 90 %; Means among oral cancer patients, 90% is caused due to tobacco chewing

EXERCISE 3.2

In a study on the role of raised serum cholesterol in coronary heart disease (CHD), 100 known cases of CHD and 100 age and sex matched healthy persons (without CHD) were studied. Previous medical records showed that 60 patients of CHD and 20 controls had the history of raised Serum Cholesterol.

1. What is the study design?
2. Construct a 2 × 2 contingency table.
3. How will you estimate the risk of CHD? Calculate the values.
4. On the basis of the above calculation, what inference can be drawn by you?
5. Why is matching important in this study design?
6. Can you calculate Relative Risk from this study design? Why / Why not?

EXERCISE 3.3

Following table shows an example from a study by Doll and Peto R that relates mortality from lung cancer and CHD in smokers and non-smokers. Calculate the missing Values in the table. Comment on the results.

Lung Cancer and CHD Mortality in Male British Physicians: Smokers v/s Non smokers

	Age adjusted death rates per 100,000		Relative Risk	Attributable Risk
	Smokers	Non Smokers		
Lung Cancer	140	10		
CHD	669	413		

Doll R, Peto R: Mortality in relation to smoking: Twenty years' observation on male British doctors. Br Med J 2:1525-1536, 1976.

EXERCISE 3.4

A survey was conducted to assess the role of physical inactivity in Type II diabetes among middle aged males working in IT industry. 75% of diabetics and 40% of non-diabetics reported to be physically inactive.

(a) What is the study design?

(b) Calculate Risk and interpret the result.

EXERCISE 3.5

In a factory of 3000 workers, 1000 workers were exposed to toxic fumes. All the workers were examined periodically for a duration of three years. During the study period, 800 of the exposed workers developed some type of lung disease, and only 40 of the non-exposed workers developed a lung disease.

1. What is the study design and why
2. Construct a 2 × 2 table
3. Calculate the incidence of lung disease in the factory workers
4. Calculate Risk values and interpret the results

The factory is located in a block of 100,000 people. If we assume that the incidence of lung disease in the rest of the population of the block is the same as that in the non-exposed factory workers, calculate Population Attributable Risk of lung disease due to exposure to toxic fumes. Interpret your findings.

STUDENT'S NOTES

STUDENT'S NOTES

STUDENT'S NOTES

STUDENT'S NOTES

STUDENT'S NOTES

STUDENT'S NOTES

STUDENT'S NOTES

Supervisor's Signature

CHAPTER 4

Association and Causation

Date:__________

Specific learning objectives: At the end of the session, Phase III (Part-1) student will be able to:

1. Know How to measure the degree or strength of association.
2. Demonstrate whether association is statistical or casual and use of Chi Square test of significance to verify association statistically.
3. To apply the Student t-test and paired t-test.

Association between two factors:

Two attributes A and B are said to be associated / related in a population of 'N' subjects, if they appear together in a greater number of cases than is expected, when they are independent.

Correlation (r): The degree and direction of relationship or association between two quantitatively measured on continuous variables is called correlation. It determines the relationship between two variables but, it does not prove that one particular variable alone causes the change in the other.

The extent of correlation varies between minus one and plus one.

Correlation is positive when two variables increase or decrease simultaneously; while correlation is negative when increase in one variable cause decrease in the other or vice versa.

Ways to measure correlation

1. Scatter Diagram
2. Pearson's Coefficient of Correlation
3. Spearman's Rank Correlation
4. Kendall's Rank Correlation

Regression: It is used to quantify the correlation between two or more variables by establishing a relationship equation. It is used to forecast or determine further values of one variable, provided the value of other variable is known.

TESTS OF SIGNIFICANCE

In statistics, a result is called statistically significant if it is unlikely to have occurred by chance. The chance probability is also called the p-value of the test. Smaller the p-value, more significant is the test.

Null hypothesis: This nullifies the claim that the experimental result is different from or better than the one already observed.

(A) Chi-square test : Prerequisites for applying this test

1. Random sample
2. Qualitative data

STEPS:

1. State the null hypothesis
2. Make the contingency tables. Note the frequency observed (O) in each class of one event both horizontally and vertically.
3. Determine the expected no. (E) in each group, where E = (Row Total × Column Total)/Grand Total
4. Find the difference between the observed and the expected frequency in each cell (O-E) and square the value obtained i.e. $(O\text{-}E)^2$
5. Calculate the χ^2 values by the formula $\chi^2 = \frac{(O\text{-}E)^2}{E}$ for each cell
6. Sum up the χ^2 values of all the cells to get the total chi-square value

   $$\chi^2 df = \frac{\Sigma (O\text{-}E)^2}{E}$$

7. Calculate degrees of freedom

   d.f. = (Column -1) (Row - 1)

8. Read the value from the probability table.
9. Decision Rule: The calculated (χ^2) is compared with the χ^2 table value and decision to reject χ^2 is taken if the calculated test statistic value is greater than the table value.

   Chi-square test is used for:

   1. Significance of Difference in Proportion.
   2. Measure of association- to test whether two or more characteristics are associated (independently) to each other.
   3. Goodness of fit- to study whether two or more independent populations are similar with respect to some characteristic.

EXAMPLE

To find out the association between hypertension and sedentary lifestyle.

Disease Status	**Sedentary Lifestyle**		
	Yes	**No**	**Total**
Hypertensive	20	10	30
Non-hypertensive	30	140	170
	50	150	200 (n)

Observed frequencies

O1 = 20, O2=10, O3=30, O4=140

Expected frequencies if Null hypothesis is true

E1= 50 × 30/200=7.5, E2=150 × 30/200= 22.5,

E3=50 × 170/200= 42.5, E4= 150 × 170/200=127.5

$$\chi^2 = \frac{\Sigma (O-E)^2}{E}$$

= (20-7.5)2/7.5 + (10-22.5)2/22.5 + (30-42.5)2/ 42.5 + (140-127.5)2/ 127.5

= 32.68 which is > 10.83 ($p<0.001$)

From Chi and square table for df =1 [{ (r-1) × (c-1)} = 1 × 1]

There is significant difference between two groups for p value of 0.001 and hence null hypothesis is rejected. Hypertension is statistically associated with sedentary lifestyle and association is highly significant.

(B) Unpaired (student) T-test:

Prerequisites for applying t-test

(i) Random samples

(ii) Quantitative data

(iii) Variable normally distributed

(iv) Sample size less than 30.

This test is applied to compare date of independent observations made on individuals of two different or separate groups or samples drawn from two populations.

STEPS:

1. Find the observed difference between means of 2 Samples (X1 - X2)
2. Calculate standard error (SE) of difference between 2 means i.e.$(\overline{X1} - \overline{X2})$
3. Calculate the t-value i.e. the ratio between the observed difference and its SE by substituting above values in the formula:

$$t = \frac{\overline{X1} - \overline{X2}}{SE}$$

$$SE = \sqrt{\frac{\sigma 1^2}{n1} + \frac{\sigma 2^2}{n2}}$$

4. Determine the pooled degrees of freedom from the formula:

$df = (n_1 - 1) + (n_2 - 1) = n_1 + n_2 - 2$

'If calculated 't' test statistic value is more than the table value at a particular degree of freedom (df) and at that particular "two tailed level of significance", we reject the null hypothesis.

EXAMPLE

Weight of girls and boys of a class VII in a school is compared. Girls' weight are 42,39,38,60 and 41 kgs. Boys of the same class weighed 38, 42, 56, 64, 68, 69, and 62 kgs. Find whether there is any difference between the weights of girls and boys?

Ho: $\mu 1=\mu 2$ (i.e) there is no significant difference between the weights of girls and boys

H1: $\mu 1 \neq \mu 2$ (i.e) there is a significant difference between weights of girls and boys

Level of significance = 5%

	Girls	Boys
Mean	44	57
Std deviation	8.12	11.49

$$t = \frac{|(\bar{x}_1 - \bar{x}_2)|}{s\sqrt{\frac{1}{n_1}+\frac{1}{n_2}}} \sim t_{(n1+n2)}\ \text{df}$$

Where

$$S^2 = \frac{\left[\sum x_1^2 - \frac{(\Sigma x_1)^2}{n^1}\right] + \left[\sum x_2^2 - \frac{(\Sigma x_2)^2}{n^2}\right]}{n_1 + n_2 - 2} = \frac{330+926}{10} = 125.6$$

$$t = \frac{44-57}{\sqrt{125.6\,(\frac{1}{5}+\frac{1}{7})}} = 1.98$$

Df = 7+5-2=10; t value from table -2.26 at 5%

Since calculated t value is lesser than t value in table, null hypothesis is accepted

No significant difference in weights of two groups

(C) Paired t-test:

It is applied to data of independent observations from one Sample only when each individual gives a pair of observations. Can be used for before-after comparisons, to compare the effect of two drugs, given to same individuals and to compare results of two different laboratory techniques.

STEP:

(i) Find the difference in each set of paired observations before and after (x1- x2 = x)

(ii) Calculate the mean of the difference ($\overline{X}$)

(iii) Work out the SD of differences and then the SE of mean from it SD/ √n

(iv) Determine 't' - value by substituting the above values in the formula

$$t = \frac{\overline{X}}{SD/\sqrt{n}}$$

(v) Calculate degrees of freedom , being only one sample it is = (n-1)

Refer 't' table

EXAMPLE*

Result of change in systolic blood pressure after giving medication in 10 patients

	PATIENT NUMBER									
	1	2	3	4	5	6	7	8	9	10
BEFORE	160	150	170	130	140	170	160	160	120	140
AFTER	140	110	165	140	145	120	130	110	120	130

Ref: Medical Statistics by K R Sundaram 2nd Edition

	Mean	S.D.
Before	150	17.00
After	131	17.13
Change	19	22.46

$t = 19\sqrt{10}/22.46$

$= 2.67$

T value from t-table at $\alpha = 0.05$ is 2.26

Since calculated value is higher, it means there is a significant difference between the two values at 5% level of significance.

EXERCISE 4.1

A study was done to investigate whether there is a relationship between survival of patients with coronary heart disease and pet ownership. A representative sample of112 patients with CHD was taken. Each of these patients was classified as having a pet or not and by whether they survived one year following their first heart attack. Of 63 pet owners, 58 survived. Of 49 non-pet owners, 37 survived. Determine statistically, if there is a significant relation between survival at one year and pet ownership.

EXERCISE 4.2

A new drug for lowering serum cholesterol was tried on 11 patients. Results after one month are given below:

	Serum Cholesterol (mg/dl)	
Patient	**Before**	**After**
1	200	201
2	231	230
3	221	215
4	250	222
5	228	222
6	237	215
7	326	296
8	235	190
9	240	205
10	265	245
11	284	208

Is there any change is Serum Cholesterol after administration of the new drug?

EXERCISE 4.3

Weight of ten randomly selected children coming for DPT Booster vaccination at a govt and private clinic is recorded. Test whether there is significant difference in the mean weight of children in these two groups.

Weight of children at Centre A (In Kg) – 10, 9, 8, 11, 12, 14, 16, 15, 12, 13

Weight of children at Centre B (In Kg) – 8, 7, 11, 13, 10, 12, 12, 12, 15, 10

EXERCISE 4.4

A study was conducted for one week in Delhi on the pollution measure PM10 and number of patients reporting asthma attacks. Comment on the correlation between these.

Day	1	2	3	4	5	6	7	8	9	10
PM10	176	179	411	297	352	261	190	379	405	352
Number of patients reporting asthma attacks	11	21	30	14	21	8	9	33	24	11

EXERCISE 4.5

If you want to test for a statistical relationship between taking Vitamin C and upper respiratory infections in a population of primary school students (ie: testing the null hypothesis of no difference in the proportion of respiratory infections in Vitamin C and placebo groups, versus the alternative of a difference in proportions), the correct statistical test is:

(a) Two-sample t-test

(b) Chi-square test

(c) Paired t-test

EXERCISE 4.6

Attack rates among the vaccinated and unvaccinated against measles are given in the table. Prove the protective value of vaccination by chi-square test.

Group	Results		
	Attacked	**Not-attacked**	**Total**
Vaccinated	10	90	100
Unvaccinated	26	74	100
Total	36	164	200

EXERCISE 4.7

Write the criteria used to assess causality. Try applying these criteria for smoking as probable cause of lung cancer.

STUDENT'S NOTES

STUDENT'S NOTES

STUDENT'S NOTES

STUDENT'S NOTES

STUDENT'S NOTES

STUDENT'S NOTES

Supervisor's Signature

CHAPTER 5

Screening: Concept, Criteria and Uses

Date:__________

Specific learning objectives: At the end of the session, Phase III (Part-1) student will be able to:

1. Understand the role of screening as an important epidemiological tool for prevention and diagnoses.
2. Know the concept of: False positives and False negatives of a test.
3. Calculate: sensitivity, specificity, predictive value of a screening test.
4. Predict the effect of prevalence on predictive value of a Test.
5. Use the properties of sensitivity and specificity to choose the most appropriate screening and diagnostic test.

Screening:

It has been defined as the search for unrecognized disease or defect by means of rapidly applied tests, examinations or other procedures in apparently healthy individuals.

A screening test is not intended to be a diagnostic test. It is only an initial examination. Those who are found to have a positive test result are referred to a physician for further diagnostic workup and treatment.

Screening test criteria :

The test must satisfy the criteria of acceptability, repeatability, and validity.

1. **Acceptability:** Since the test is to be performed on individuals who are apparently healthy, it is important that the test should be acceptable. This will help to achieve greater coverage and co-operation.
2. **Repeatability:** This means that the test must give consistent results when repeated more than once on the same individual or materials under the same conditions.
3. **Validity:** It refers to what extent the test accurately measures which it aims to measure. Validity expresses the ability of a test to correctly distinguish those who have the disease from those who do not. In simple words how close are the test results to those of the gold standard.

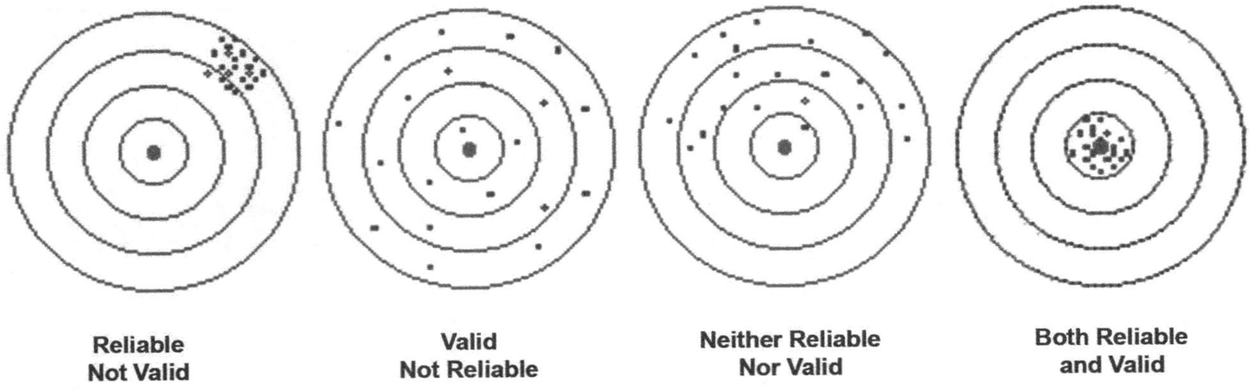

Validity has two components:

(a) Sensitivity

(b) Specificity

Diagnostic Test:

Use of clinical and/or laboratory procedures to confirm or refute the existence of disease in patients presenting with signs and symptoms presumed to be caused by the disease; When a sick persons goes to a clinician(s), he examines and advises a battery of tests to reach a conclusion about the final diagnosis.

"A diagnostic test" is generally taken to mean a test performed in a lab.

Name some diagnostic tests. Comment which all are lab tests and which are not?

____

____

____

____

Study the figure and define **LEAD TIME.** Can there be any difference in actual and perceived lead time?

(Instructors to discuss in relation to lead time bias)

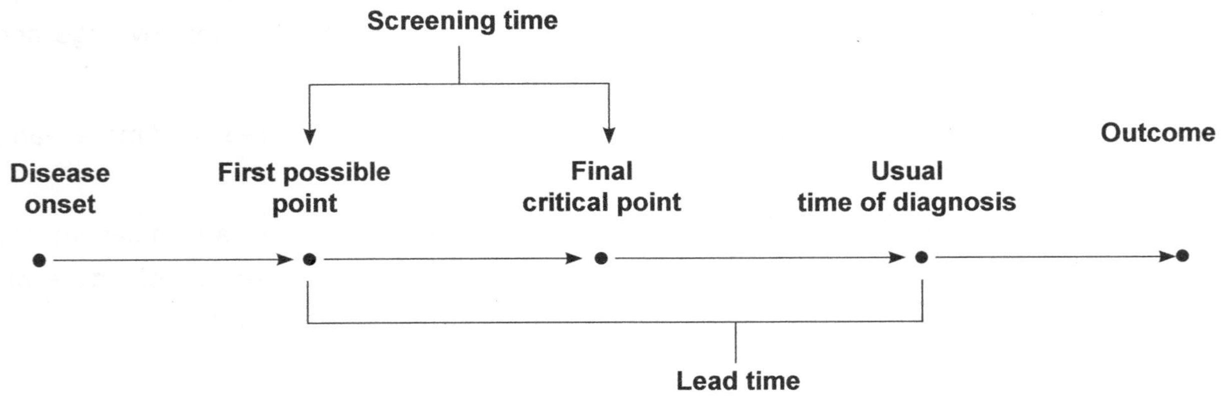

Gold Standard

A gold standard is defined as the most accurate diagnostic feature of the disease in question. Thus it is that diagnostic criteria, which, as per current knowledge, can be assumed to be 100 percent accurate in diagnosis of that particular disease / health attribute.

- Doesn't exist for all diseases
- May not be practical due to cost, labor or invasiveness

Name the commonly used screening tests and gold standard for following diseases

Carcinoma cervix ____________________

Cholera ____________________

Typhoid Fever ____________________

U.T.I.

Gold standards are difficult to define for some diseases andmay be dynamic as some of them may be redefined by subsequent knowledge, but they do help to clarify the usefulness of diagnostic test.

We can of course arbitrarily define a certain test as a gold standard and measure other tests against it.

Validity (accuracy) of a test:

It is ability of a test to indicate those who have the disease and those who don't. In other words, it is the relationship between a test's results and the true diagnosis.

To assess the validity of a test, we need a group of subjects, each of whom should be subjected to both the tests - the test under evaluation and the gold standard test.

By comparing the test results with the gold-standard, we determine the sensitivity and specificity of a screening test; which are measure of Validity.

Table 1:

		Disease Present	Disease Absent	
Test	Positive	True Positive a	False Positive b	a+b
	Negative	False Negative c	True Negative d	c+d
		a+c	b+d	

Here, presence or absence of disease is determined by the result of Gold Standard

Test has given correct answer when it is Positive in the presence of disease negative in the absence of disease i.e., test is correct when it gives the same result as gold standard and incorrect when its result differs from that of the gold standard test.

Which, out of the four categories in the given table, are misleading for the epidemiologist:

(i) ____________________

(ii) ____________________

Sensitivity is defined as proportion of subjects with disease who have a positive test result for a disease.

A sensitive test would rarely miss ____________________

Write the Formula of Sensitivity =

Specificity is defined as proportion of subjects without disease who have a negative test result.

A specific test will rarely miss ____________________

Write the Formula of Specificity =

Percentage of False Positives =

Percentage of False Negatives =

Predictive value

However, the clinicians' interest is truly not in knowing sensitivity or specificity, but rather to know if patients has tested positive on a Test, what are his chances of really having the disease? Or if he has tested negative, what are the chances that he really does not have the infection?

Probability of disease, given the results of a test, is called the predictive value of the test.

Positive predictive value is the probability of disease in a patient with positive test result

Write formula for Positive Predictive Value =

Negative predictive value is the probability of not having the disease when the test result is negative.

Write Formula for Negative Predictive Value =

The Likelihood Ratios

Since Positive Predictive Value, which is of concern for clinicians in practice, depends on the prevalence of the target condition in the population, which is generally not accurately known. Hence To overcome this problems, the concept of likelihood ratios has been developed.

Positive Likelihood Ratio

LR+ = Sensitivity / (1- Specificity)

Interpretation: The ratio of the likelihood of a positive test result occurring in patients with disease (true positive) to the likelihood of a positive test result in patients without disease (false positive)

Negative Likelihood Ratio

LR- = (1-Sensitivity)/ Specificity

Interpretation:

____

For Continuous variables, a cut-off point has to be decided to label the test result as positive or negative, or, in other words a person as diseased or non-diseased

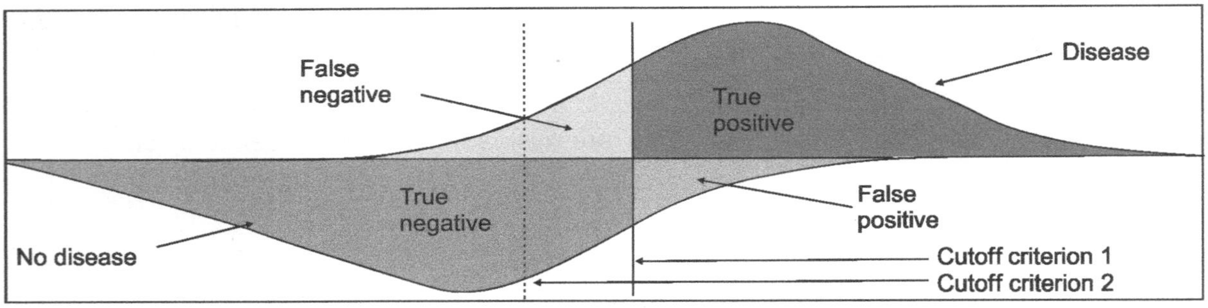

In general, as:

Sensitivity increases (lower threshold), false-positive test results will increase, Specificity increases (higher threshold), false-negative test results increase.

GOOD TO KNOW........

1. Administration of more than one test for a given disease / health attribute

Sequential testing (Tests in series)

When Two screening tests are applied in serial (sequentially) one after the other, by taking people who test positive on the first test for the second test greatly increase the specificity and positive predictive value increase, but net sensitivity decreases.

Simultaneous testing (Tests in parallel)

When two tests are applied in parallel (simultaneously) and the person is considered as positive if any one or both of the tests are positive, this leads to an increase in net sensitivity but a decrease in net specificity.

2. ROC Curve

Receiver operating characteristic (ROC) curves are a graphical depiction of a test's performance

- Y axis: sensitivity
- X axis: 1-specificity
- The higher the curve, the better the test

EXAMPLE

Following are the results of Visual Inspection with Acetic Acid in 100 women with already diagnosed dysplasia by cervical biopsy. VIA was also done for 500 age-matched women without cervical cancer. (Here – VIA- Screening Test; Biopsy – Gold Standard) Study the 2 x 2 table and answer the below mentioned questions.

Cervical Biopsy		**Dysplasia**	**No Dysplasia**	**Total**
VIA	Positive	96 (a)	250 (b)	346
	Negative	04 (c)	250 (d)	254
Total		100	500	600

Percentage of False Positives = b/(b + d) × 100

= 250/500 × 100 = 50%

Percentage of false Negatives – c/(a + c) × 100

= 4/100 × 100= 4%

Predictive value of a positive test = a/(a + b) × 100

= 96/346 × 100 = 27.7%

Predictive value of a negative test = d/(c + d) × 100

= 250/254 × 100 = 98.4%

Sensitivity of VIA as compared to Cervical Biopsy = = a/ (a + c) × 100

= 96/100 × 100 = 96%

Specificity of VIA as compared to Cervical Biopsy = d/(b + d) × 100

= 250/500 × 100

= 50%

EXERCISE 5.1

Mention the Screening tests used in common practice for following population groups

1. Antenatal mothers
2. Newborns
3. Post-menopausal women

Discuss the diagnostic tests for the conditions that you would screen for.

EXERCISE 5.2

A screening test for Breast cancer was administered to 400 women with biopsy proven breast cancer and 400 women without breast cancer. The test results were positive for 100 women with breast cancer and 50 women without cancer.

- Prepare 2 × 2 table for the above given situation?
- What is the sensitivity and specificity of the test?
- Calculate positive and negative predictive value of the test.

EXERCISE 5.3

A new ELISA test is introduced and the results are compared with the definitive test Western Blot (Gold Standard). Serum from 10000 positive Western Blot samples were tested with the new test kits and 9900 were found to be positive. Serum from 10000 negative western blot samples were also tested and 9900 were found to be negative.

5.3.1 Calculate sensitivity and specificity of the new ELISA test

5.3.2 ***Furthermore, the new ELISA was used to test three different populations of one lakh each with HIV prevalence of 0.1, 1 and 10 percent respectively. Construct 2*2 tables for screening these three populations and comment on predictive value of test in these cases.

***Optional Question

EXERCISE 5.4

Pneumonia in under-five children requires antibiotic therapy to prevent deaths. Chest X-ray is the gold standard to diagnose pneumonia in children, but facilities are not available at the community level. Training of ANMs to diagnose pneumonia through increased respiratory rate was proposed and study conducted to assess the validity of using respiratory rate. Following results were obtained 37 of the 149 children with cough and fever had positive chest X-ray and 27 of these had increased respiratory rate. On the other hand112 patients had negative chest X-ray and 77 of these did NOT have increased respiratory rate.

5.4.1 Prepare 2 × 2 table for the above given situation?

5.4.2 What is the sensitivity and specificity of using respiratory rate as a screening tool for pneumonia?

EXERCISE 5.5

In a district hospital of Haryana , TMT (screening test) and coronary angiography (Gold standard) were done for 1000 patients. Following results were obtained.

Test	CHD Present	CHD Absent	Total
TMT Positive	180	400	580
TMT Negative	20	400	420
Total	200	800	1000

Serum Cholesterol test (Screening) and coronary angiography (Gold standard) were also compared for 1000 patients and following results were obtained.

Test	CHD Present	CHD Absent	Total
High Serum Cholesterol	100	80	180
Normal Serum Cholesterol	100	720	820
Total	200	800	1000

Calculate and comment upon the findings of both tables and draw conclusions. Which test would you prefer for screening and why.

EXERCISE 5.6

A home drug screening test kit is currently being developed. The cut-off level is initially set at 4 mg/uL, which is associated with a sensitivity of 92% and a specificity of 97%. How might the sensitivity and specificity of the test change if the cut-off level is changed to 2 mg/uL?

(a) Sensitivity = 90%, specificity = 99%
(b) Sensitivity = 92%, specificity = 97%
(c) Sensitivity = 95%, specificity = 98%
(d) Sensitivity = 97%, specificity = 96%
(e) Sensitivity = 100%, specificity = 97%

EXERCISE 5.7

A screening camp was organized for diabetes in Nangal Raya, Delhi Cantt.

Adult men over the age of 45 years were screened using a single random blood glucose test. Subsequently, all of them were subjected to Glucose Tolerance Test for confirming presence or absence of diabetes. The results are shown in the table below. Study and answer the following questions.

Number of positive and negative tests at specified blood glucose levels in 560 diabetic/ non-diabetic men

Blood Glucose Level (mg%)	Diabetes (n=60)		Non-diabetes (n=500)		Sensitivity	Specificity
	Test + ve	Test - ve	Test +ve	Test -ve		
80	60	0	494	6		
90	55	5	463	37		
100	52	2	371	129		
110	50	5	253	247		
120	50	8	152	348		
130	45	10	80	420		
140	42	18	35	465		
150	35	25	10	490		
160	29	31	7	493		
170	27	33	3	497		
180	25	35	1	499		
190	21	39	1	499		
200	16	44	0	500		

(a) Observe the sensitivity and specificity for each blood glucose level and comment on the pattern that emerges.

(b) Discuss the relation of sensitivity to specificity and the choice that needs to be made for an appropriate test.

STUDENT'S NOTES

STUDENT'S NOTES

STUDENT'S NOTES

STUDENT'S NOTES

Supervisor's Signature

CHAPTER 6

Epidemic Investigation

Date:____________

Specific learning objectives: At the end of the session, Phase III (Part-1) student will be able to:

1. Describe and demonstrate the steps in the Investigation of an epidemic of a communicable disease.
2. Classify and analyse the data of epidemic investigation in terms of distribution viz time, place, person.
3. To understand the determinants viz agent, host and environment factors.

Epidemic

An epidemic is defined as the unusual occurrence in a community or region of disease, specific health related behaviour or other health related events clearly in excess of "expected occurrence".

Type of epidemics

There are three major types of epidemics, let us recollect how they occur by giving one example of each.

(A) Common-source epidemics:

- (i) Single source or point source epidemics: e.g., epidemic of food poisoning.
- (ii) Continuous or multiple source epidemics: e.g., epidemic of gastroenteritis in a village after consumption of water from a common well.

(B) Propagated Epidemics: e.g., outbreak of measles

(C) Slow epidemic: e.g., diabetes, obesity

A graph of time distribution of epidemic cases is called the epidemic curve. The epidemic curve suggests:

(a) A time relationship with exposure to a suspected source

(b) A cyclical or seasonal pattern suggestive of a particular infection

Disease pattern can be described by the time of its occurrence. There are three kinds of trends in disease occurrence

- i. Short term fluctuation
- ii. Periodic fluctuation
- iii. Long term or secular trends.

Short term fluctuation

In a "point source" epidemic

(i) The epidemic curve rises and falls rapidly with no secondary waves.

(ii) Clustering of cases within a narrow interval of time

(iii) All cases develop within one incubation period

A point source may have a single exposure or a multiple exposure.

A propagated epidemic is infectious in origin and can result from person-to-person transmission of an infectious agent.

Periodic Fluctuation

Seasonal Trend: Mostly seen with communicable diseases, e.g., measles, varicella, upper respiratory tract infections etc.

Cyclical trend: Diseases occurring in cycles over short period of time. Both communicable and non-communicable diseases may show periodic fluctuation, e.g., influenza.

Long term or secular trend

Changes in the occurrence of disease over a long period of time, e.g., coronary heart disease, tobacco related cancer.

The objectives of an epidemic investigation are:

(a) To describe and quantify epidemic in terms of time, place and person.

(b) To determine agent, host and environmental factors that are responsible for occurrence of disease

(c) To identify the cause, source of infection and modes of transmission for an effective control of epidemic.

(d) To make recommendations to prevent recurrence.

The Steps in an epidemic investigation are as follows:

1. Verification of diagnosis
2. Confirmation of the existence of an epidemic
3. Defining the population at risk
4. Rapid search for all cases and their characteristics
5. Data analysis
6. Formulation of hypothesis
7. Testing of hypothesis
8. Evaluation of ecological factors
9. Further investigation of population at risk
10. Writing the report

EXERCISE 6.1

In the city X, there was an epidemic of cholera in 2019. A total of 30 patients were reported from sector 20 to sector 42. A list of these patients is as follows. Draw a spot map showing sector wise distribution of cholera patients. Comment on the distribution in the spot map.

S. No.	Sector	S. No.	Sector	S. No.	Sector
1	29	11	39	21	35
2	20	12	31	22	34
3	29	13	32	23	29
4	29	14	33	24	20
5	30	15	34	25	30
6	20	16	30	26	31
7	42	17	31	27	42
8	39	18	32	28	20
9	29	19	42	29	29
10	20	20	34	30	30

EXERCISE 6.2

Two days after a bout of heavy rainfall that flooded the area, there was a sudden outbreak of gastroenteritis on 18 October 2019 in Uttam Nagar area of West Delhi. The cases presented in the nearby Health Centre with presenting complaints of diarrhea, vomiting and abdominal pain. The day-wise distribution of the cases coming to the OPD were as follows:

Date	No. of case
18.07.19	1
19.07.19	3
20.07.19	92
21.07.19	76
22.07.19	46
23.07.19	24
24.07.19	10

1. Draw an epidemic curve for the outbreak
2. If contamination of water is considered as the source of epidemic:
   (a) Calculate the median value of incubation period.
   (b) What is the type of epidemic as per this epidemic curve?

EXERCISE 6.3

Cases of a particular disease appeared in a given community. Day-wise incidence of new cases for a period of two weeks is given below. Draw appropriate diagram and write interpretation citing reasons.

Day	Cases	Day	Cases	Day	Cases	Day	Cases
1	Zero	5	9	9	16	13	2
2	3	6	10	10	13	14	1
3	5	7	11	11	8	15	Zero
4	7	8	14	12	5		

EXERCISE 6.4

In December 2003, an outbreak of gastroenteritis occurred among tenth-grade students who had participated in a city-wide field trip. Half of the students travelled from December 2 to December 7 (Tour A); the other half traveled from December 3 to December 8 (Tour B), The itineraries were similar. Although teachers and other adult chaperones accompanied the students on both tours, no adult reported illness. In addition, no illness was reported among students who did not go on the field trip, and no cases of *E. coli* O157 were reported in the community that week.

A line listing of 26 persons with symptoms of abdominal pain and/or diarrhea is presented below. Using the information in the line listing, develop a case definition that you might use for the outbreak investigation. [Note that persons infected with *E. coli O157* typically experience severe abdominal cramps, bloody diarrhea, and low grade fever after a 1-to 8-day incubation period (usually 2-4 days)].

Table: Line listing of 26 Persons with Symptoms - School District A, December 2003								
Patient #	**Grade and School**	**Age**	**Sex**	**Tour**	**Onset Date**	**Severe Abdominal Pain**	**Frequency (Diarrhoea)**	**Stool Testing**
1.	10-1	17	M	A	Dec. 8	Y	3	Not Done
2.	10-1	16	F	A	Dec. 6	N	1	Negative
3.	10-2	16	M	A	Dec. 10	Y	2	*E. coli* O157
4.	10-2	17	F	A	Dec. 8	Y	3	Not done
5.	10-2	16	F	A	Dec. 5	Y	8	*E. coli* O157
6.	10-2	16	M	A	Dec. 6	Y	3	Not done
7.	10-3	17	M	A	Dec. 7	Y	4	Not done
8.	10-3	17	F	A	Dec. 8	Y	2	*E. coli* O157
9.	10-3	16	F	A	Dec. 7	Y	3	Negative
10.	10-4	17	F	A	Dec. 7	Y	2	*E. coli* O157
11.	10-4	16	M	A	Dec. 8	Y	3	Not done
12.	10-4	16	M	A	Dec. 9	Y	3	Negative
13.	10-5	16	F	A	Dec. 8	Y	3	Not done
14.	10-6	17	F	B	Dec. 8	Y	3	*E. coli* O157
15.	10-6	16	F	B	Dec. 9	Y	2	Negative
16.	10-7	17	F	B	Dec. 6	Y	3	Not done
17.	10-7	17	F	B	Dec. 7	Y	5	*E. coli* O157
18.	10-7	16	F	B	Dec. 8	Y	2	Negative
19.	10-8	17	F	B	Dec. 6	Y	5	*E. coli* O157
20.	10-8	17	F	B	Dec. 7	Y	3	Negative
21.	10-9	16	M	B	Dec. 8	Y	2	Not done
22.	10-9	16	F	B	Dec. 7	Y	3	Negative
23.	10-9	16	F	B	Dec. 7	Y	3	*E. coli* 0157
24.	10-10	17	F	B	Dec. 9	Y	3	*E. coli* 0157
25.	10-10	17	M	B	Dec. 7	N	1	Negative
26.	10-10	16	M	B	Dec. 6	Y	3	Not done

EXAMPLE

Consider the data regarding outbreak of gastroenteritis among 105 students of a hostel block where 60 students reported ill after consumption of food from the mess. Details about meals consumed were obtained and tabulated as follows. Study-Attack rate for various meals and comment.

Date	Meal	Ate Meal			Did Not Eat Meal		
		Number Ill	**Attack rate (%)**	**Total**	**Number Ill**	**Attack Rate (%)**	**Total**
10/9	Breakfast	30	**50**	60	30	**66.6**	45
10/9	Lunch	35	**50**	70	25	**71.5**	35
10/9	Dinner	58	**68.2**	85	2	**10**	20

EXERCISE 6.5

Following table shows the data from an investigation of an outbreak of *Salmonella* Typhimurium gastroenteritis following a company's holiday banquet in December 2003. Approximately 135 persons attended the party, and out of 116 who were interviewed, 57 (49%) met the case definition. Based on this, answer the following questions:

(a) Calculate food-specific attack rates for those who did and did not eat each of the 9 items served only at this banquet.

(b) Which item shows the highest attack rate?

(c) Is the attack rate lowest among persons not exposed to that item?

(d) Were most of the 57 case-patients exposed to that food item?

Food Items Served	Number of Persons who ate Specified Food				Number of Persons who did not eat Specified Food				Risk Ratio
	Ill	Not Ill	Total	Attack Rate	Ill	Not Ill	Total	Attack Rate	
Meat	53	28	81		4	31	35		
Ravioli	43	35	78		14	24	38		
Cajun sauce*	19	11	30		37	48	85		
Pesto cream*	37	29	66		19	30	49		
California rolls*	21	14	35		34	44	78		
Mushrooms*	32	26	58		24	31	55		
Broccoli*	34	30	64		23	28	51		
Carrots*	34	30	64		23	28	51		
Potatoes*	39	41	80		17	17	34		

* Excludes: One or more persons with indefinite history of consumption of that food.

EXERCISE 6.6

The medical officer of a town received a telephone call on 12th December that there were many cases of nausea, vomiting, diarrhea and abdominal pain among persons staying in a guest house premises. On visiting the guest house, it was found that many cases have occurred on the night of 11th December till the morning of 12th December. There was a destination engagement party on the evening of 11th December for which the guests had come to stay in the guest house. On further investigation the M/O found a total of 50 persons had dinner in the party, out of which 30 suffered from gastrointestinal symptoms. Clinically, illness consisted of nausea, vomiting, diarrhea and abdominal pain. None had fever. The illness was of acute onset. Based on this information, answer the following questions:

(a) Discuss application of steps of investigating an epidemic to the above setting.

(b) Discuss case definition, epidemiological case sheet, line listing of cases, population at risk and formulation of hypothesis.

Table gives information on the age and sex of persons who had dinner in the party, time of food consumption, onset of symptoms and food items eaten at the party.

Table: Persons who had dinner on 11th September in the party (DNK refers to do not know)

S. No.	Age (years)	Sex	Time of dinner	Date of onset	Time of onset	Biryani	Paratha	Aloo Gobhi	Dal Fry	Custard
1.	18	M	7:30pm	11th	11:00pm	Y	N	Y	N	Y
2.	20	F	8:30pm	12th	00:15am	N	Y	Y	N	Y
3.	31	M	9:00pm	12th	02:00am	N	Y	N	Y	N
4.	42	M	DNK	Well	--	Y	Y	Y	Y	N
5.	27	M	7:30pm	Well	--	Y	Y	Y	Y	N
6.	51	F	DNK	12th	01:00am	N	Y	N	Y	Y
7.	23	M	9:30pm	12th	00:45am	N	N	Y	Y	Y
8.	61	F	8:00pm	12th	00:30am	Y	Y	N	Y	Y
9.	21	F	7:30pm	Well	--	N	Y	Y	Y	N
10.	58	F	DNK	12th	01:00am	Y	N	N	Y	Y
11.	57	M	11:00pm	12th	02:00am	Y	N	Y	N	Y
12.	19	F	8:00pm	11th	11:30pm	N	Y	Y	Y	Y
13.	20	M	7:30pm	Well	--	Y	N	Y	Y	Y
14.	22	F	DNK	Well	--	N	Y	N	Y	N
15.	23	F	9:00pm	12th	01:30am	N	Y	Y	N	Y
16.	25	M	DNK	11th	10:45pm	Y	Y	Y	N	N
17.	21	F	DNK	Well	--	N	Y	Y	N	Y
18.	26	F	8:30pm	11th	11:45pm	Y	Y	N	Y	N
19.	20	M	DNK	Well	--	Y	Y	N	Y	Y
20.	319	M	7:30pm	Well	--	Y	N	Y	Y	N
21.	24	M	9:30pm	12th	02:15am	N	Y	N	Y	N
22.	41	F	11:30pm	12th	03:45am	N	N	Y	Y	Y
23.	24	F	DNK	Well	--	Y	Y	Y	Y	Y
24.	28	F	7:30pm	12th	02:30am	N	Y	Y	N	Y
25.	23	M	10:30pm	25th	04:15am	Y	Y	N	Y	Y
26.	19	F	7:00pm	Well	--	N	Y	Y	Y	N

Contd.

Contd.

27.	33	M	9:00pm	Well	--	Y	Y	Y	Y	N
28.	51	F	8:00pm	12th	02:15pm	Y	N	N	Y	Y
29.	43	F	11:00pm	12th	04:30am	Y	N	Y	N	Y
30.	29	F	9:30pm	12th	03:45am	N	Y	Y	Y	Y
31.	27	M	8:00pm	Well	--	Y	N	Y	Y	N
32.	36	M	DNK	11th	11:45pm	Y	Y	Y	N	Y
33.	34	F	10:00pm	12th	04:45am	N	Y	N	Y	Y
34.	27	M	11:00pm	Well	--	N	Y	Y	Y	Y
35.	31	F	8:00pm	12th	00:45am	Y	Y	N	Y	Y
36.	59	M	10:30pm	12th	02:15am	Y	N	N	Y	Y
37.	55	F	7:30pm	Well	--	Y	N	Y	Y	N
38.	43	F	DNK	Well	--	Y	N	Y	Y	N
39.	24	F	10:00pm	12th	05:00am	N	Y	N	Y	Y
40.	51	M	DNK	11th	11:45pm	N	N	Y	Y	Y
41.	26	M	9:30pm	Well	--	N	Y	Y	Y	Y
42.	50	M	DNK	Well	02:00am	Y	Y	N	Y	Y
43.	39	F	DNK	Well	--	Y	Y	Y	Y	N
44.	25	F	9:00pm	12th	03:00am	N	Y	Y	Y	Y
45.	40	M	7:00pm	12th	00:30am	N	Y	Y	N	Y
46.	27	F	8:30pm	Well	--	Y	N	Y	Y	N
47.	22	M	DNK	Well	--	N	Y	N	N	N
48.	29	F	7:30pm	12th	02:00am	Y	Y	Y	Y	Y
49.	37	F	DNK	12th	05:30am	Y	Y	Y	N	Y
50.	45	M	8:00pm	Well	--	N	Y	Y	Y	N

(c) Compute the data obtained and tabulate by age, sex, symptoms and type of foods taken.

(d) Calculate food-specific attack rates to make comparisons and draw conclusion.

(e) Draw an epidemic curve for graphical representation of data.

(f) Interpret the epidemic curve.

(g) Calculate the range of incubation period from available data and determine the median incubation period of the outbreak.

(h) Based on food-specific attack rates, which food item(s) are likely to be the source of infection?

(i) What are the likely micro-organisms to cause this food poisoning?

(j) Discuss the investigations that should be carried out for the food handlers.

(k) Assuming one of the cooks tested positive for Staph aureus on throat culture, give your provisional hypothesis for source of infection.

STUDENT'S NOTES

STUDENT'S NOTES

STUDENT'S NOTES

STUDENT'S NOTES

STUDENT'S NOTES

STUDENT'S NOTES

Supervisor's Signature

CHAPTER 7

Presentation of Data

Date:__________

Specific learning objectives: At the end of the session, Phase III (Part-1) student will be able to:

1. Classify types of data and various scales used in statistical measurements.
2. Enumerate methods for presentation of data.
3. Understand the various methods for graphical presentation of data.
4. Apply the appropriate methods of graphical presentation for the given data.

Statistics: It means a measured or counted fact or piece of information stated as a figure such as height of a person, birth of a baby etc.

Biostatistics: It is the term used when tools of statistics are applied to the data that is derived from biological sciences such as medicine. It is also called as biometry.

Variable: A characteristic that changes with respect to a person, place, time or any other factor(s). e.g. Height, Weight, Blood Pressure etc

Types of data :

There are two types of data:

1. Qualitative
2. Quantitative

Qualitative or discrete data

There is only one variable that is the number of persons having a particular characteristic. The magnitude or size of the characteristic does not vary. In other words, the various groups for this data are classified by counting the individuals having the same characteristic or attribute and not by measuring the size. These take discrete values. They can be measured on **Nominal** or **Ordinal scale.**

Nominal Scale: The variables can be placed into categories. These don't have a numeric value and therefore, cannot be added, subtracted, divided or multiplied. These also have no order, and nominal scale of measurement only satisfies the identity property of measurement, e.g., Blood Groups – we count only the number of people with each blood group (A, B, AB, O).

Ordinal Scale: The variables have some order and are measured in terms of magnitude, or rank. Ordinal scales give us relative order, but does not give any information regarding difference in magnitude between the categories. The ordinal scale has the property of both identity and magnitude, e.g., Socioeconomic class as measured by Modified Kuppuswamy scale.

Quantitative or continuous data

The quantitative data has a magnitude. In such classification, there are two variables- the magnitude of the characteristic and the frequency. The groups are divided on the size of characteristic and number of individuals in each sub-group. These can take continuous or discrete values. The characteristic is measured either on an **interval** or on a **ratio** scale, e.g. – Height of individuals. Magnitude of height is done as measurement on a scale and frequency is number of individuals in each measurement level of height.

Interval Scale: An interval scale has ordered numbers with meaningful divisions, the magnitude between the consecutive intervals are equal. Interval scales do not have a true zero i.e In Celsius scale, 0 degrees does not mean the absence of heat but 40°C is hotter than 10°C.

Ratio Scale: The ratio scale of measurement is similar to the interval scale in that it also represents quantity and has equality of units with one major difference: zero is meaningful. The true zero allows us to know how many times greater one case is than another. For length, zero cm means there is no length.

EXERCISE 7.1: Classify the following as qualitative or quantitative data and mention the scale used for measurement in each.

(1) Blood Pressure of patients coming to Medicine OPD

(2) Weight of students in a class

(3) Family Size

(4) Temperature reading of inbound passengers in an airport

(5) Fasting blood sugar

Methods of Presentation of Data

There are two main methods of presentation of frequencies of a variable

Tabulation

For qualitative data, making frequency distribution tables is easy as only the frequency varies, and the characteristic remains discrete 1. For quantitative data, magnitude of variable and frequency both have to be presented in the frequency distribution table.

EXERCISE 7.2: Prepare frequency distribution tables for the following:

1. Height of students in your batch
2. Gender distribution of your batch
3. BMI distribution by Gender for your batch

Graphical presentation of data

Simple and useful method by which data can be presented. Presentation of quantitative, continuous or measured data is done by graphs. Commonly used graphs are:

(1) **Histogram:** Graphical presentation of frequency distribution in which variable is represented on X-axis while frequency is presented on Y-axis. Frequency of each group forms a rectangular column.

(2) **Frequency polygon:** Area diagram of frequency distribution developed over a histogram. Obtained by joining the mid point of class-intervals at the height of frequency by straight lines.If the class intervals are very narrow, frequency polygon forms a frequency curve.

(3) **Line chart:** It is a frequency polygon presenting variations by a line. It shows the trend of an event occurring over a period of time. It is useful for understanding fluctuation or change in an event over a period of time.

(4) **Scatter diagram:** It is a graphical presentation to show the nature of correlation between two variables. It gives pictorial representation of how change in one variable influences the other variable.

Presentation of qualitative, discrete, data is done by diagrams and those in common use are:

(1) **Bar diagram:** This method is adopted for visual comparison of the magnitude of different frequencies in discrete data. The length of bar is directly proportional to the frequency of the variable. Bar diagrams can be simple, multiple or proportional.

(2) **Pie diagram:** In this the frequencies of the groups are shown in a circle. Here, frequency of a variable is denoted by the degree of angle and area of the sector of circle representing that variable.

(3) **Pictogram:** This is a simple method used to represent the frequency of occurrence of events using pictures so that they are easily understandable. Each pictures represent one unit.

(4) **Spot map:** This shows geographical distribution of frequencies of a characteristic. A dot or point indicates one unit of occurrence.

(5) **Chloroplethic map:** Differences in a variable across different geographic units is represented by colouring the area with different shades of same color.

EXCERSISE 7.3: Discuss the diagrams suitable to different types of data, given below.

(a) A report on 1,82,827 deaths during 2010-2013 was prepared by the Registrar General's office based on SRS data. The age distribution of deaths was as follows:

Age Group	Number of Deaths	Percentage (%)
Less than 1 year	18,885	10.3
1-14 years	7263	3.8
15-69 years	91,391	49.9
>/= 70 years	65,288	35.7
Total	1,82,827	100

(b) Distribution of heights of 200 medical students, measured at the time of admission with a scale with least count of 0.1 cm, is given in the table below. Comment on type of data and scale of measurement. Present the data by suitable diagram and comment.

Height (in cm)	Number of students	Percentage (%)
140.0-144.9	7	3.5
145.0-149.9	15	7.5
150.0-154.9	24	12
155.0-159.9	63	31.5
160.0-164.9	58	29
165.0- 169.9	21	10.5
170.0-174.9	10	5
175.0-179.9	2	1
Total	**200**	**100**

EXERCISE 7.4: Find out month-wise cases and deaths due to COVID-19 in India during the year 2020 and represent using a suitable diagram. Also, draw Ogive curve for the same.

EXERCISE 7.5: Compare the change in Total Fertility Rate and Maternal Mortality Ratio (per 100,000 live births) over the years by drawing a suitable diagram and discuss.

Year	1951	2001	2005	2021	2015	2017	2018
TFR	6.0	3.1	2.9	2.5	2.3	2.2	2.2
MMR	NA	301	254	178	130	122	113

EXERCISE 7.6: A study was conducted to find out whether gestational age has any relation with birth weight of infants. The findings recorded for 15 infants born during July 2021 were recorded as follows.

Infant ID	Gestational Age (Completed Weeks)	Birth Weight (Kg)
1	34	1.8
2	36	2.0
3	29	1.4
4	40	2.8
5	35	3.1
6	42	3.8
7	40	3.2
8	37	2.6
9	40	3.2
10	38	2.9
11	38	3.4
12	41	3.6
13	39	3.3
14	41	3.2
15	38	2.0

Find out the relationship between gestational age and birth weight diagrammatically.

STUDENT'S NOTES

STUDENT'S NOTES

STUDENT'S NOTES

STUDENT'S NOTES

STUDENT'S NOTES

Supervisor's Signature

CHAPTER 8

Measures of Central Tendency and Dispersion

Date:____________

Specific learning objectives: At the end of the session, Phase III (Part-1) student will be able to:

1. Understand the concept of average or central value.
2. Interpret how other values are dispersed around this value.
3. Calculate mean, median, mode, mean deviation and standard deviation from a given data.
4. Understand the concept of normal distribution and skewness of data.

Average: Value of a characteristic is the one central value around which all other observations/values are dispersed.

Mean: Implies arithmetic average for a set of observations; which is obtained by summing up all the observations and dividing the total by the number of observations. Most commonly used measure of central tendency.

Median: When all the observations of a variable are arranged in either ascending or descending order, the middle observation is known as median. It is a better indicator of central value when one or more of the lowest or the highest observations are wide apart or not so evenly distributed.

Mode is the most frequently occurring value of observation in a given data.

Range: A range defines the normal limits of a biological characteristic. For a given set of observations, range is simply the difference between highest and lowest value.

Mean Deviation: It is the arithmetic mean of the deviations of the observations from the arithmetic mean ignoring the sign of these deviations.

MD = $\Sigma \mid X - \bar{X} \mid / n$

Where, $\mid X - \bar{X} \mid$ indicates the difference between the value of the observations and the arithmetic mean; n refers to total number of observations.

Variance = $\dfrac{\Sigma \mid X - \bar{X} \mid^2}{n-1}$

Standard Deviation: It is the square root of the average of the squared deviation of the observations from the arithmetic mean. The deviation from mean is squared in standard deviation.

$$s = \sqrt{\frac{\Sigma (x - \bar{x})^2}{n - 1}}$$

To get an unbiased estimate of population standard deviation from small sample, denominator becomes n-1.

Percentiles: Centiles or percentiles are values in a series of observations arranged in ascending order of magnitude which divide the distribution into 100 equal parts. 50th percentile will have 50% observations on either side. Similarly there can be quartiles or quintiles or deciles.

Normal distribution: (also known as Gaussian distribution) is a continuous probability distribution. The shape of frequency curve is smooth, symmetrical and bell shaped.

Relationship between mean median and mode - Mode = 3 Median – 2 Mean

Skewness:

Positive Skewed (Right tailed): – Mean > Median > Mode

Negative Skewed (Left tailed): – Mean < Median < Mode

Symmetric (Normal): – Mean = Median = Mode

Characteristics of Normal Curve

1. Mean, median and mode ____________________
2. Three simple relationships are

   mean ± 1SD which covers ____________________ of the observations,

   mean ± 2SD covers____________________ of the observations and

   mean ± 3SD covers____________________ of the observations.
3. Area under the curve ____________________
4. It has two inflections. The central part is ____________________ while at the points of

   inflection, the curve changes from____________________ to ____________________

NORMAL CURVE

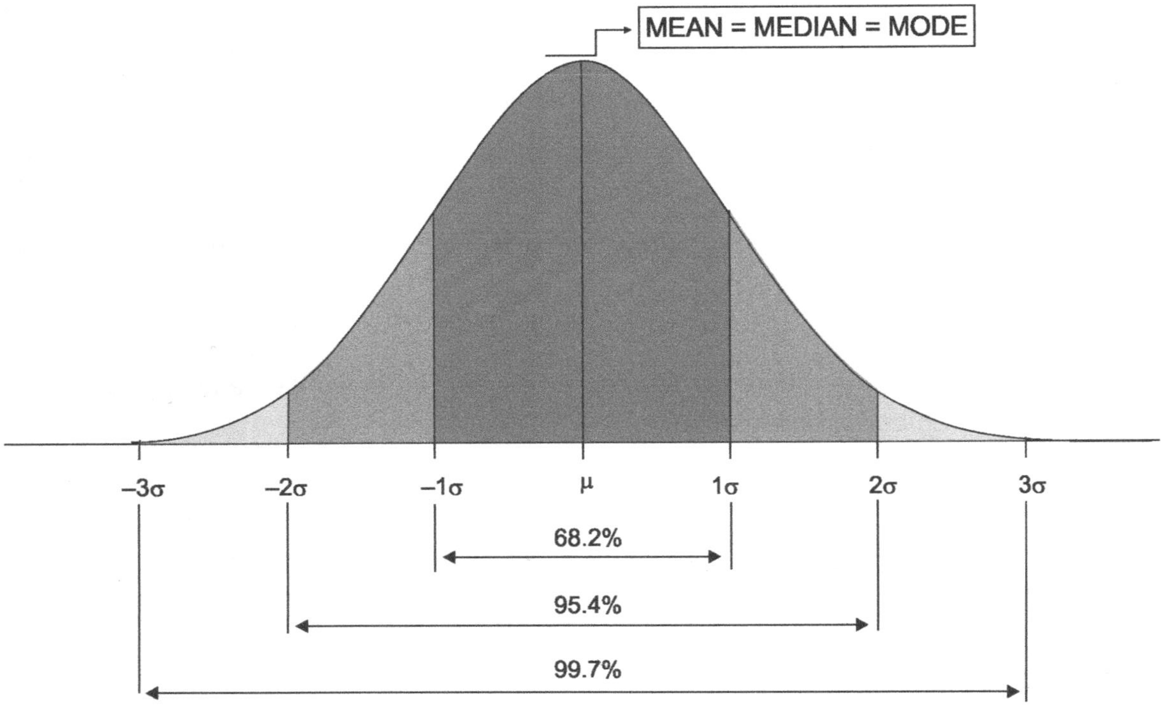

The standard normal distribution is a normal distribution with a mean of zero and standard deviation of 1. In general, the standardized value (standard normal deviate (S.N.D.) tells how many standard deviations below or above the mean, the original value is, and is calculated as follows:

$$\text{Z-score} = \frac{\text{Value} - \text{mean}}{\text{Standard deviation}}$$

Coefficient of variation: It is used to compare variability in different variables that otherwise are not comparable and is expressed as standard deviation divided by the mean times 100%.

$$CV = \frac{SD}{\text{Mean}} \times 100$$

EXAMPLE:

Respiratory rate among 9 individuals was found to be 22, 23, 24, 20, 16, 17, 18, 19 and 21.Find the mean respiratory rate of healthy adults per minute when respiratory rate among 9 individuals was found to be 22, 23, 23, 20, 16, 17, 18, 19 and 21.

$$\text{Mean} = \frac{\text{Sum of Obversations}}{\text{Number of Observations}}$$

= (22+ 23+24+20+16+17+18+19+21) / 9

= 20

Resp Rate (X)	**Mean Deviation** $\lvert X - \bar{X} \rvert$	**Square of Mean Deviation** $\lvert X - \bar{X} \rvert^2$
22	+2	4
23	+3	9
24	+4	16
20	0	0
16	-4	16
17	-3	9
18	-2	4
19	-1	1
21	+1	1

$$S.D.^2 = \frac{\Sigma \lvert X - \bar{X} \rvert^2}{n-1}$$

= (4+9+16+0+16+9+4+1+1) / (9 -1) = 60/8 = 7.5

S.D = $\sqrt{7.5}$ = 2.74

EXAMPLE – MEAN FOR GROUPED SERIES

When the number of observations is large, the data is arranged in groups as per the characteristic value and frequency distribution table is prepared first. Find the value contributed by each group separately and multiply the mid value of group with its frequency. Total these product values and then divide by the total number of observations in the sample. This mean is called weighted mean.

Average salary of 40 (f1) Female Bankers = Rs 40,000 (*x*1) per month

Average Salary of 60 (f2) Male Bankers = Rs 50,000 (*x*2) per month

Total monthly Income of 40 female bankers (f1*x*1) = 40 * 40,000 = Rs 1,600,000

Total monthly income of 60 male bankers(f2*x*2) = 60 * 50,000 = Rs 3,000,000

Average Income = {(f1x1) + (f12x2)} / (x1+x2)

= (1,600,000 + 3,000,000) / 100 = Rs 46,000/-

*In case of frequency distribution tables of grouped data, mid-point of the class interval is considered the value for that group.

EXERCISE 8.1

What are the appropriate measures of central tendency for the following data. State reason.

(a) Age in years of 10 Acute Flaccid Paralysis cases in a district during a year
4, 5, 3, 4, 6, 7, 3, 5, 8, 4

(b) Duration of anosmia (in days) in 10 patients after recovery from COVID
9, 7, 8, 10, 64, 5, 6, 9, 28, 14

EXERCISE 8.2

Birth weights (in kg) of 10 new born babies are given below:

Weight: 2.3, 3.6, 3.2, 3.4, 3.4, 2.7, 3.3, 3.5, 3.2, 2.0;

Calculate all the measures of central tendency for this data.

EXERCISE 8.3

Mid-Upper arm circumference (MUAC) (in cm) of 15 male children aged 4 years is given below:

14, 12, 11, 10, 12, 10, 13, 11, 14, 11, 12, 12, 12, 14, 12

Calculate mean and Standard Deviation for the above set of values. Based on this, what will be the normal limits of MUAC for children in this age group?

EXERCISE 8.4

1. Define co-efficient of variation and write its significance.
2. Following infant mortality rates per 1000 live births were reported by 5 CHCs in each of the 3 districts in a state. Which of these 3 districts show lowest and highest variation in IMR?

   A - 27, 28, 40, 32, 30 B - 32, 27, 35, 36, 29 C - 26, 30, 20, 35, 32

EXERCISE 8.5

Calculate mean, median and mode for the following data

Height of Students (cm)	Number of students
145-150	4
151-155	8
156-160	18
161-170	21
171-175	6

EXERCISE 8.6

A large study of serum cholesterol levels in patients with diabetes mellitus reveals that the parameter is normally distributed with a mean of 220 mg/dl and standard deviation of 10 mg/dl.

(a) What proportion of patients have Serum Cholesterol between 210-230 mg/dl?

(b) What would be considered normal range of Cholesterol for patients of diabetes mellitus?

EXERCISE 8.7

Suppose a random sample of 200 boys aged 17-18 years was chosen and the height of these 200 boys was recorded. The sample mean height was 160 cm, and the sample standard deviation was 7 cm. If the height of the given sample is normally distributed, which interval below includes approximately 95% of the heights of 17-18-year-old boys?

(a) 153 to 167 cm. (b) 146 to 174 cm.

(c) 139 to 181 cm. (d) 150 to 160 cm.

STUDENT'S NOTES

STUDENT'S NOTES

STUDENT'S NOTES

STUDENT'S NOTES

Supervisor's Signature

CHAPTER 9

A. Sampling: Methods and Application

Date:____________

Specific learning objectives: At the end of the session, Phase III (Part-1) student will be able to:

1. Understand sampling, identify sampling frame and sampling units.
2. Determine sample size for a given research / survey.
3. Understand types of sampling and draw a sample from given set of observations.
4. Find the sample statistic for a given variable and compare with population parameter.
5. Understand concept of cluster in a population.
6. Identify and locate clusters in study population.
7. Understand the concept and importance of Standard error in estimating confidence interval for population parameters.

SAMPLING:

Objectives of sampling:

1. Estimation of population parameters (Mean, proportion etc) from the sample statistics.
2. To test the hypothesis about the population from which the sample(s) is drawn.

To be able to get correct results for the above, the sample should be representative of the population from which it is chosen. A representative sample should have:

1. Precision, which implies the size of the sample
2. Unbiased character

SAMPLING FRAME: Is a listing of members of the universe from which the sample is to be drawn.

Sampling Methods:

A. Probability Sampling: In this, each unit has an equal chance of being drawn in the sample.

1. **Simple random sampling:** This is done by assigning a number to each of the units in the sampling frame. A table of random numbers is then used to determine which units are to be included in the sample. Used when population is small and homogenous.

2. **Systematic random sampling:** This is done by picking every k^{th} (e.g. 5th or 10th) unit at regular interval. The sampling units are numbered first. Then for a 10% sample, a random number is

selected between 1 and 10; e.g., 3. Then every 10th number is selected from that point, i.e, 3, 13, 23, 33 etc. Used for field studies when the population is large, scattered and not homogeneous.

3. **Stratified random sampling:** This method involves classifying the population into distinct groups called strata. Then sample is drawn from each stratum using simple random method so that each portion of the sample represents corresponding stratum of the universe. This method is useful when one is interested in analyzing the data by a certain characteristic of the population viz. religion, socio-economic strata.

4. **Multi stage sampling:** This method refers to the sampling procedures carried out in several stages using random sampling techniques. This is employed in large surveys. e.g. In the first stage, districts are chosen using simple random sampling (or any other probability sampling method) in all the states, followed by choosing required no. of talukas, villages and households randomly in the chosen bigger units. Effective in primary data collection from geographically dispersed population.

5. **Multi phase sampling:** In this method, required information is collected from the bigger sample and additional information from the smaller sub sample; either at the same time or some time later. e.g. In a TB survey, mantoux test may be done in all cases of the sample in the first phase, in the second phase X-ray of the chest may be done in mantoux positive cases and in those with clinical symptoms, while sputum may be examined in X-ray positive cases in the third phase only.

6. **Cluster sampling:** In this method, the population is divided into different groups called clusters. A group of sampling units occurring in close approximation, is known as a cluster. A cluster is heterogeneous and usually representative of the population. Each of these clusters is considered as a sampling unit. In this sampling technique, few such (usually 30) clusters are selected, and samples are drawn from each cluster. It is, therefore, a modification of systematic sampling methodology. WHO recommends this method for assessing the coverage of Immunization services in developing countries; e.g., Extended Coverage Evaluation Surveys, employed the 30 cluster technique and examined 7 children encountered consecutively, from each cluster thereby evaluating a total of 210 children for the study. The advantages of this type of sampling are:

   (a) It does not require a detailed sampling frame, only village wise total population is required.

   (b) It is quick and economic way of assessment.

The drawbacks of this method are:

(a) There is lack of precision due to heterogeneity within the clusters.

(b) Inter cluster comparison is not possible.

(c) Chance of least-representative sample.

B. Non Probability Sampling:

1. **Convenience Sampling:** This is a type of sample which is simply available to the researcher by virtue of its accessibility, e.g., Lucas (1997) conducted a study among university students to determine the extent and kind of part-time employment among them. Data was collected from the same college where the author was working as a lecturer and students were selected purposively based on availability rather than randomly.

2. **Quota Sampling:** In this method, predetermined number of sampling units are selected from every sub-group (known as quotas) of the population. However, unlike a stratified sample, the sampling of individuals is not carried out randomly, and the final selection is left to the interviewer. It has been extensively used in commercial research including market research and political opinion polling.

3. **Snowball Sampling:** In this method, the researcher makes initial contact with a small group of people who are relevant to the research topic and then uses this to establish contact with others, e.g., Becker's (1953) study on marijuana users.

EXERCISE 9.1

To assess the prevalence of anaemia amongst the students, a group of 90 students were examined in a govt. school of rural area and their haemoglobin level (Hb gm %) was assessed. The observations thus made are tabulated (See Table 1). Read the table and answer the following questions.

Table 1: Level of haemoglobin (Hb.=gms%) among government school students belonging to different socioeconomic class

Hb. Conc. (gm%)											
Socio-economic Class	**S. No. of Students**	**1**	**2**	**3**	**4**	**5**	**6**	**7**	**8**	**9**	**10**
Upper	1-10	10	9.5	8.5	11.5	8	9.5	9	12	10	14
	11-20	11	9.5	9.5	10.5	8	9	9	9.5	9	8
	21-30	9	10	7	8	7	9.5	9.5	9	6.5	13
Middle	1-10	12.5	9.5	11.5	4	9.5	10	10	11	10	8
	11-20	8	9	10	10	7	10.5	9	8	9.5	9.5
	21-30	7	9	9.5	9	13	7.5	9.5	12	10.5	8
Lower	1-10	9.5	10	5	11.5	9	10	11.5	10	11.5	6
	11-20	7.5	5.5	12	10.5	11	11.5	10	9.5	11	10
	21-30	8.5	9.5	9	11	8	8	11	11	10	11.5

1. Find out the average (Mean) and standard deviation of haemoglobin level among the students.
2. Find out the number and percentage of students suffering with anaemia, considering the normal haemoglobin level at 11.00 gms %.
3. Draw a sample size of 20% from the given population by:
   (a) Simple Random method
   (b) Systematic Random Method
   (c) Stratified Random method (using socioeconomic classes as strata)
4. Calculate the mean value of haemoglobin level in each sample and compare it with the true value.
5. Find out the precentage of students suffering with anaemia in each sample and compare it with the true value.
6. Calculate standard error for mean hemoglobin level using values obtained in the previous question.

7. Calculate the minimum size of the sample (Sample size) required to assess the prevalence of anaemia amongst the students at 95% confidence limit with a error of 10% and 20% respectively.

EXERCISE 9.2

Define simple random sampling. Divide yourselves into two groups and select a sample containing 20% students of your batch using

1. Random number table
2. Lottery method

Now calculate the measures of Central tendency for height and weight for your batch and represent the relationship diagrammatically.

CLUSTER SAMPLING

Steps of cluster sampling (for identification of clusters for data collection)

1. List all towns, villages and wards of cities of the district with their population.
2. Calculate cumulative population of the area (district) and divide the same by 30. This gives the sampling interval.
3. Select a random number less than or equal to sampling interval having same number of digits. This forms the first cluster.
4. Random number plus sampling interval. Gives the population of 2nd cluster.
5. Second cluster + sampling interval = 3rd cluster.
6. 3rd cluster + sampling interval = 4th cluster and so on.
7. Last or 30th cluster = 29th cluster+ sampling interval.

All houses with population are numbered. The first house for survey in each cluster should be randomly selected with the help of random number table or number on a currency note. Before starting house to house survey, define the age group(e.g.12-23 months) and vaccinations that you wish to include in your survey.

Now survey houses, starting with the randomly selected house till you get 7 fully vaccinated children. Thus, 210 such children will be found in 30 clusters.

$$\text{Coverage} = \frac{210}{\text{Eligible Children of surveyed houses}} \times 100$$

EXERCISE 9.3

In a district 'X' there are 60 villages with a total population of 3,30,000. The village-wise distribution of population has been given in the Table 2. Complete the table and identify the villages where the clusters fall by 30 cluster sampling technique. Write the steps that you use for identification of these clusters using the step-guide given above?

Table 2: CLUSTER IDENTIFICATION FORM (SAMPLE FORMAT) - CITIES, TOWNS AND VILLAGES OF DISTRICT "A"							
S. No	Name	Population	Cumulative population	S. No	Name	Population	Cumulative population
1	Haripura	11623		31	Makanpur	2652	
2	Rampur	2990		32	Dinaj	35000	
3	Nurpur	5826		33	Balau	3954	
4	Chopal	3339		34	Paragpur	2115	
5	Jangat	2203		35	Taruwala	507	
6	Sadhuwala	4341		36	Deola	3516	
7	Pipri	1044		37	Gopalpur	14402	
8	Totapur	885		38	Sadwar	3105	
9	Urag	2962		39	Indoor	4176	
10	Niwach	3234		40	Durganagar	1919	
11	Durgapur	1520		41	Bagipar	3261	
12	Uwach	3267		42	Chadiah	4270	
13	Hathnikund	3053		43	Jugnu	3301	
14	Naithal	58000		44	Udain	3250	
15	Kalibari	2207		45	Bajipur	4670	
16	Fatehpur	1355		46	Nagadh	757	
17	Jagatpur	833		47	Paonta	12037	
18	Mewa	4118		48	Surti	2155	
19	Aut	2782		49	Mianwali	3702	
20	Shamshi	3285		50	Manpur	2262	
21	Andheri	4416		51	Pakki	791	
22	Bauli	3188		52	Nagaiah	3468	
23	Barthin	1179		53	Kamroa	4338	
24	Bhartal	612		54	Agroha	3930	
25	Sitapur	3193		55	Abunagar	2112	
26	Majra	17808		56	Sindhupur	2953	
27	Sataun	3914		57	Uratpur	2198	
28	Budhpur	15006		58	Shimle	9891	
29	Tarapur	9584		59	Nagrota	3154	
30	Sappan	4225		60	Ratlam	2575	

B. Standard Error

It is a measure of the variability that would occur while drawing repeated samples of the sample size from the same universe of observations, i.e. shows variations that occur in samples by chance. Standard error of mean varies directly with the standard deviation and inversely as the square root of the sample size.

Standard error of mean is given by:

SE ($\bar{x}$) = *SD/√n, where SD = Standard deviation; n = number of observations.*

Application of Standard Error: To find out the confidence limit within which the population mean would lie at specified level of significance. To test whether the sample mean is drawn from population with known population mean (μ). Confidence interval for population mean:

95% confidence limits for population mean = ($\bar{X}$-1.96* SE ($\bar{X}$), $\bar{X}$+1.96* SE ($\bar{X}$)) or ($\bar{X}$ ± 1.96* SE ($\bar{X}$))

99% confidence limits for population mean= ($\bar{X}$- 2.58* SE ($\bar{X}$), $\bar{X}$+2.58* SE ($\bar{X}$)) or ($\bar{X}$± 2.58* SE ($\bar{X}$))

Where SE referes to standard error and $\bar{X}$ refers to sample mean.

EXAMPLE: A healthcare company is interested in estimating the average charge for a standard patient visit to a physiotherapist in Delhi. Data is collected from 16 randomly selected physiotherapist and the following are calculated – Mean charge: Rs 2550; SD of charges: Rs 200. Assuming the charges are normally distributed for all physiotherapists in Delhi, estimate a 95% confidence interval for the mean amount charged by physiotherapists in Delhi.

Solution: Standard Error of charges = SD/ √N = 200/ √16 = 200/4 = 50

95% confidence interval of charges = Mean charges ± 1.96 (S.E.) = 2550 ± 1.96 (50)

= Rs 2550± 98 = [Rs 2452 – Rs 2648]

EXERCISE 9.4

The results are reported from a study performed on a random sample of 100 deliveries at a large teaching hospital. The sample mean birth weight is reported as 2800 gms, and the sample standard deviation is 150 gms. The researchers did not report 95% confidence interval for the population birth weight. Calculate the same for all deliveries of the hospital.

EXERCISE 9.5

The mean height of sample of 100 students in a medical college is 150 cm with SD of 10 cm. What would be the estimate of mean height of the population with 95% and 99% confidence?

EXERCISE 9.6

In a sample of 15 individuals the mean Hemoglobin is 14.5 g% and SD is 1.5. How would you test whether the sample is drawn from a population having mean Hemoglobin is 13.8 g?

STUDENT'S NOTES

STUDENT'S NOTES

STUDENT'S NOTES

STUDENT'S NOTES

STUDENT'S NOTES

Supervisor's Signature

CHAPTER 10

Public Health Planning: Logistic Management

Date:___________

Specific learning objectives: At the end of the session, Phase III (Part-1) student will be able to:

1. Discuss the use of epidemiology in health service planning.
2. Calculate logistic requirement for vaccines and other supplies for delivery of MCH services.

Vaccine Requirement: Vaccine requirement needs to be calculated, while planning for immunization activity both as a part of routine immunization services provided at health centre or for various reach out activities.

Vaccine requirement = Total no. of beneficiaries X no. of doses required for the vaccine X WMF. Where WMF is the wastage multiplication factor.

Number of beneficiaries can either be counted by ANM / ASHA worker through house to house survey; or estimated using birth rate and infant mortality rate of the area. These give annual estimates which are divided by 12 to get monthly estimates of beneficiaries.

Vaccine Wastage: Wastage of vaccine depends on multiple factors, e.g., vaccine characteristics like type of vaccine (live or attenuated), reuse of vaccine for subsequent sessions (as per open vial policy), number of doses in each vial, vaccine packaging and handling in the field).

Wastage multiplication factor (WMF): This is used to estimate vaccine logistics. It is calculated using the equation: 100 divided by [100 – (wastage rate %)].

E.g., if wastage rate is 15%, then WMF is 100/ [100-15] 100/85 = 1.18.

	No. of Doses	Permissible Wastage (%)	WMF
Hep B	1	10	1.11
BCG	1	50	2
DPT	2 booster	10	1.11
OPV	3+2 booster	10	1.11
Rota	3	25	1.33
IPV	2	10	1.11
Pentavalent	3	10	1.11
MR / JE	2	25	1.33
PCV	3	10	1.11
TT/ Td	2	10	1.11

EFFICACY VERSUS EFFECTIVENESS

A. Vaccine efficacy

The extent to which a vaccine prevents disease among vaccinated persons under ideal conditions. It is influenced by:

1. Ability of vaccine to induce an immunologic response in the host; and
2. Persistence of immunity in the host.

Determination is ideally based on a double blind randomized vaccine trial with placebo in which both groups have the same inherent risk of disease.

B. Vaccine effectiveness

The extent to which a vaccine prevents disease among vaccinated persons in a community setting. Most studies of vaccine efficacy are really measuring vaccine effectiveness. It is usually not based on randomized trials. Assessment is most often based on non-experimental (or observational) studies.

Vaccine efficacy is generally reported as a relative risk reduction (RRR). It uses the relative risk (RR)—i.e., the ratio of attack rates with and without a vaccine—which is expressed as 1–RR.

$$VE = \frac{ARU\text{-}ARV}{ARU} \times 100$$

VE – Vaccine Efficacy

ARU – Attack Rate among Unvaccinated people

ARV– Attack Rate among Vaccinated People

Or **Efficacy** = (1 - Risk Ratio) × 100

Where RR is the relative risk of developing the disease for vaccinated people compared to unvaccinated people.

Community Effectiveness CE = PPV × VE (PPV – Proportion of Population Vaccinated).

EXERCISE 10.1

As In-charge Medical Officer of PHC Rampur, you are required to estimate the yearly requirement for Reproductive and Child Health Services (RCH). The population of the sub centre Sitapuri in your area is 6400. Health worker (F) of the area has just started her annual community needs assessment for RCH services through household survey. Compute the following estimates for planning RCH activities at this sub-centre for the coming year. Use the following information as a guideline.

S. No.	Expected RCH related events in the area	Probable number
1.	Total expected Pregnancies	(Pop. * Birth Rate) + Preg Wastage
2.	Total expected Deliveries	Population * Birth Rate
3.	Antenatal registration (for requirement of ANC visits, IFA and TT does)	As in Row 1
4.	High risk ante-natal case (for preparedness at PHC and FRU)	10% of total pregnancies
5.	Pregnant women suffering with anemia	Min 50% or through latest NFHS Data for the state
6.	High risk neonates (for preparedness at PHC and FRU)	15% of total live births
7.	Infants for vaccine requirement calculation	Population * Birth Rate
8.	No. of Children below 2 yr. (for requirement of DPT/ OPV booster, MR-II and Vitamin A doses)	(Population * Birth Rate) – Infant Deaths
9.	No. of children below 6 yr.	13% of total population

EXAMPLE

You are posted as a MOI/Cof PHC Ujjwa. A sub centre Dhansa is catering to a population of 5000, the birth rate of the area is 25 and the IMR is 43 per 1000 live births.Calculate the annual vaccine requirement for immunization of pregnant women and pentavalent vaccine for infants, for the sub centre.

Solution

Number of pregnant women = Population * Birth Rate + Pregnancy wastage

= 5000* 25 per 1000 + 10% pregnancy wastage

= 125 + 10% pregnancy wastage

≈ 138

Number of Td doses required in a year = Total no of beneficiaries X no of doses required for the vaccine X WMF

= 138 * 2 * 1.11

= 307 doses

Quarterly requirement of doses = 307/4= 77 doses

Yearly Pentavalent vaccine doses required = Number of infants * Number of doses* WMF

= (Population*Birth Rate) * 3 *1.11

= [5000 * (25/1000)] * 3 *1.11

= 417 doses

EXERCISE 10.2

The PHC X, which is located on outskirts of Delhi covers population of 1,30,000. It has 6 sub centres. One of the sub centre, Bijian covers a population of approximately 20,000. The infants of Bijian suffered with an average of 3.5 attacks of diarrhoea during the year and the children in the age group of 1-5 years, also suffered with 2.5 attacks per year. Each episode of diarrhoea in both the age groups lasted for 3 days. As a medical officer of the PHC.

(a) Calculate annual requirement of ORS packets for Bijian.

(b) If the endemicity of diarrhoea is similar at other health centres, find out the total requirement of ORS for the PHC X for the year.

EXERCISE 10.3

Given below is the total population covered by a PHC. The 6 villages covered are as follows:

Village A	6,000
Village B	3,500
Village C	1,500
Village D	5,000
Village E	500
Village F	2,000

You are the medical officer in-charge of the PHC. As stated in the National Health goals, there should be 100%, coverage of antenatal women, in which immunization against tetanus and iron and folic acid prophylaxis is included. As reported from the previous year statistics, about 60% women in your area are anaemic. You have to estimate the annual requirement for the above mentioned services. Enumerate steps you would undertake to achieve this objective.

EXERCISE 10.4

Following are the results of field-trial of an inhalational (aerosol-based) COVID-19 vaccine.

Groups	Had COVID-19 during follow up		Total
	Yes	No	
Vaccinated	24		12,419
Unvaccinated	106		12,221

- Complete the table and calculate the protective efficacy of the vaccine.
  *Optional – Discuss the concept and calculate ARR (Absolute Risk Reduction) and NNV (Numbers needed to vaccinate).

STUDENT'S NOTES

STUDENT'S NOTES

STUDENT'S NOTES

STUDENT'S NOTES

STUDENT'S NOTES

STUDENT'S NOTES

STUDENT'S NOTES

Supervisor's Signature

ANNEXURE I

Table of 't'

Probability of larger Value of 't'

DF	0.10	0.05	0.02	0.01	0.01
1.	6.31	12.71	3.82	63.66	636.62
2.	2.92	4.30	6.97	9.93	31.60
3.	2.35	3.18	4.54	5.84	12.92
4.	2.13	2.78	3.75	4.60	8.61
5.	2.02	2.57	3.37	4.03	6.87
6.	1.94	2.45	3.14	3.71	5.96
7.	1.90	2.37	3.00	3.50	9.41
8.	1.86	2.31	2.90	3.36	5.04
9.	1.83	2.26	2.82	3.25	4.78
10.	1.81	2.23	2.76	3.17	4.59
11.	1.80	2.20	2.72	3.11	4.44
12.	1.78	2.18	2.68	3.06	4.32
13.	1.77	2.16	2.65	3.U1	4.22
14.	1.76	2.15	2.62	2.98	4.14
15.	1.75	2.13	2.60	2.95	4.07
16.	1.75	2.12	2.58	2.92	4.02
17.	1.74	2.11	2.57	00	3.97
18.	1.73	2.10	2.55	2.88	3.92
19.	1.73	2.09	2.54	2.86	3.88
20.	1.73	2.09	2.53	2.85	3.85
21.	1.72	2.08	2.52	2.83	3.82
22.	1.72	2.07	2.51	2.82	3.79
23.	1.71	2.07	2.50	2.81	3.77
24.	1.71	2.06	2.49	2.80	3.75
25.	1.71	2.06	2.49	2.79	3.73
26.	1.71	2.06	2.48	2.78	3.71
27.	1.70	2.05	2.47	2.77	3.69
28.	1.70	2.05	2.47	2.76	3.67
29.	1.70	2.05	2.46	2.76	3.66
30.	1.69	2.04	2.46	2.75	3.65
40.	1.68	2.02	2.42	2.70	3.55
60.	1.67	2.00	2.39	2.66	3.45
120.	1.66	1.98	2.36	2.62	3.47
00 (infinity)	1.96	2.33	2.58	3.29	

The table gives the probability of observing the highest 't' value by chance at particular degrees of freedom. The probability of observing value of 't' greater then 2.95 at 15 degrees of freedom is 0.01 or 1%.

ANNEXURE II

Table of $\chi 2$ -Probability (p)

DF	0.50	0.10	0.05	0.02	0.01	.005	.001
1.	0.45	2.71	3.84	5.41	6.64	7.88	10.83
2.	1.39	4.61	5.99	7.82	9.21	10.60	13.82
3.	2.37	6.25	7.82	9.84	11.34	12.64	16.27
4.	3.36	7.78	9.49	11.67	13.28	14.86	18.47
5.	4.35	9.24	11.07	13.39	15.09	16.75	20.51
6.	5.35	10.65	12.59	15.03	16.81	18.55	22.46
7.	6.35	12.02	14.07	16.62	18.48	20.28	24.32
8.	7.34	13.36	15.51	18.17	20.09	21.96	26.13
9.	8.34	14.68	16.92	1968	21.67	23.59	27.88
10.	9.34	15.99	18.31	21.16	23.21	25.19	29.59

ANNEXURE III

Table of Random Numbers

76	58	30	83	64	87	29	25	58	84	86	50	60	00	25
47	56	91	29	34	05	87	31	06	95	12	45	57	09	09
10	80	21	38	84	90	56	35	03	09	43	12	74	49	14
00	95	01	31	76	17	16	29	56	63	38	78	94	49	81
07	28	38	07	61	11	16	35	27	03	78	86	72	04	95
20	26	36	31	62	68	69	86	95	44	84	95	48	46	45
31	56	34	19	09	79	57	95	36	59	14	93	87	81	40
98	40	07	17	81	22	45	44	84	11	24	62	20	42	31
24	33	45	77	58	80	45	67	93	82	78	70	16	08	24
01	31	60	10	39	53	58	47	70	93	85	81	56	39	38
50	78	13	69	36	37	68	53	37	31	71	26	35	03	71
90	78	50	05	62	77	79	13	57	44	59	60	10	39	66
46	72	60	18	77	55	66	12	62	11	08	99	55	64	57
47	21	61	88	32	27	80	30	21	60	10	92	35	36	12
12	73	73	99	12	49	99	57	94	82	96	88	57	17	91
23	54	20	83	85	23	86	66	99	07	36	37	34	92	09
65	76	36	95	90	18	48	27	45	68	27	23	65	30	72
37	55	85	78	78	01	48	41	19	10	35	19	54	07	73

B. Research Methodology

Chapter 11

Introduction to Research Methodology

Date:____________

The goal of research is to establish facts or principles through careful and systematic investigation in a particular area. Ultimately, the result of such investigation is to improve the health of the population.

In general, following are the basic steps to conduct a research

1. **Identifying data needs:** This depends on the interest of the investigator, importance of the health condition and already available evidence. Scientific Research may be exploratory (to find out something new) or confirmatory (to prove or disprove something for which we already have some clues). It may also be classified as theoretical or applied research.
2. **Formulating the research question:** It should spell out very clearly what the investigator wants to know. It should focus on only one aspect at a time and should be unambiguous and clearly understood.
3. **State objectives of the study:** Clearly defined in scientific terms, use only a single verb and can be defined as primary or secondary.
4. **Outlining a one-page concept paper** describing research methodology (type of study, method of data collection, sample size), ethical considerations and framing dummy tables.
5. **Plan data analysis:** Appropriate methods like specific software depending on the kind of analysis and statistical tests that would be required to answer the research question. Commonly used software's are Excel, Epi-info, SPSS, R etc.
6. **Prepare tools for data collection:** Key variables of the study, how will they be measured and unit of measurement. Questionnaires, interview schedules, measurement instruments like lab tests. Validity and reliability of instruments to be ensured.
7. **Data collection:** Standardization of data collection procedures very important especially in case of multi-centric research projects.
8. **Data analysis:** Using appropriate statistical tools like tabulation and testing for statistical significance. Issues like confounding, effect modifiers, crossover / missing data to be identified and appropriately addressed.
9. **Drawing conclusions** that are valid.
10. **Prepare recommendations** for alleviation of health problem.

REPORT WRITING

Preparing the report and/ or publication of research in a scientific journal is also important for dissemination of the findings.

Following are the general headings used for this purpose:

1. **Title:** Should be concise and yet sufficiently descriptive and informative.
2. **Summary (Abstract):** A structured summary should contain the following subheadings: background, novelty, objectives, methods and expected outcomes.
3. **Keywords:** Five to Six keywords that best describe the project.
4. **Abbreviations:** Only standard abbreviations should be used in the text. List of abbreviations may be given as a list.
5. **Background / Introduction:** State the background information to adequately present the problem, its magnitude and impact; urgency of the need for a solution; amenability of the problem to investigation; and how the research question may help in filling in the existing knowledge gap related to the problem.
6. **Literature review:** Review of existing available scientific literature pertaining to the research question to build justification for the current research project.
7. **Study objectives:** Define the objectives clearly and in measurable terms; mention as primary and secondary objectives if necessary. Do not write too many objectives.
8. **Methodology:** Include the following subheads.
    i. **Study design:** whether descriptive, analytical, experimental, operational, a combination of these or any other. In case of Intervention studies, a detailed description of Intervention should be given. The use of quantitative and qualitative methods may be specified if any.
    ii. **Study population:** 'Who' and 'how' the study participants will be selected: inclusion and exclusion criteria, rules for discontinuation, definitions of cases, controls and lost to follow up etc.
    iii. **Sample size:** Sampling method and sample size estimation should be described in detail with references where needed; data from pilot studies can also be used for sample size calculation.
    iv. **Data collection and statistical analysis plan:** Describe the key variables of the study, how will they be measured and unit of measurement. Specify comprehensively the data collection methods and tools as relevant to the study objectives. Briefly discuss validity, reliability and standardization of the tool used.
9. **Results:** Findings to be presented in a lucid manner using tables, graphs or diagrams. Unnecessary repetition of findings intexts and tables/diagrams to be avoided.
10. **Discussion:** Discuss the findings of your study and compare it with already available scientific literature.
11. **Conclusions:** Draw inferences from the results and discussion.
12. **Recommendations:** That can help alleviate the problem.
13. Limitations of the study.
14. Conflict of interest and Financial Support.

STUDENT'S NOTES

Supervisor's Signature

CHAPTER 12

Exercise: Conducting A Research Study (Project)

Date:____________

Specific learning objective: At the end of the session, Phase III (Part-1) student will be able to:

1. Design and execute a simple research; preferably a cross sectional study design.

Duration of the Project:

Number of students and Roll numbers in the group assigned:

Name of Faculty Incharge/ Supervisor(s):

Identified area of work:

Research Question:

Research Objectives (preferably three)

1.

2.

3.

Hypothesis:

Methodology:

Implementation Plan:

Reflection:

(Report of the Project to be submitted separately along with the master-chart to faculty in-charge)

Remarks of Supervisor:

(Grading to be done on the basis of punctuality, regularity, clarity of concepts and team-work)

Supervisor's Signature and Date:

Hints and Answers to Exercises

2.2

1. Proportion
2. Rate – Disease specific
3. Ratio
4. Proportion
5. Ratio

2.3

(a) Attack Rate = 20/800 * 100 = 2.5%

(b) Incidence = 10266674 / 1380004385 * 1000 = 7.439 cases per 1000 population

2.4 Duration = 0.004 / 0.0008 = 5 years

2.5 Secondary attack rate

Households without access to sanitary latrine – 29.3%, 13.10%, 11.52%, 15.82%

Households with access to sanitary latrine – 5.69%, 4.16%, 3.14%, 3.88%

2.6.2 SAR = 4/12 * 100 = 33.3%

2.7 Cumulative Incidence can only be calculated if all the persons are observed throughout the period of study

Incidence density = No. of cases / Person years of observation

= 4 / 25 person years = 160 per 1000 person years

2.8.1 Period prevalence = 10/20 × 100 = 50%

2.8.2 Cumulative Incidence = 8/20 × 1000 = 400/1000 at risk population

2.10

1. $\frac{90}{99000} \times 1000$ = 0.90 deaths per 1000 population
2. Incidence = 6 cases per 1000 population
3. Age specific death rate (0-14 years) = 0.55 deaths per 1000 population of 0-14 years age
   Age specific death rate (15-44 years) = 1.19 deaths per 1000 population of 15-44 years age
   Age specific death rate (45+ years) = 0.51 deaths per 1000 population of 45+ years age
4. Case fatality rate = 15%

2.11 a

2.12 c

2.13 Increase in both cases

2.14 c

2B.1

Crude Birth Rate = 3.33 births per 1000 population; IMR = 50 per 1000 Live Births

Perinatal Mortality Rate = (4+2)/202 * 1000 = 29.7 per 1000 births

2B.2 IMR = 48 per 1000 Live births; Neonatal Mortality Rate = 32 per 1000 LB

Post Neonatal Mortality Rate = 16 per 1000 LB; Perinatal Mortality Rate = 41 per 1000 LB

2B.3 Crude Birth Rate = 20 births per 1000 population; IMR= 30 per 1000 Live Births; Neonatal Mortality Rate = 5.6 per 1000 LB; Perinatal Mortality Rate = 32 per 1000 LB; Post Neonatal Mortality Rate = 10 per 1000 LB

3.1.4 Cohort

3.1.5 Cohort

3.1.6 Retrospective Cohort study

3.1.7 Case control

3.1.8 Randomised Control Trial (Field trial)

3.1.9.1 Descriptive

3.1.9.2 Case Control

3.1.9.3 Cohort

3.1.9.4 Randomized Control Trial

3.2 Case control study; Odds Ratio = 5

3.3 Lung Cancer RR = 14; AR = 92%

CHD RR= 1.61; AR= 38.2%

3.4 Odds Ratio = 4.5

3.5 Relative Risk = 40

4.1

	Survival after 1year of CHD	Non-survival after 1 year of CHD	Total
Pet owner	58	5	63
Non-pet owner	37	12	49
Total			112

χ^2 = 5.97 df = 1 Table χ^2 = 3.84. Hence there is significant relation between survival at one year and pet ownership.

4.2 Paired t-test should be applied. t-value= 3.42, table t-value at 10 degrees of freedom and 5% significance is 2.23. Hence, null hypothesis is rejected and there is significant change in serum cholesterol after administration of the new drug.

4.3 Mean x = 120/10=12 Mean y = 110/10 = 11

x	$x-\bar{x}$	$(x-\bar{x})^2$	y	$y-\bar{y}$	$(y-\bar{y})^2$
10	-2	4	8	-3	9
9	-3	9	7	-4	16
8	-4	16	11	0	0
11	-1	1	13	2	4
12	0	0	10	-1	1
14	2	4	12	1	1
16	4	16	12	1	1
15	3	9	12	1	1
12	0	0	15	4	16
13	1	1	10	-1	1
$\sum$ = 120		$\sum$ = 60	$\sum$= 110		$\sum$ = 50

$$s = \sqrt{\frac{\Sigma(x-\bar{x})^2 + \Sigma(y-\bar{y})^2}{n_1+n_2-2}}$$

$$S = \sqrt{(60+50)}/18 = 2.47$$

$$t = \frac{|x-y|}{S\sqrt{\frac{1}{n1}+\frac{1}{n2}}}$$

$$= \frac{12-11}{2.47 * \sqrt{2}}$$

= 0.928; which is less than t value in table for df = 18 (2.10090), hence null hypothesis id accepted and there is no significant difference between mean of two groups.

4.4 **r = 0.39, hence there is positive correlation between pollution measure PM10 and asthma attacks.**

4.5 **Chi-square test**

4.6 O1 = 10 O2 = 90 03 = 26 O4 = 74

E1 = 18 E2 = 77 E3 = 18 E4 = 77

χ^2 = 9.31 df=1 , tabulated χ^2 = 3.84. Hence the null hypothesis is rejected and measles vaccine has protective value.

5.2 Sensitivity = 25%; Specificity= 87.5%; PPV= 66.6%; NPV= 53.8%

5.3 Sensitivity = 99% Specificity= 99%

5.4 Sensitivity= 72.9% Specificity= 68.7%

5.6 a; sensitivity decreases while specificity increases

5.7 At lower level of cut-off, sensitivity is high but by increasing the cut-off level sensitivity decreases while the inverse happens for specificity

At 80 mg/dl Sensitivity =100%; specificity = 1.2%

At 90mg/dl Sensitivity = 91.6%; Specificity = 7.4%

6.4 Since attack rate is highest in those who consumed dinner and lowest in those who did not consume dinner, most likely the critical exposure occurred due to consumption of dinner

6.5 Scan the column of attack rates among those who ate the specified items and consider the three criteria listed on the previous page.

Attack rate for those who ate specific foods (in order)

65.4%, 55.1%, 63.3%, 56.1%, 60%, 55.2%, 53.1%, 53.1%, 48.85

Attack rate in those who did not eat specific food item

11.4%, 36.8%, 43.5%, 38.8%, 43.6%, 43.6%, 45.1%, 45.1%, 50.1%

Risk Ratio for various foods (in order of table)

5.7, 1.5, 1.5, 1.4, 1.4, 1.3, 1.2, 1.2, 1.0

Highest attack rate for meat for those who consumed

Lowest attack rate for meat for those who did not consume

8.3 Mean = 12 cm S.D. = 1.3; 95% of value will lie between 12 ± 2.6 cm

8.6 (a) 68.2% (b) 200-240 mg/dl

8.7 b

9.4 95% confidence limits for birth weight = [2800 ± (1.96) (15)] = [2800 ± 29.4 grams]

9.6 95% confidence interval for population mean= 14.5 ± 0.74; which includes 13.8, therefore sample is drawn from the population.

Section V

Visits to Institutions of Public Health Importance

Section V: Visits to Institutions of Public Health Importance

S. No.	Public Health Institute Visited	Signature of Supervisor	Grade
1.			
2.			
3.			
4.			
5.			
6.			
7.			
8.			
9.			
10.			
11.			
12.			
13.			
14.			
15.			
16.			
17.			
18.			
19.			
20.			

S. No.	Proposed Public Health Institutes for Visit and Competency Covered	Specific Learning Objectives of the Visit	Preparatory Reading
1.	Water Treatment Plant : CM 3.2	1. To discuss the importance of disinfection and purification of water 2. To describe water purification and quality monitoring on a large scale i.e. public water supply.	1. Steps of water purification in water treatment plant 2. Differentiate between Rapid & Slow sand filters? (Structure & Mechanism)
2.	Sewage Treatment Plant : CM 3.4	1. To discuss the importance of safe excreta disposal and sanitation barrier. 2. To elicit the functioning of a sewage treatment plant.	1. Parts of sewage treatment plant and processing of sewage in each of these steps. 2. Methods of effluent disposal in sewage treatment plant.
3.	Industrial Visit : CM 11.3, 11.4	1. Enumerate and describe specific occupational health hazards, their risk factors and preventive measures 2. Describe the principles of ergonomics in health preservation	1. Various occupational health hazard their risk factors and preventive measures 2. Significance of ergonomics in prevention of occupational hazards.
4.	Anganwadi : CM 5.6	1. To enumerate the beneficiaries and services provided by Anganwadi. 2. To discuss the organisational pattern of ICDS scheme. 3. To describe the role of ICDS in health of children.	1. Organizational pattern and records maintained in ICDS scheme. 2. Beneficiaries and services provided by Anganwadi. 3. Nutritional content of diet provided to various groups through ICDS.
5.	Subcentre : CM 17.5	1. To describe public health care delivery system in rural areas. 2. To enumerate the services provided at Subcentre/PHC/CHC/UHTC	1. Healthcare delivery system in rural/urban areas. 2. Manpower available, records maintained and services provided at Subcentre/PHC/CHC/UHTC. 3. Indian Public Health Standards
6.	Primary Health Centre (PHC)/ Rural Health Training Centre (RHTC) : CM 17.5		
7.	Community Health Centre (CHC) : CM 17.5		
8.	Urban Health Training Centre (UHTC) : CM 17.5		

9.	Milk Processing Unit (MILK DAIRY) : CM 5.7,5.8	1. To discuss the concept and importance of milk hygiene. 2. To explain the collection, processing and distribution of milk at the Mother Dairy Plant. 3. To describe methods of pasteurization.	1. Milk borne diseases. 2. Methods and importance of pasteurization of milk. 3. Tests for pasteurized milk.
10.	Malaria Clinic/Entomology Lab: CM 8.1	1. To explain the concept of integrated vector control. 2. To discuss various vector control activities.	1. Methods for vector control 2. Various insecticides , their mode of action & dosage in which they are used. 3. Indoor residual spraying
11.	Immunization Clinic : CM 10.5, PE19.1,19.3, 19.4	1. Enumerate National Immunization Schedule. 2. Describe various injection techniques. 3. Explain AEFI	1. National Immunization Schedule 2. AEFI and investigation of a case of AEFI
12.	DOTS Centre : CM 8.3, PE 34.3, 34.4	1. To describe diagnosis and treatment of TB patents under NTEP 2. To elicit organizational structure of NTEP	1. Diagnostic algorithm for diagnosis of tuberculosis under NTEP 2. Treatment schedules for tuberculosis under NTEP
13.	Blood Bank : CM 7.2	1. To discuss the concept of blood safety & voluntary blood donation. 2. To describe the blood storage, testing and precautions observed in a blood bank.	1. Process of collection, storage, fractionization of blood in the blood bank. 2. Various blood borne diseases
14.	Integrated Counselling and Testing Centre : CM 8.1, 8.3	1. To enumerate services provided by Integrated counseling and Testing Centres. 2. To do counseling for HIV / AIDS patients	1. Types of ICTC. 2. Services provided at ICTC 3. Counselling in HIV/AIDS testing.
15.	CSSD	1. To enumerate various disinfection and sterilization techniques used in hospital. 2. To describe the importance and functioning of the central supply and sterilization division.	1. Function of CSSD in hospital. 2. Hospital acquired infections.
16.	Biomedical Waste Management Facility : CM 14.1, 14.2, 14.3	1. To enumerate categories of biomedical waste 2. To describe the procedures followed in biomedical waste management and laws related to it.	1. Types of waste generated in hospitals, collection, segregation & their methods of disposal?

17.	School Health Clinic : CM 10.2	1. To discuss the concept and relevance of school Health services in community Health. 2. To enumerate components of School Health Services.	1. Components of school health services. 2. Structure of school health services in your state
18.	Old Age Home : CM 12.1, 12.2	1. To enumerate social and medical problems of the elderly population 2. To discuss social security services for the elderly	1. Common problems of the elderly people. 2. Social security services available for the elderly.
19.	Non-Governmental Agency (NGO) : CM18.1, 18.2	1. To describe the concept of international health 2. To describe roles of various health agencies including NGOs	Role of NGOs in improving health of the community
20.	Any Other Visit		

How to Document Field/ Clinic Visit

1. **Competencies identified**
2. **Identify the Public Health Institute to be visited**
3. **Components of visit:**
   a. Pre-planned activity
   b. Learner to visit center in small groups
   c. A briefing session to be provided
   d. Objective should be to make learner understand organization, team work, services provided
   e. Learner observes services provided and record maintenance in various public health institutions
   f. Learner interacts with team members
   g. A debrief of learning done is provided
   h. Learner writes a summary of observation and reflection
4. **Criteria for successful completion of visit**

   Activity completed and documented in logbook

   Summary of observations placed in manual
5. **Assessment of the activity** – Grading
6. **Documentation of activity in manual** – Required

Visit Number:

Date:____________

Name of the Institution Visited:

Supervisor's Signature

Visit Number:

Date:____________

Name of the Institution Visited:

Supervisor's Signature

Visit Number:

Date:______________

Name of the Institution Visited:

Supervisor's Signature

Visit Number:

Date:____________

Name of the Institution Visited:

Supervisor's Signature

Visit Number:

Date:______________

Name of the Institution Visited:

Supervisor's Signature

Visit Number:

Date:________________

Name of the Institution Visited:

Supervisor's Signature

Visit Number:

Date:__________

Name of the Institution Visited:

Supervisor's Signature

Visit Number:

Date:______________

Name of the Institution Visited:

Supervisor's Signature

Visit Number:

Date:____________

Name of the Institution Visited:

Supervisor's Signature

Visit Number:

Date:________________

Name of the Institution Visited:

Supervisor's Signature

Visit Number:

Date:____________

Name of the Institution Visited:

Supervisor's Signature

Visit Number:

Date:____________

Name of the Institution Visited:

Supervisor's Signature

Visit Number:

Date:__________

Name of the Institution Visited:

Supervisor's Signature

Visit Number:

Date:____________

Name of the Institution Visited:

Supervisor's Signature

Visit Number:

Date:____________

Name of the Institution Visited:

Supervisor's Signature

Visit Number:

Date:__________

Name of the Institution Visited:

Supervisor's Signature

Section VI

Spots

Chapter 1

Nutrition

Date:____________

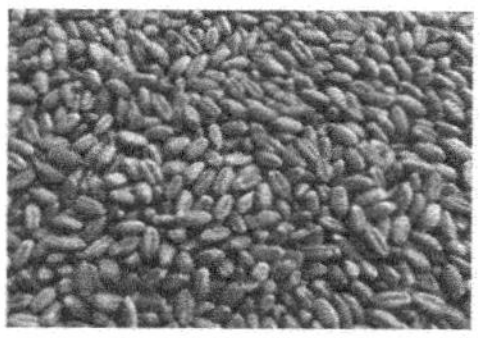
A. Wheat

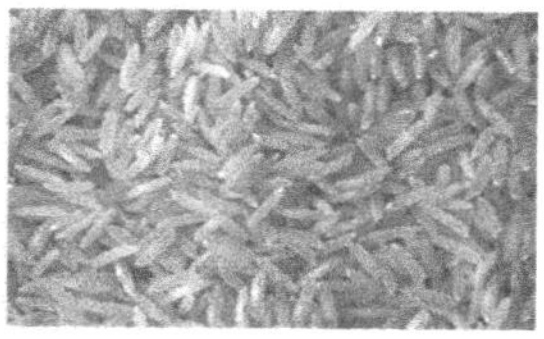
B. Rice

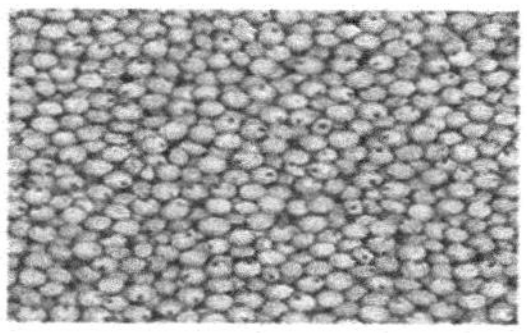
C. Jawar

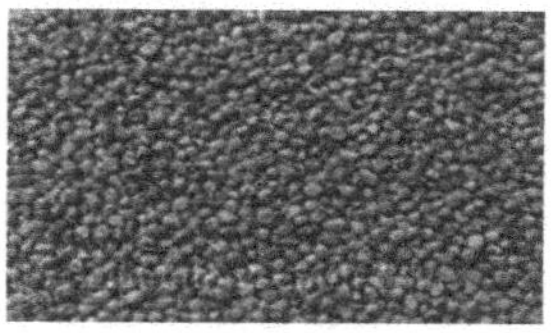
D. Bajra

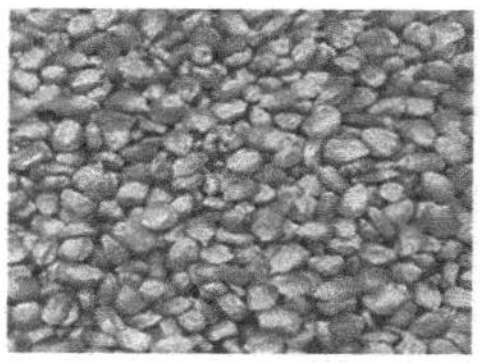
E. Maize

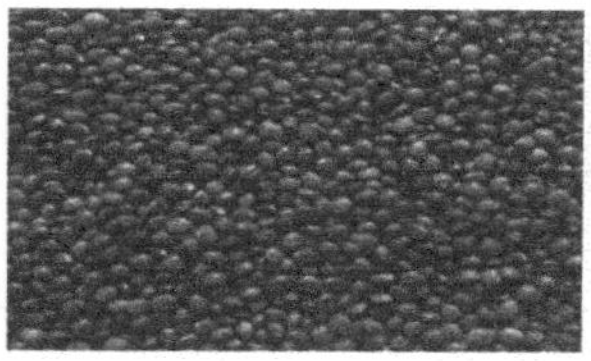
F. Ragi

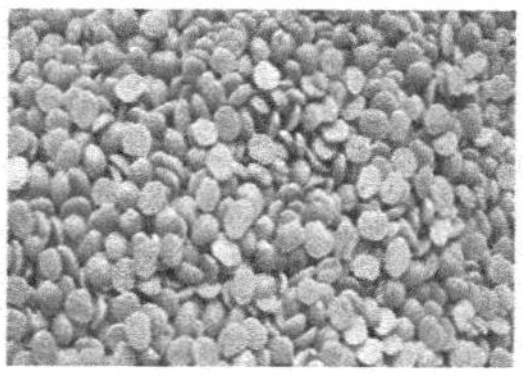
G. Arhar Dal/ Tuvar Fal

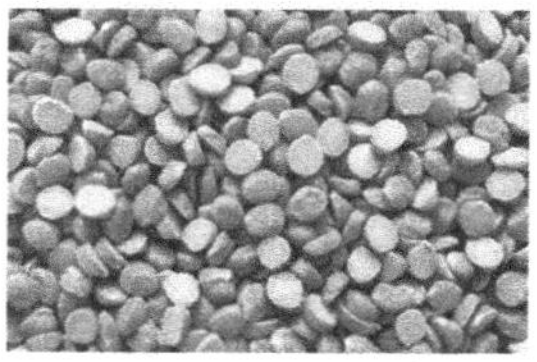
H. Bengal Gram (Chana Dal)

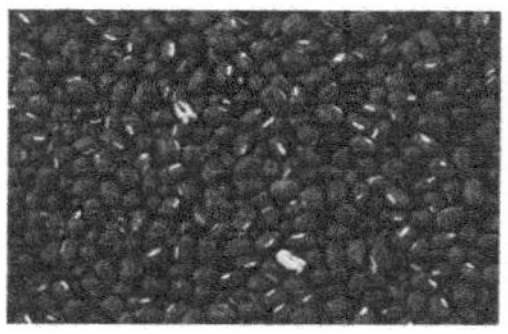
I. Black Gram (Urd Dal)

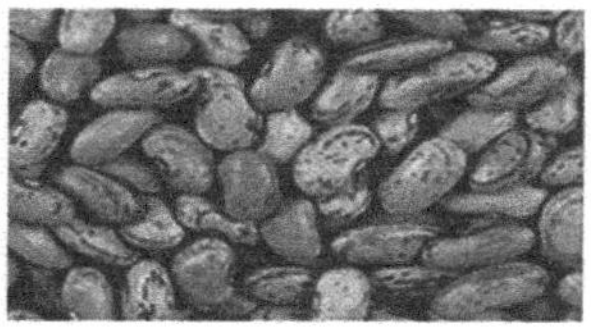
J. Rajmah

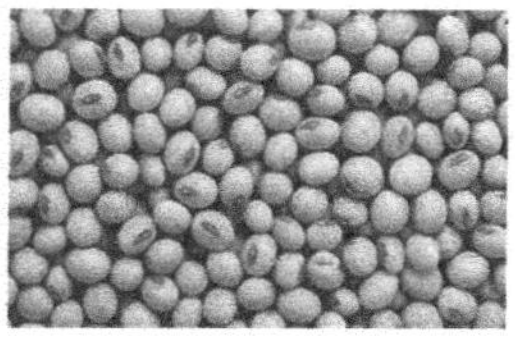
K. Soyabean

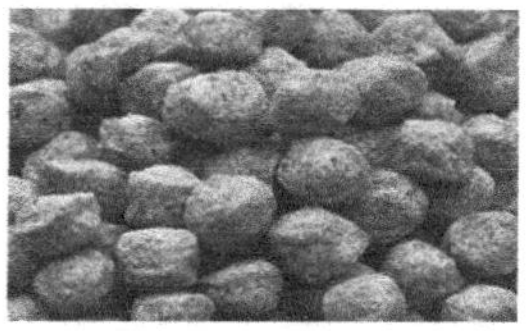
L. Soya Chunks

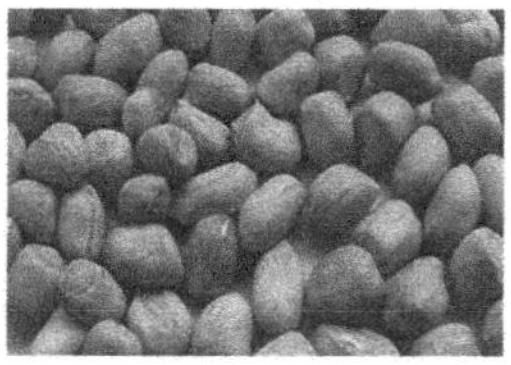
M. Groundnut

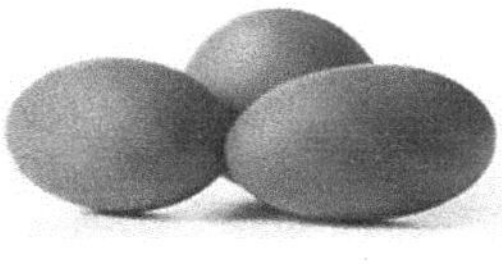
N. Eggs

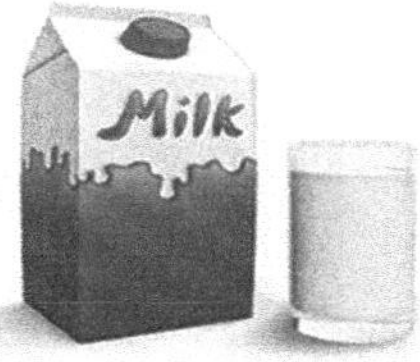

O. Milk

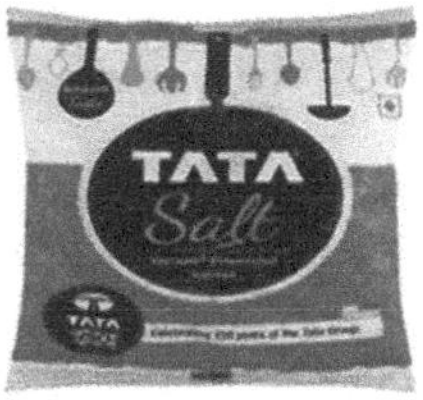

P. Iodized Salt

Suggested spots:

1. Parboiled Rice
2. Brown Rice
3. Chickpeas
4. Green Gram (Dal)
5. Coffee/Tea
6. Fruits and Vegetables
7. Nuts and Dry fruits
8. Sugar
9. Oil
10. Fish
11. Meat
12. Sooji

FREQUENTLY ASKED QUESTIONS

Questions Common to all Nutrition Related Spots

1. Identify the spot.
2. Mention the food group it belongs to.
3. Mention the important nutrients available in the given spot.
4. What is the calorie content per 100 gm?
5. What should be the recommended daily intake for a moderate working adult?
6. What is the public health importance of the given spot?

Questions Specific to Various Food Groups					
Cereals	**Pulses**	**Nuts and Dry fruits**	**Fruits**	**Vegetables**	**Miscellaneous**
1. What are the limiting amino acids in this group? 2. Between wheat and rice, which has better NPU. 3. What are the advantages and disadvantages of parboiling of rice? 4. Why ragi is a suitable weaning food? 5. Which antinutritional factors are present in millets? 6. Name the vitamins deficient in most of the cereals and millets. 7. Consumption of highly polished rice leads to which nutritional deficiency disorder? 8. Excessive use of jowar leads to which nutritional disorder?	1. What are the limiting amino acids in this group? 2. What is supplementary action of proteins? 3. What is reference protein? 4. What is daily protein requirement for an adult and an infant? 5. Name two processes by which nutritive value of pulses can be improved. 6. What is Indian multipurpose food? Mention its purpose.	1. Groundnuts are prone to be contaminated by which fungus? 2. What is the protein content of groundnuts? 3. Among all nuts which is the richest source of iron?	1. Name 2 fruits rich in Vitamin C 2. Name 2 fruits rich in Vitamin A 3. Name 2 fruits recommended for diabetics 4. Name 2 fruits to be avoided by diabetics	1. Name important Nutrients present in most of Green Leafy Vegetables (GLVs). 2. Name important nutrients present in most of roots and tubers. 3. Name the vegetable having highest folic acid content	1. Name the vitamin and mineral deficient in milk. 2. Name methods of pasteurization 3. Why egg protein is considered the best? 4. Why egg should not be eaten raw? 5. How much cholesterol is provided by an egg? 6. Name an infection that occurs due to consumption of contaminated eggs. 7. Name 2 diseases in which consumption of eggs needs to be avoided. 8. Name the chemical compound used for iodization of salt in India. 9. What are the precautions for salt storage. 10. What are the recommended iodine content at production and consumer level?

STUDENT'S NOTES

Supervisor's Signature

CHAPTER 2

Contraceptives

Date:_____________

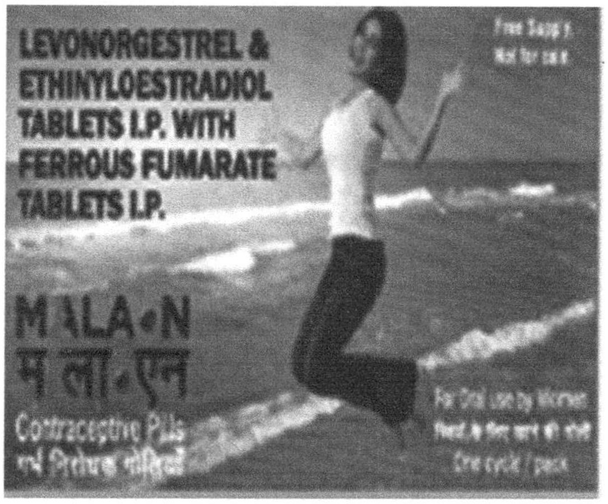

A. Mala-N

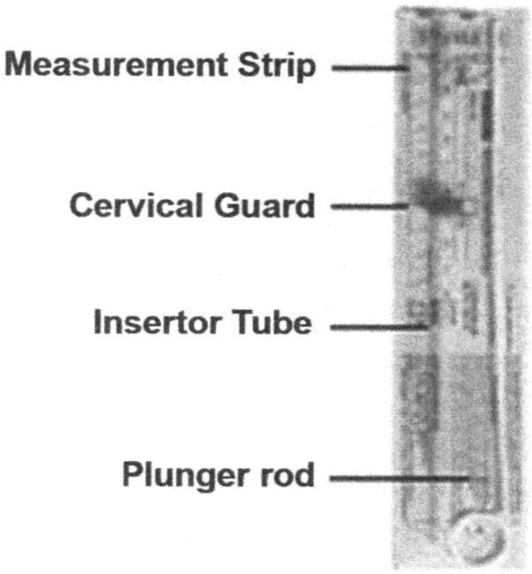

B. Copper T-380 A

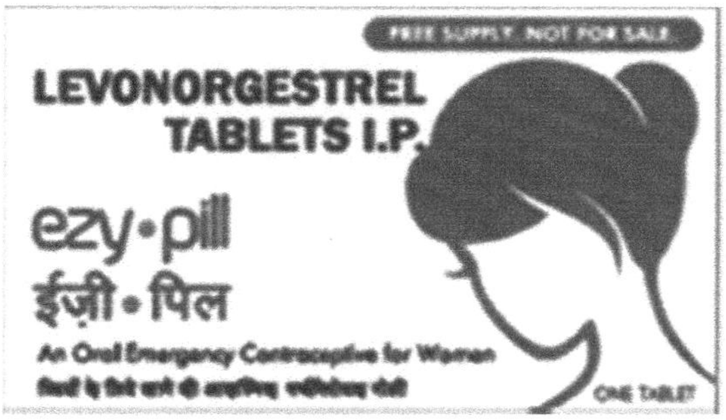

C. Ezy pill

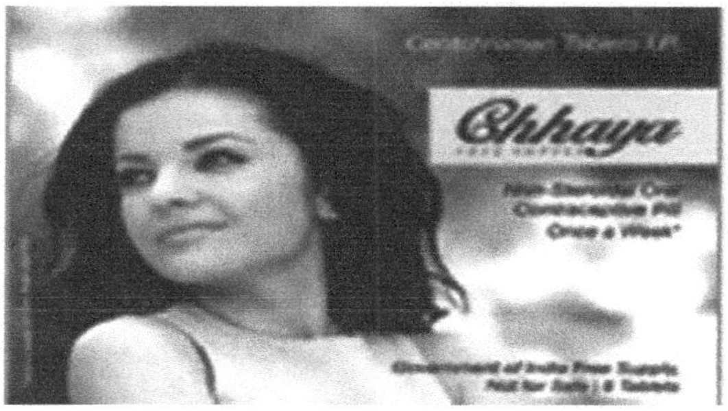

D. Chhaya

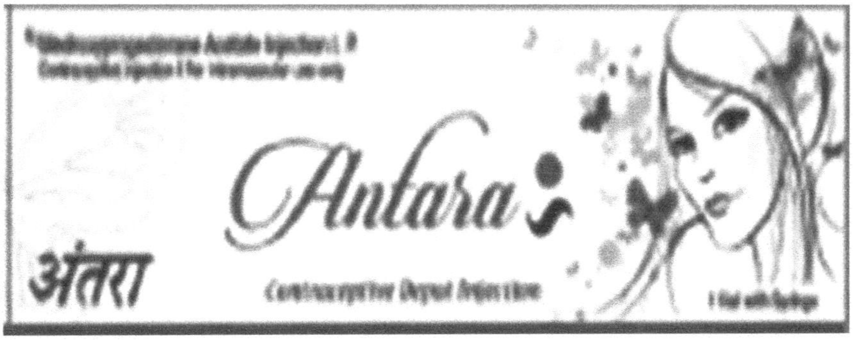

E. Antara

Suggested spots:

Male condom, diaphragm, vaginal pessary, female condom, lippes loop, Mirena, Copper T-375, vaginal sponge

FREQUENTLY ASKED QUESTIONS

1. What are the advantages, disadvantages, side effects and contraindications (absolute and relative) of the given contraceptive?
2. What is the failure rate of the given contraceptive?
3. What is the effectiveness of the given contraceptive?
4. What is the mechanism of action of the given contraceptive?
5. What is the dose schedule for the given contraceptive?
6. What are the non-contraceptive benefits of the given contraceptive?
7. What is lactation amenorrhea?
8. What should be done if a woman misses 3 or more pills in the first or second week of starting the pills
9. What should be done if a woman misses one pill in the fourth week?
10. Name two methods used to measure contraceptive efficacy.
11. What are the indications for removal of IUCD?
12. How should the given contraceptive be prescribed to a woman after 2nd trimester abortion?

STUDENT'S NOTES

Supervisor's Signature

CHAPTER 3

Maternal and Child Health

Date:______________

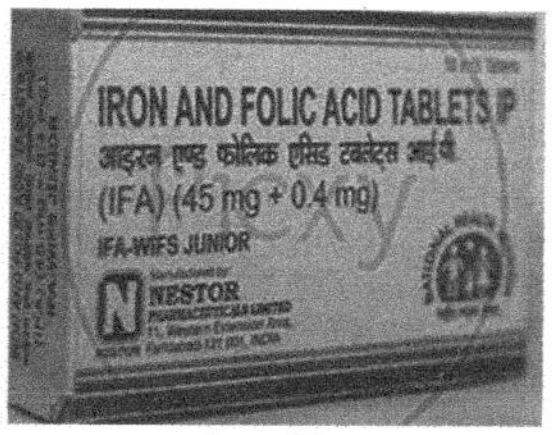

A. IFA small

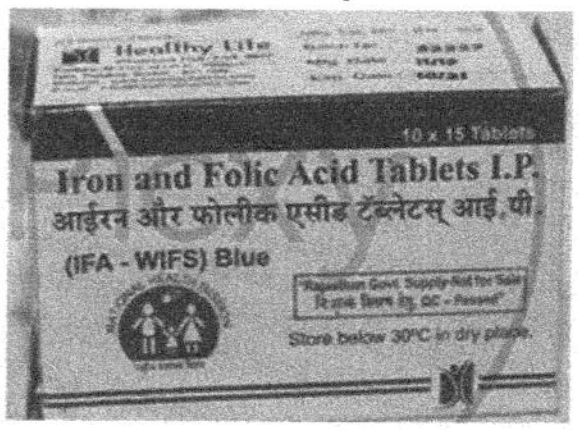

B. IFA Blue

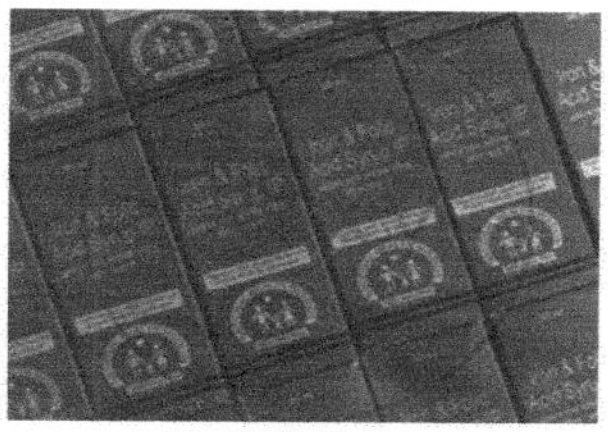

C. IFA Syrup

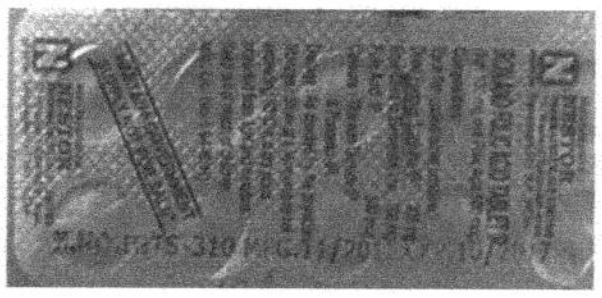

D. IFA Large

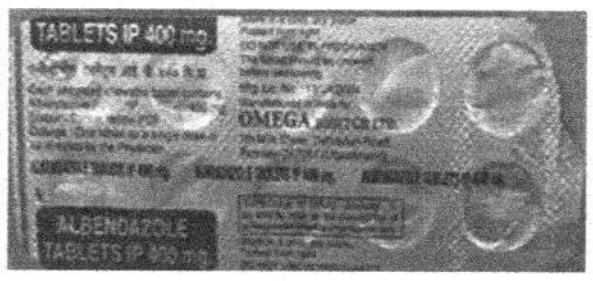

E. Albendazole Tablet

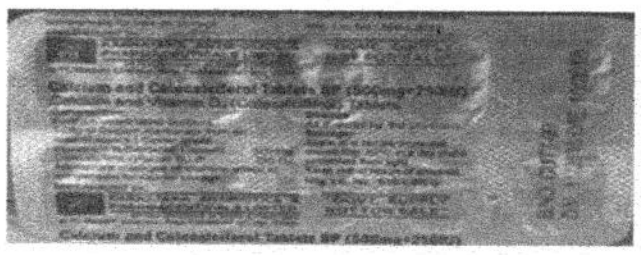

F. Calcium with
Vitamin D Tablets

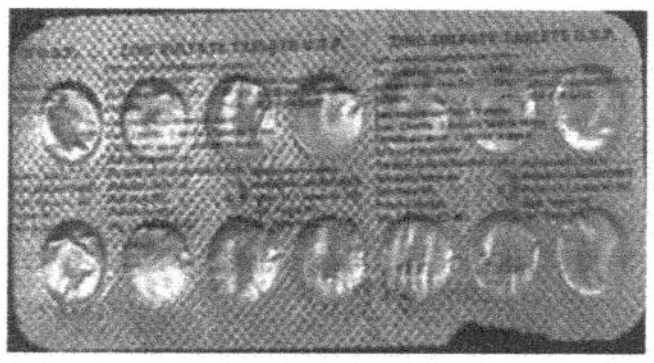

G. Zinc Sulphate Tablets

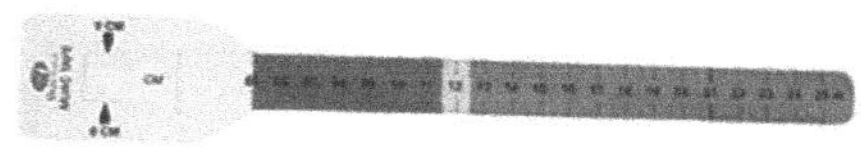

H. Shakir Tape

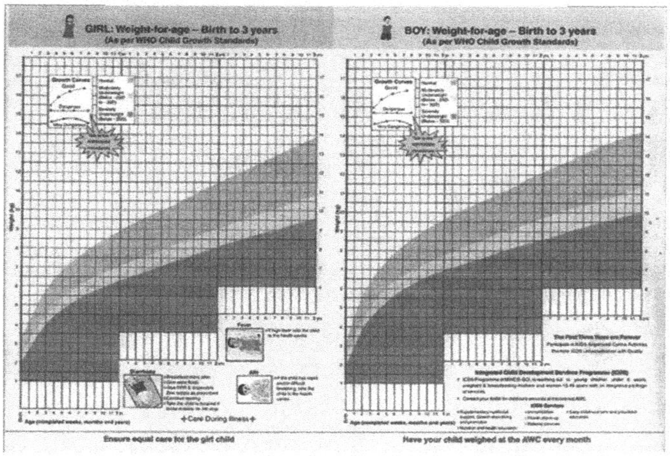

I. Growth Chart

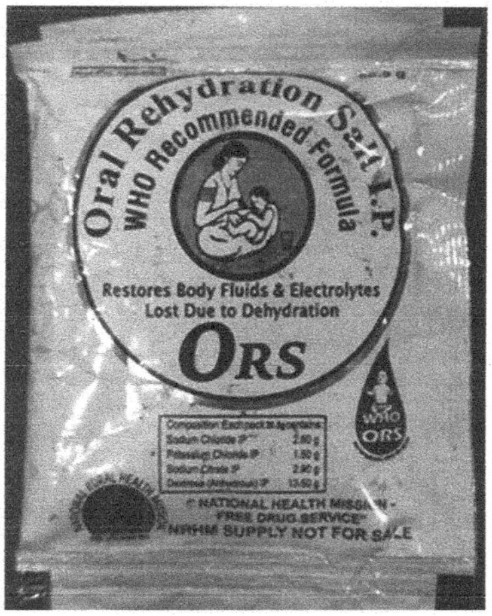

J. Oral Rehydration Salt

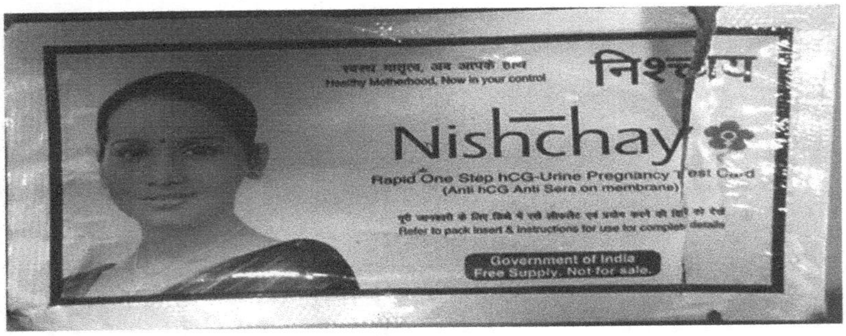

K. hCG Urine Pregnancy Test Card

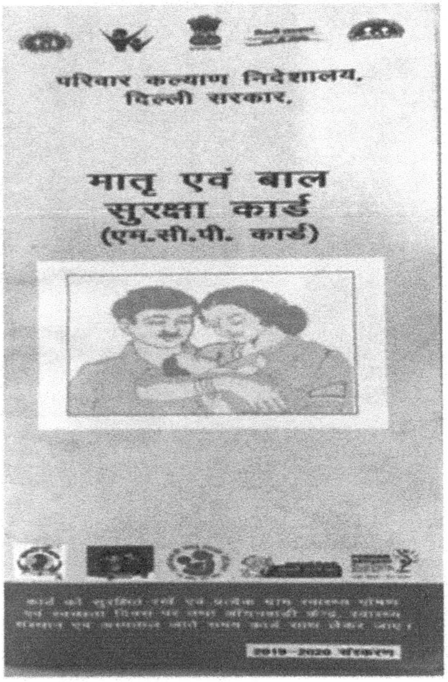

L. Mother and Child Protection Card

Suggested spots:

1. Infantometer
2. Disposable delivery kit

Frequently Asked Questions

Iron and folic acid (IFA) Tablets	Albendazole Tablets	Calcium with Vitamin D Tablets	Zinc Tablets	Shakir Tape	Growth Chart	Oral Rehydration Salt	hCG Urine Pregnancy Test Card	Mother and Child Protection Card (MCP Card)
1. What is the composition of IFA tablets? 2. What is the prophylactic dose of IFA tablets for children, adolescent girls, pregnant and lactating mothers? 3.Under which national health programme IFA tablets are being distributed?	1.What are the indications for its use? 2.What is the dose schedule in pregnancy? 3.What is the dose schedule under the IFA supplementation programme. 4.When National Deworming Day is celebrated?	1.What is the composition of this tablet? 2.Who are the beneficiaries? 3.What is the dose schedule in pregnancy and lactation? 4.Name the national health programme under which this drug is used. 5.Name two food items advised to be avoided along with this tablet. 6.What is the rationale behind adding Vitamin D to calcium?	1.What are the indications for its usage? 2.What is the dose? 3.What are the advantages?	1.What is its use? 2.How do you interpret your observations in reference to various color zones?	1.What are its uses? 2.Name the health care worker responsible to maintain this chart. 3.What is the interpretation of different directions of growth curve (Flat, downwards, upwards)? 4.What do the different coloured areas of the chart indicate (green, orange and yellow areas)? 5.Up to what age health workers are supposed to maintain the growth card? 6.What is the responsibility of the health worker if she discovers the direction of the growth chart as downwards?	1.What is its composition? 2.How do you prepare ORS? 3.Once prepared, for how long the solution can be used? 4.What is its mechanism of action? 5.At Village level, who can provide this pack to beneficiaries?	1.What is its use? 2.Name the national health programme responsible for distribution of these kits. 3.What is the objective of introducing this kit. 4.Name the lowest level of health care delivery system where these kits are available. 5.How do you interpret the results?	1.To whom MCP card is given? 2 Enlist 4 uses of this card? 3.What is the ideal time for issuing an MCP card? 4. Enlist the health services -components covered under this card.

STUDENT'S NOTES

Supervisor's Signature

CHAPTER 4

Vaccine And Vaccine Related Spots

Date:____________

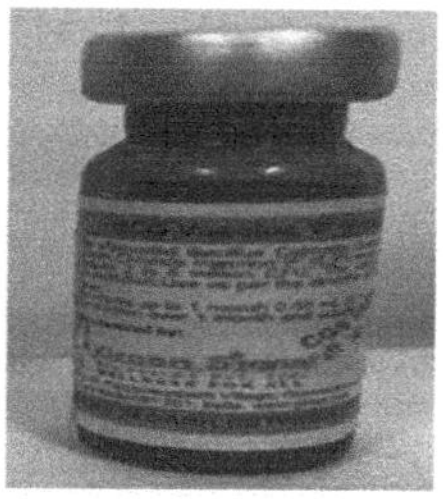

A. BCG vaccine

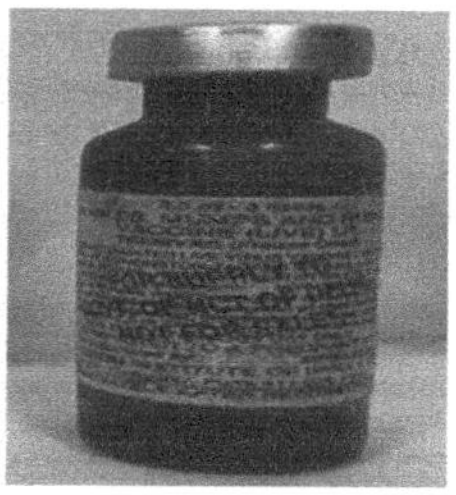

B. Measles mumps rubella vaccine

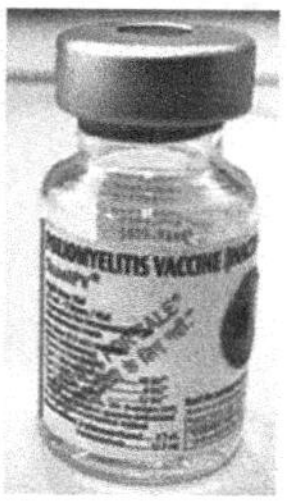

C. Oral polio vaccine

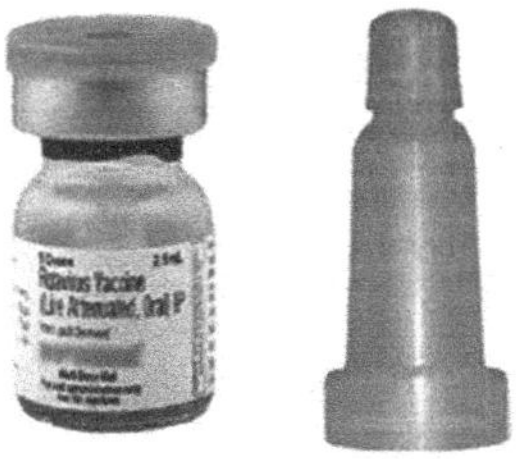

D. Rotavirus vaccine

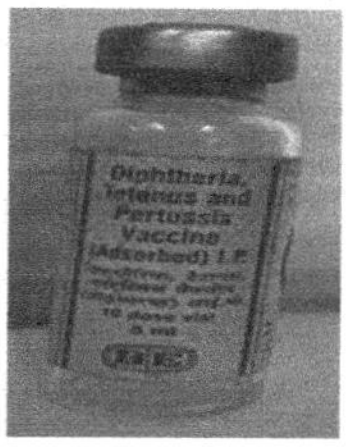

E. DPT vaccine

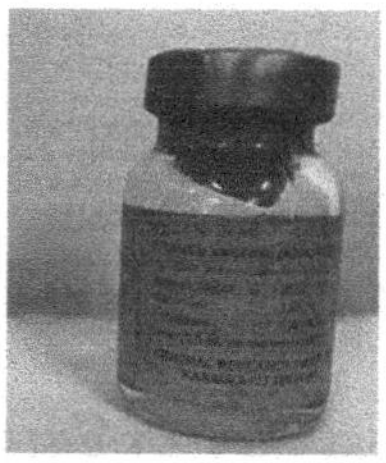

F. Tetanus toxoid vaccine

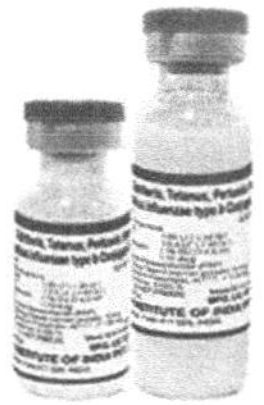

G. Pentavalent vaccine

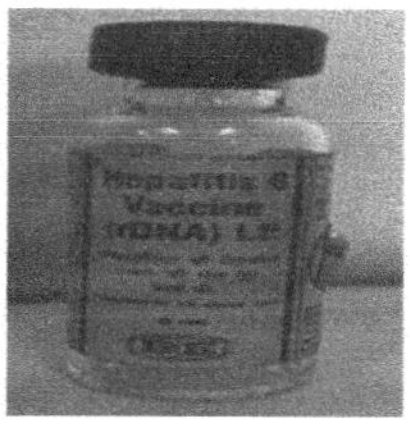

H. Hepatitis B vaccine

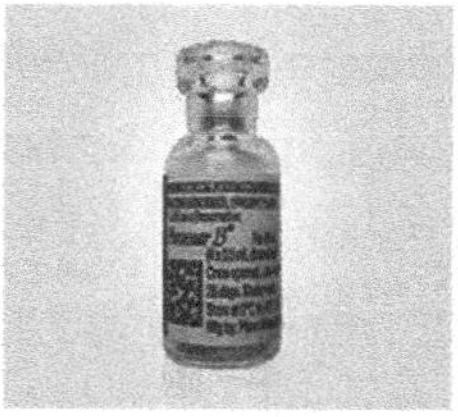

I. Pneumococcal conjugate vaccine

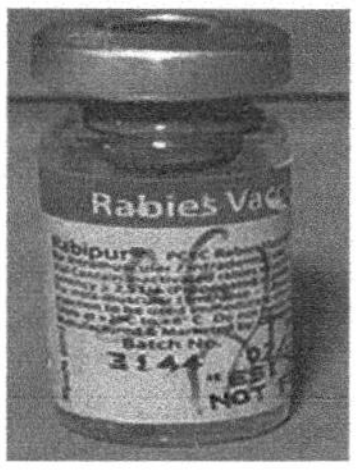

J. Anti-Rabies vaccine

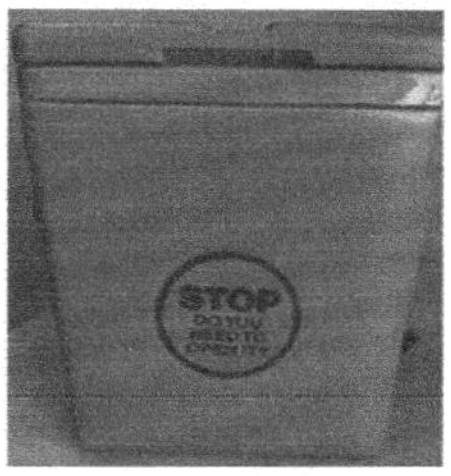

K. Vaccine carrier

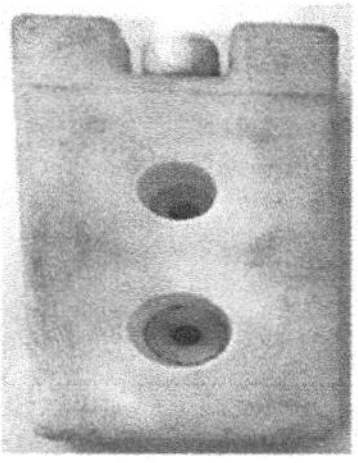

L. Ice pack

Suggested spots:
fIPV vaccine, Measles Rubella vaccine, Japanese encephalitis vaccine, Covaxin, Covishield, Vitamin A, Diphtheria and Tetanus vaccine, Typhoid polysaccharide vaccine, Measles, Varicella vaccine, ice pack, day carrier, deep freezer, ice-lined refrigerator, dial thermometer, Stem thermometer, tuberculin syringe, auto-disabled syringe, distilled water, normal saline, hub cutter

Frequently Asked Questions

Common Questions for Vaccines

1. What is the type, dose, route, site of administration and schedule of the given vaccine?
2. What is the recommended temperature for storage of this vaccine?
3. What is 'Open vial policy'?
4. Name any four vaccines to which open vial policy is applicable?
5. Write any two adverse reactions to the given vaccine.
6. Mention any two contraindications to the given vaccine.
7. Name two light sensitive, freeze sensitive, heat sensitive vaccines.
8. What precautions should be taken while administering BCG?
9. Which strain is used for production of given vaccine?
10. Which test is done to confirm if the vial has been damaged by freezing?
11. What is the adjuvant used in the given vaccine?
12. What is the diluent used for reconstitution for the given vaccine?
13. Why is the given vaccine kept in amber colored bottles?
14. Interpret the vaccine vial monitor of the given vaccine.
15. What is the indication for administration of the given vaccine? (Rabies)
16. Name the regimen for intradermal administration for the given vaccine. (Rabies)
17. What is the difference between cap used for rotavirus and oral polio vaccine? (rota)
18. Why is the given spot pink colored?

Common Questions for Vaccine Related Spots

1. Identify the spot.
2. Write the public health importance of the given spot.
3. Which type of thermometer is recommended by WHO
4. Which vaccine should be kept on the top-most shelf, bottom shelf, side of the refrigerator?
5. How frequently should the temperature of the refrigerator be checked?
6. Mention any two precautions for handling the given spot.
7. What is conditioning of ice pack? (ice pack)
8. Which vaccine should not be kept in holes in an ice pack? (ice pack)
9. What is 'hold over time' for a cold chain equipment?
10. What is the recommended procedure for safe disposal of the given spot?
11. Comment on the growth curve of the given child.

STUDENT'S NOTES

Supervisor's Signature

CHAPTER 5

Entomology

Date:____________

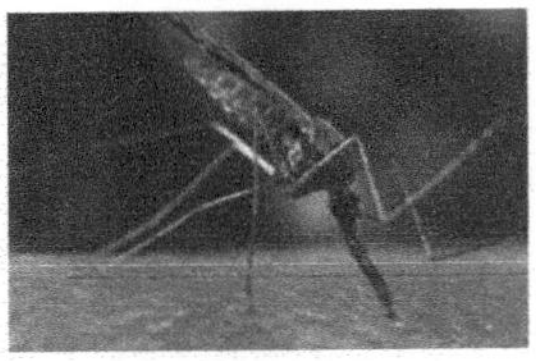

A. Anopheles mosquito

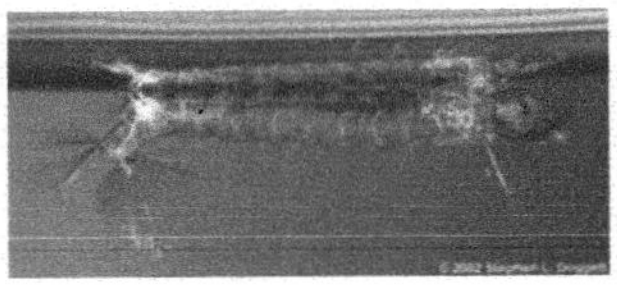

B. Anopheles larva

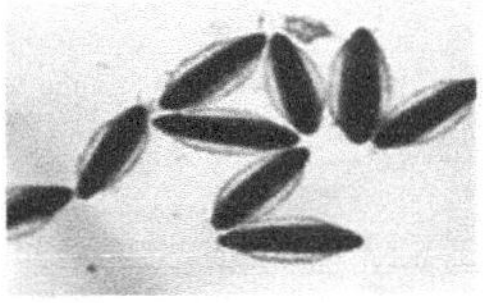

C. Eggs of Anopheles

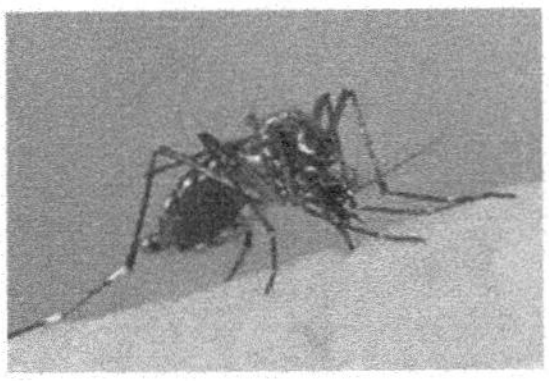

D. Aedes mosquito

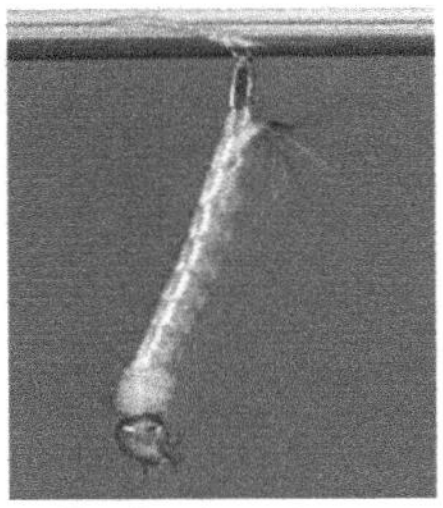

E. Aedes larva

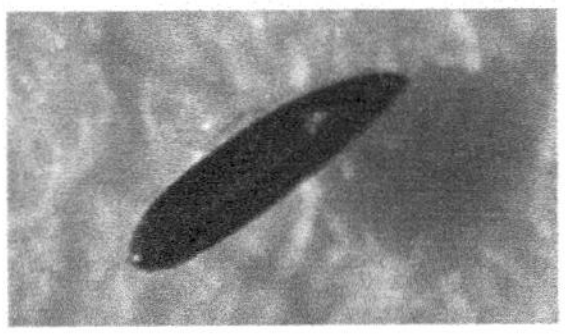

F. Eggs of Aedes

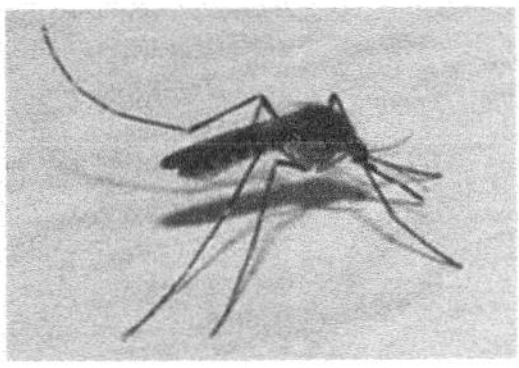

G. Culex mosquito

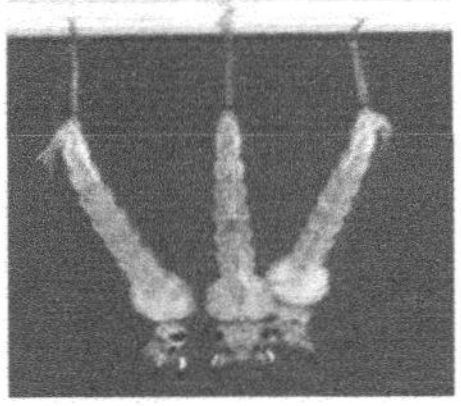

H. Culex larva

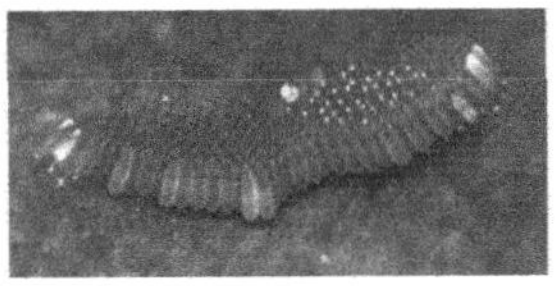

I. Eggs of Culex

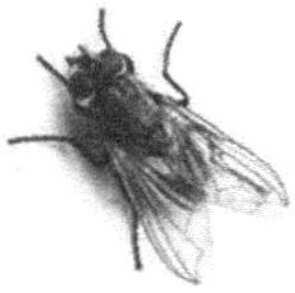

J. Housefly

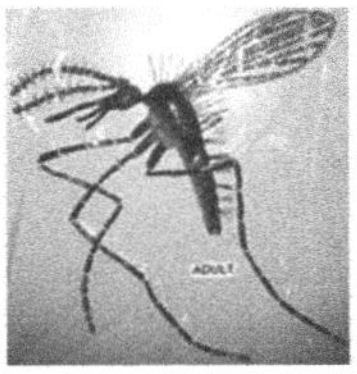

K. Sandfly

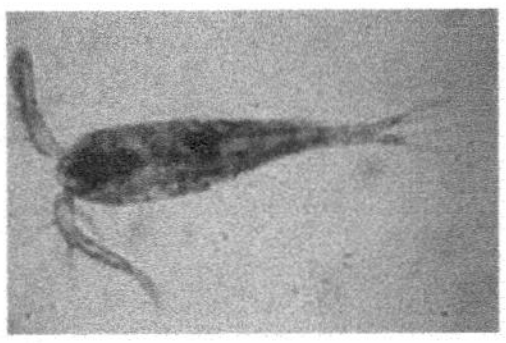

L. Cyclops

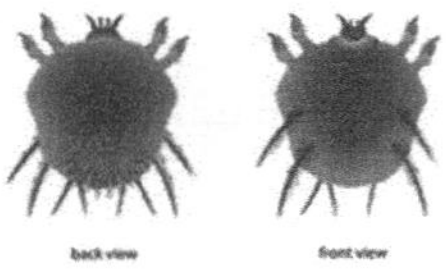

M. Itch mite

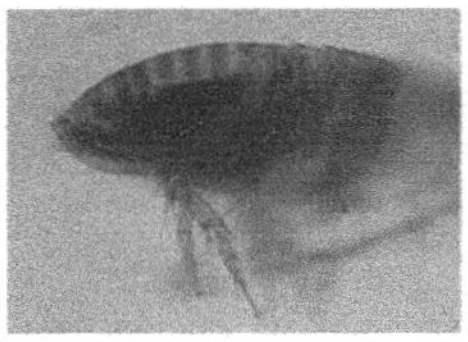

N. Cyclops

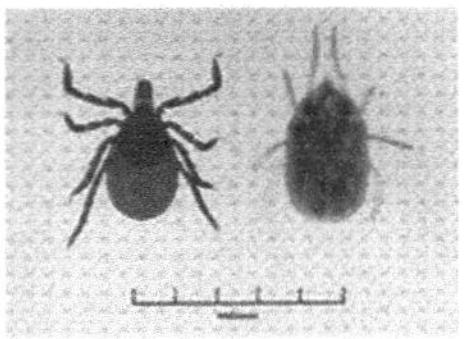

O. Hard tick (L), Soft tick (R)

Suggested spots:
Pupa of Anopheles, Culex and Aedes, Louse.

Frequently Asked Questions

Questions Common to All Entomology Spots

1. Identify the given spot.
2. Write two identifying features of the given spot.
3. What are the diseases transmitted by the given vector?
4. What is public health importance of the given spot?
5. What are the prevention and control measures for the given spot.
6. What is the breeding site of the given spot?
7. What is the flight range of the given spot?
8. What are the feeding and biting habits of the given spot?

Questions Specific to Various Vectors

1. What is Aedes aegypti index? (Aedes)
2. How is the nit attached to the strand? (Louse)
3. Name three factors that favour the spread of lice. (Louse)
4. Name some flea indices used in flea surveys. (Rat flea)
5. What is the public health importance of flea indices? (Rat flea)
6. What is the permanent measure to control guineaworm disease?
7. What is the mechanism of disease transmission for the given spot? (Housefly)

STUDENT'S NOTES

Supervisor's Signature

CHAPTER 6

Insecticides

Date:__________

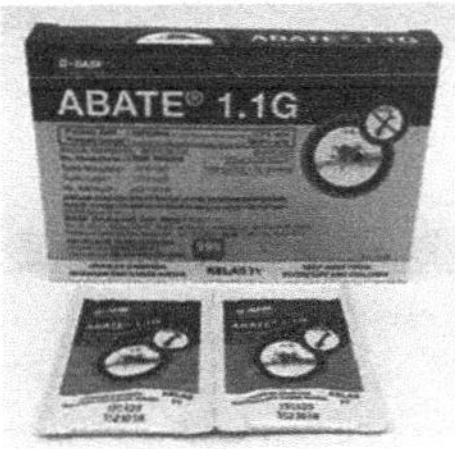

A. Abate

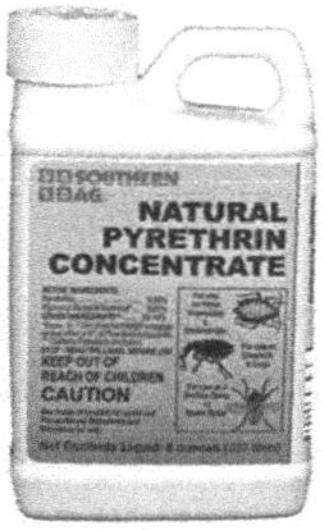

B. Pyrethrum

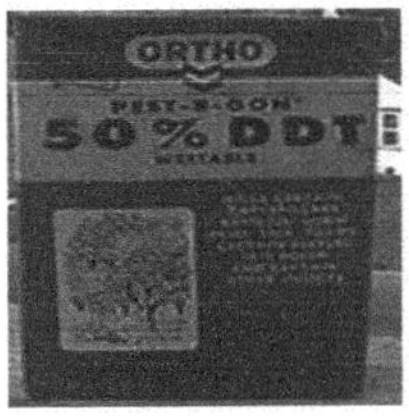

C. DDT

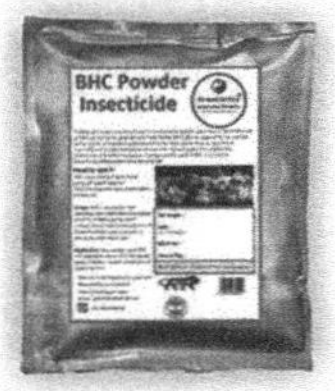

D. BHC

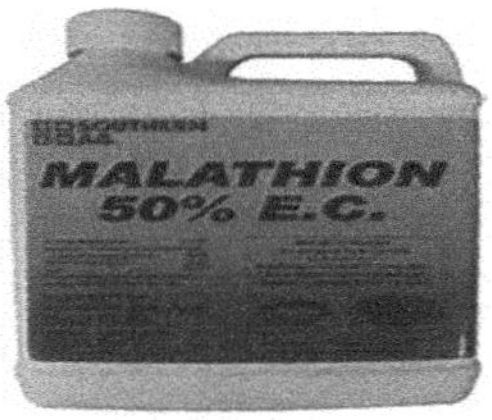

E. Malathion

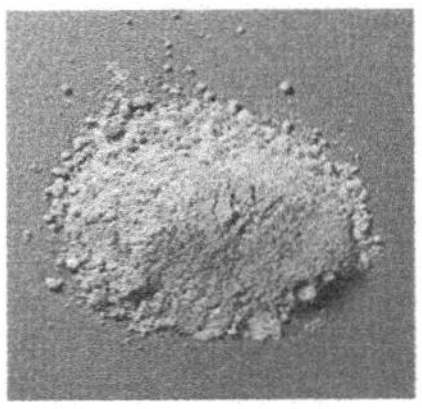
F. Paris Green

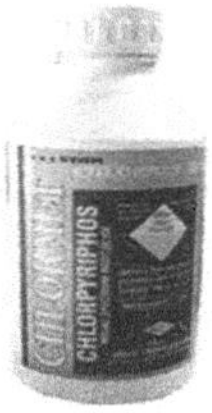

G. Chlorpyriphos

Suggested spots:

Rodenticide powder.

FREQUENTLY ASKED QUESTIONS

1. Identify the given spot.
2. Name two vectors against which the chemical is used.
3. Write the mechanism of action of the given spot.
4. What is the dose of the given spot?
5. Write the mode of application of the given spot.
6. What are the side effects and antidote for the given spot?

STUDENT'S NOTES

Supervisor's Signature

CHAPTER 7

Environment

Date:______________

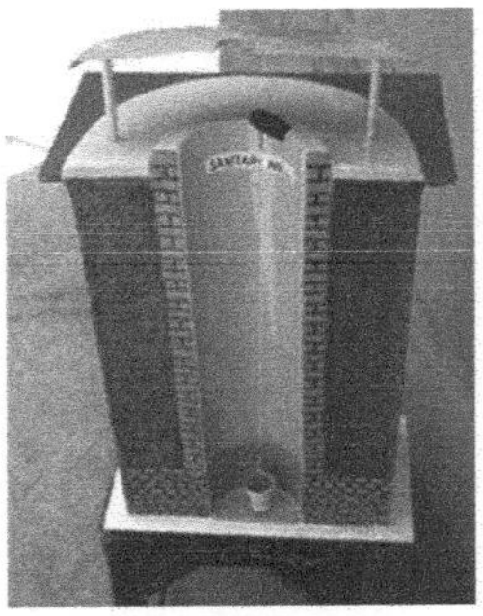

A. Sanitary well

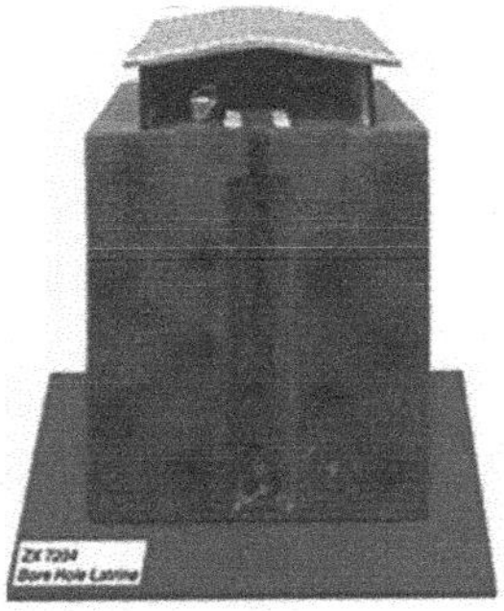

B. Bore hole latrine

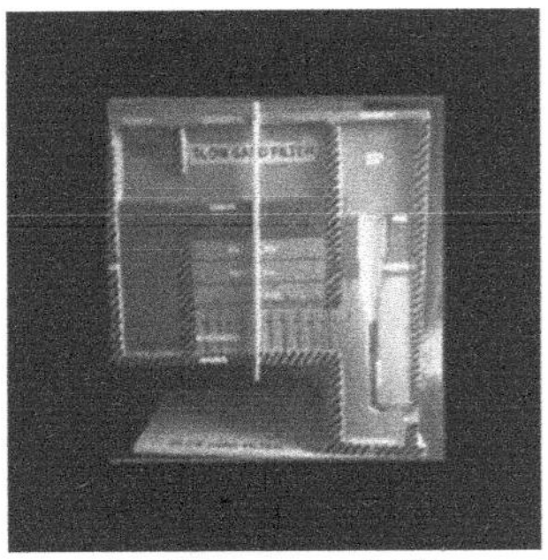

C. Slow sand filter

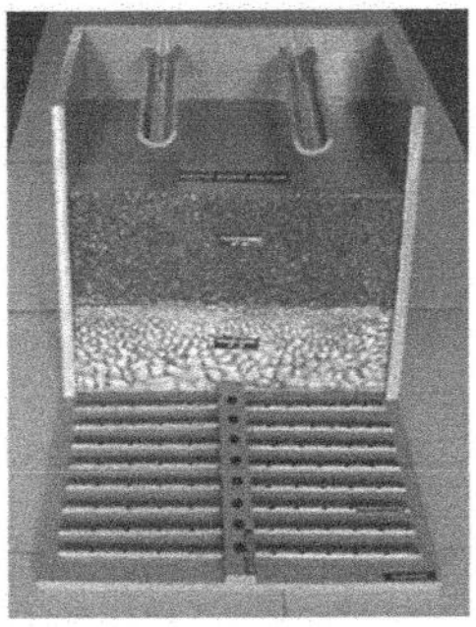

D. Rapid sand filter

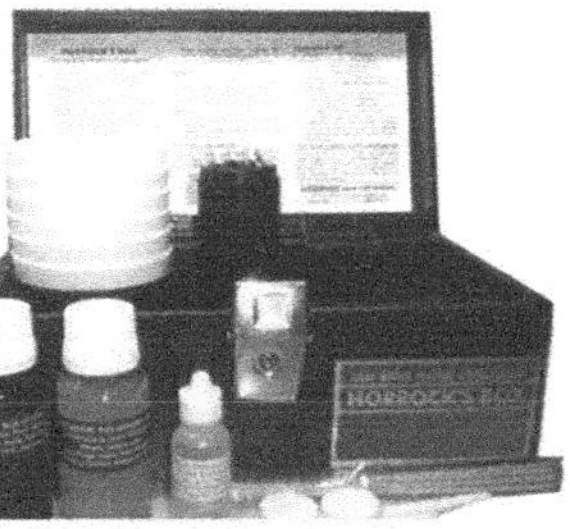

E. Horrocks apparatus

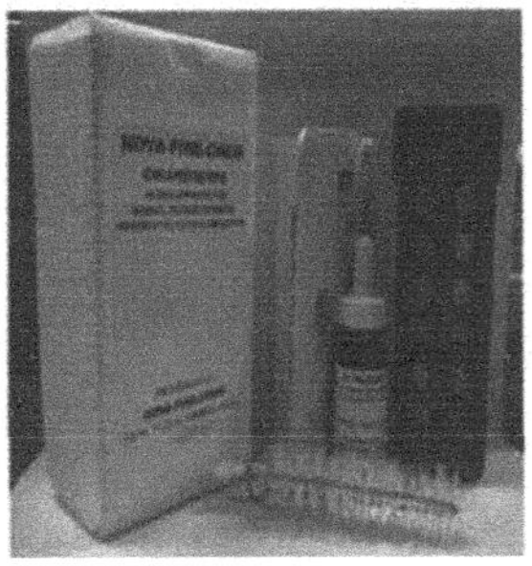

F. Chloroscope

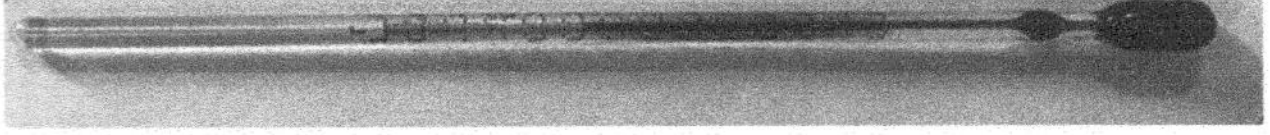

G. Kata thermometer

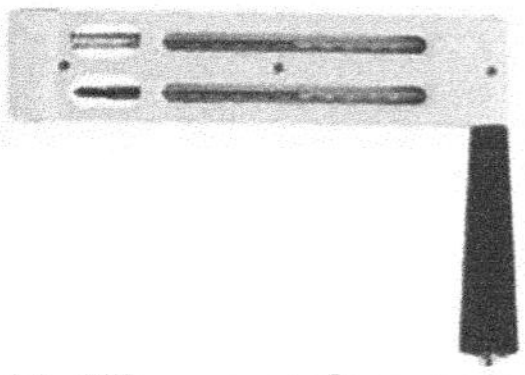

H. Sling psychrometer

Suggested spots:
Minimum and maximum thermometer, trench latrine.

FREQUENTLY ASKED QUESTIONS

1. Identify the given spots and write two identifying features.
2. What is the public health importance of the given spot?
3. Write any two advantages/ disadvantages of the given spot.

STUDENT'S NOTES

Supervisor's Signature

CHAPTER 8

Antisepsis and Disinfection

Date:____________

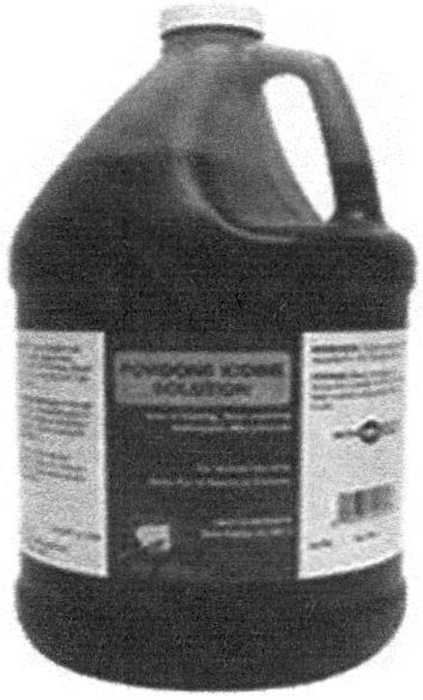

A. Povidone iodine

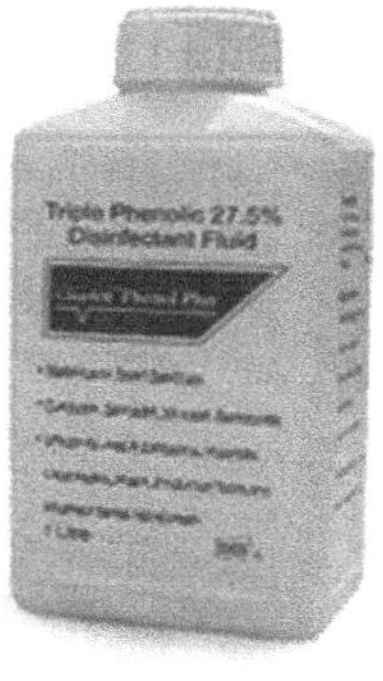

B. Crude Phenol

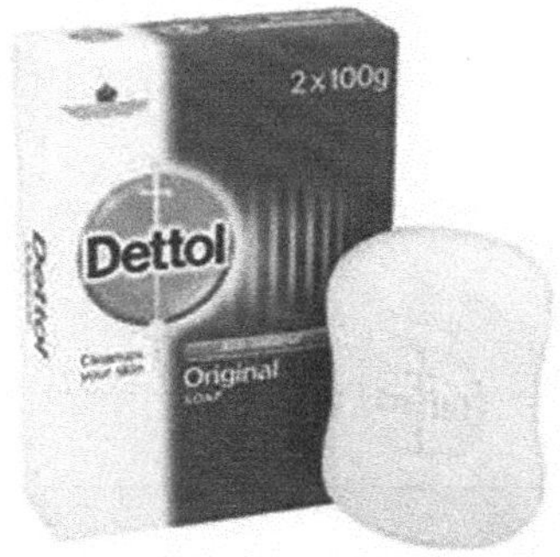

C. Soap

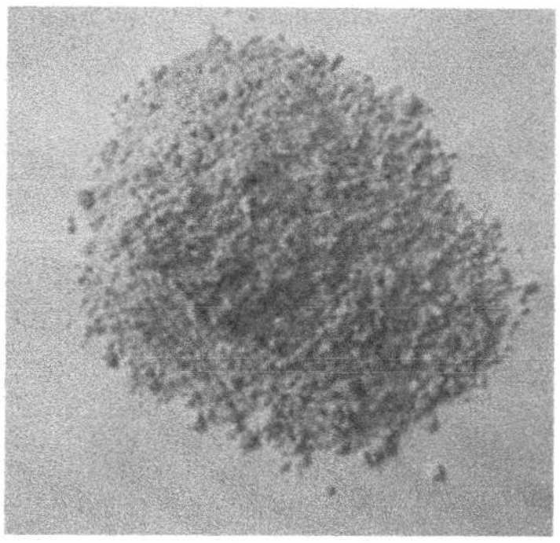

D. Bleaching powder

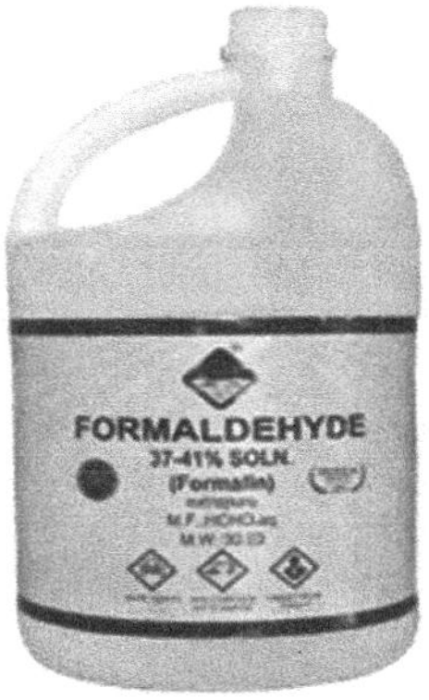

E. Formalin

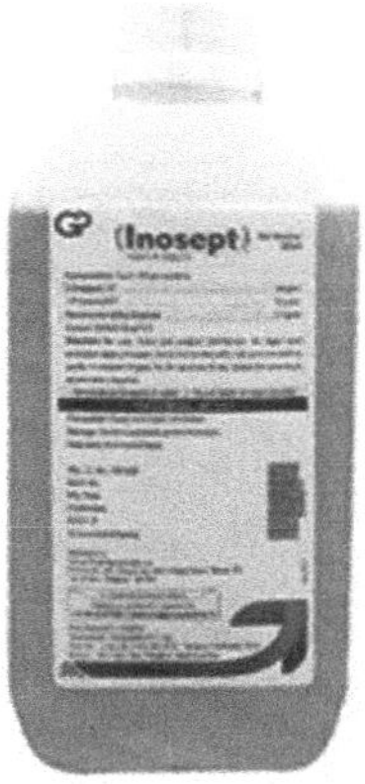

F. Alcohol hand rub

Suggested spots:
Savlon, Dettol.

FREQUENTLY ASKED QUESTIONS

1. Identify the spot and write its constituents.
2. What is the mechanism of action of the given spot?
3. What is the difference between antiseptic and disinfectant?
4. What is the public health importance of the given spot?

STUDENT'S NOTES

Supervisor's Signature

CHAPTER 9

National Health Programmes

Date:__________

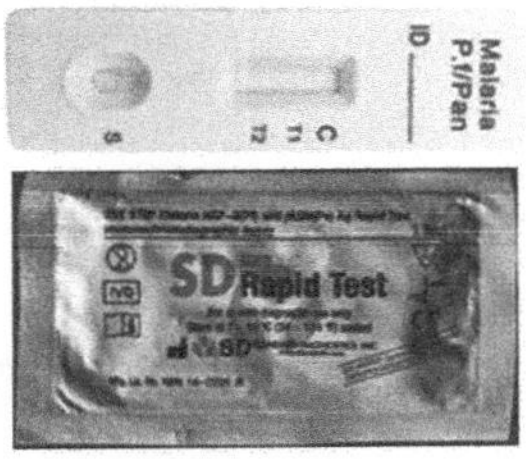

A. Rapid detection kit (RDT)– Malaria

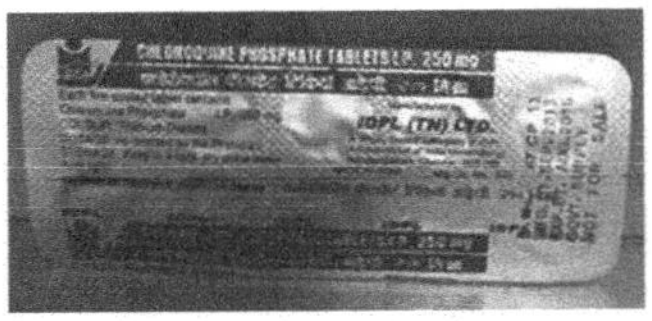

B. Chloroquine

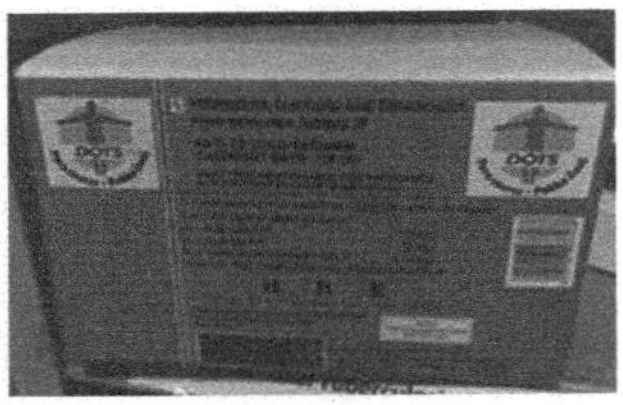

C. DOTS regimen box

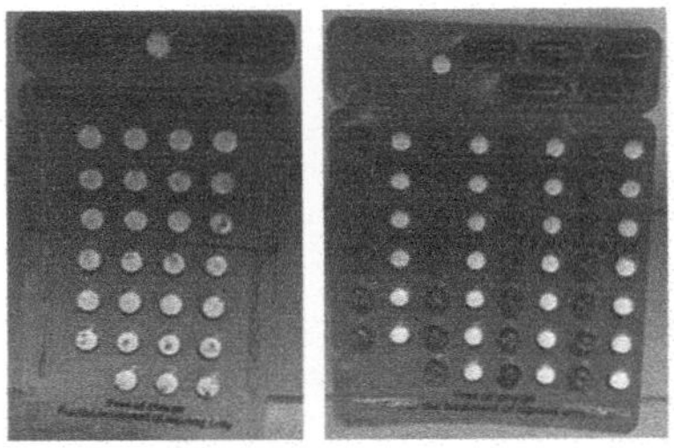

D. MDT for Leprosy (Paucibacillary (L); Multibacillary (R)

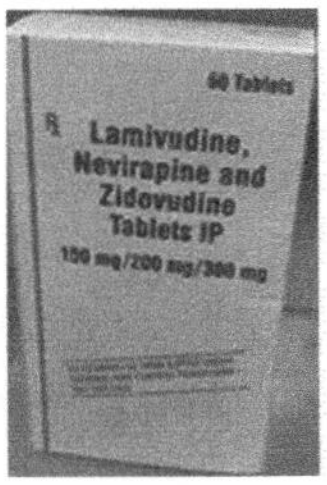

E. Lamivudine, nevirapine and Zidovudine tablets

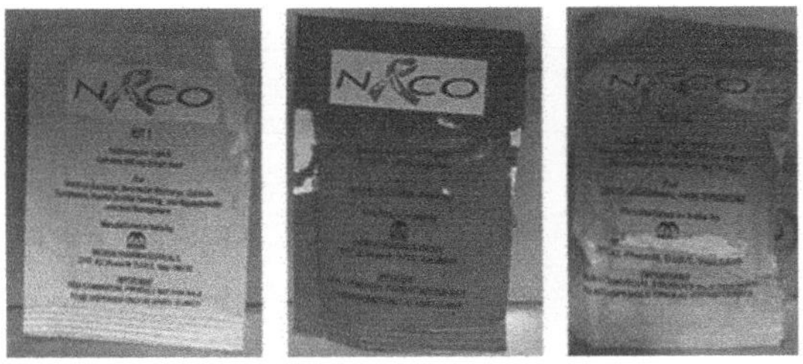

F. Kits used in syndromic management of STI/RTI's

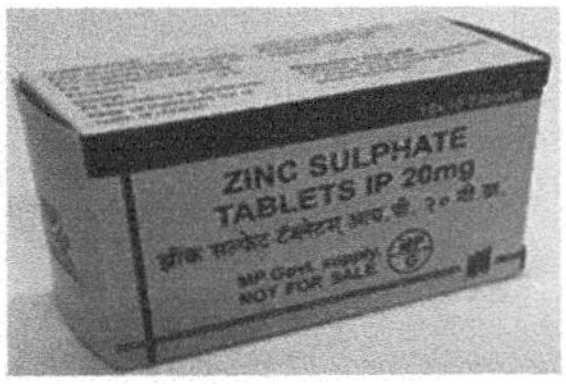

G. Zinc tablets

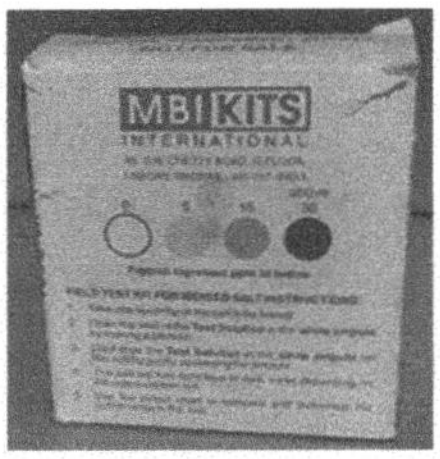

H. MBI Kit for testing of iodine

Frequently Asked Questions

Questions Common to National Health Programs

1. Name the national health program under which this medicine is used?
2. Write the indications and side effects of this drug.
3. Name the disease/syndrome in which this kit is used?
4. Mention the drug present in the given spot along with its dosage.
5. What is the public health importance of the given spot?

Specific Questions

1. What is the recommended concentration of iodine at production and consumer level in the salt? (iodised salt)
2. What is the mode of administration of MDT for PB and MB leprosy? (MDT for leprosy)
3. What is the importance of top row and the rest of the blisters in the pack? (MDT for leprosy)
4. Which issue does DOTS plus strategy address?
5. What is the interpretation if (a) only one line appears (b) two lines appear (C) no line appears? Rapid Diagnostic Test (RDT) (RDT kit for malaria)
6. What are the advantages of RDT over microscopy for malaria? (RDT kit for malaria)
7. What are the disadvantages of RDT over microscopy for malaria? (RDT kit for malaria)

STUDENT'S NOTES

Supervisor's Signature

Volume 3

Practical Manual & Logbook in Community Medicine

(Based on Latest CBME)

(Includes Family Adoption Programme)

Revised and Updated

Authors

Dr. Priya Arora
Professor, Community Medicine
Army College of Medical Sciences
New Delhi

Dr. Pooja Goyal
Professor & Head, Community Medicine
ESIC Medical College and Hospital
Faridabad, Haryana

Dr. Shveta Lukhmana
Associate Professor, Community Medicine
VMMC and Safdarjung Hospital
New Delhi

Dr. Abhishek Singh
Associate Professor, Community Medicine
SHKM Government Medical College
Mewat, Haryana

Foreword By

- **Col. (Dr) Puja Dudeja**
- **Dr. Abhishek V. Raut**
- **Dr. Prasanna Mithra P.**
- **Dr. Avijit Roy**

Peepee Publishers and Distributors Private Limited®

Practical Manual & Logbook in Community Medicine (Based on Latest CBME)

Published by
Pawaninder P. Vij and Anupam Vij

Peepee Publishers and Distributors Private Limited
Head Office: 160, Shakti Vihar, Pitam Pura, Delhi-110 034 (India)

Correspondence Address:
7/31, First Floor, Ansari Road, Daryaganj
New Delhi-110 002 (India)

Ph: 41512412, 9811156083

e-mail: peepee160@yahoo.co.in

e-mail: peepee160@gmail.com

www.peepeepub.com

join us on facebook.com/pp.publishers

LM-03

First Edition: 2022

Revised and Updated: 2025

ISBN: 978-81-9651-878-3

Contents

Volume 3

Section VII: Self Directed Learning (SDL)

Section VIII: Logbook

Section VII

Self Directed Learning (SDL)

Chapter 1

Introduction

The goal of medical education is to create a medical professional who is a clinician, leader, and lifelong learner. Lifelong learning is essential to endure rapidly growing medical knowledge.

Professional wise teaching hours allotted for SDL in Community Medicine.

Professional	Self directed learning (hours)
First Prof	5
Second Prof	10
Third Prof (Part 1)	5

Source: "Regulations on Graduate Medical Education (Amendment), 2019"

What is Self Directed Learning (SDL)?

Self-directed learning is "a process in which individuals take the initiative, with or without the help of others, in diagnosing their learning needs, formulating goals, identifying human and material resources for learning, choosing and implementing appropriate learning strategies, and evaluating learning outcomes." (Malcom Knowles, 1975).

Why SDL is Required: To keep students engaged and to learn at their own pace.

Self Directed Learning Activities

- Setting own learning goals
- Identifying appropriate learning resources
- Selecting appropriate learning strategies
- Selecting important from unimportant
- Integrating material from different resources
- Time management
- Monitoring achievement of learning outcomes
- Monitoring effectiveness of own study habits

Suggested Learning Aids: Hardcopy, digital accessibility, content control, location free (mobile learning)

Suggested Teaching-Learning Methods: Problem based learning, Role play, debate, student directed seminars, panel discussions

Suggested Assessment Methods: Participation in the activity, Reflection, Case scenarios that test problem solving.

Chapter 2

Self Directed Learning (SDL)

SDL No.	Topic	Hours Allotted	Competency	Supervisor's Signature with Date	Grade
2.1					
2.2					
2.3					
2.4					
2.5					
2.6					
2.7					
2.8					
2.9					
2.10					
3.1					
3.2					
3.3					
3.4					
3.5					
3.6					
3.7					
3.8					
3.9					
3.10					
3.11					
3.12					
3.13					
3.14					
3.15					
3.16					
3.17					
3.18					
3.19					
3.20					

SDL 2.1

Name of Facilitator: ____________________ Date: ____________

Time Allotted: ____________________ Competency: ____________

Topic: ____

Exercise given: ____

Details of activity: ____

Reflection:

Supervisor's Signature

SDL 2.2

Name of Facilitator: ______________________ Date: ______________

Time Allotted: ______________________ Competency: ______________

Topic: ____

Exercise given: ______________________________________

Details of activity: ___________________________________

Reflection:

Supervisor's Signature

SDL 2.3

Name of Facilitator: ______________________ Date: ______________

Time Allotted: ______________________ Competency: ______________

Topic: ____

Exercise given: ____

Details of activity: ____

Reflection:

Supervisor's Signature

SDL 2.4

Name of Facilitator: ______________________ Date: ______________

Time Allotted: ______________________ Competency: ______________

Topic: ____

Exercise given: ____

Details of activity: ____

Reflection:

Supervisor's Signature

SDL 2.5

Name of Facilitator: ______________________ Date: ______________

Time Allotted: ______________________ Competency: ______________

Topic: ____

Exercise given: ______________________________________

Details of activity: ____________________________________

Reflection:

Supervisor's Signature

SDL 2.6

Name of Facilitator: ______________________ Date: ______________

Time Allotted: ______________________ Competency: ______________

Topic: ____

Exercise given: ______________________________________

Details of activity: ____________________________________

Reflection:

Supervisor's Signature

SDL 2.7

Name of Facilitator: ______________________ Date: ______________

Time Allotted: ______________________ Competency: ______________

Topic: ____

Exercise given: ____

Details of activity: ____

Reflection:

Supervisor's Signature

SDL 2.8

Name of Facilitator: ______________________ Date: ______________

Time Allotted: ______________________ Competency: ______________

Topic: ____

Exercise given: ____

Details of activity: ____

Reflection:

Supervisor's Signature

SDL 2.9

Name of Facilitator: ______________________ Date: ______________

Time Allotted: ______________________ Competency: ______________

Topic: ____

Exercise given: ____

Details of activity: ____

Reflection:

Supervisor's Signature

SDL 2.10

Name of Facilitator: ______________________ Date: ______________

Time Allotted: ______________________ Competency: ______________

Topic: ____

Exercise given: ____

Details of activity: ____

Reflection:

Supervisor's Signature

SDL 3.1

Name of Facilitator: ______________________ Date: ______________

Time Allotted: ______________________ Competency: ______________

Topic: ____

Exercise given: ____

Details of activity: ____

Reflection:

Supervisor's Signature

SDL 3.2

Name of Facilitator: ______________________ Date: ______________

Time Allotted: ______________________ Competency: ______________

Topic: ____

Exercise given: ____

Details of activity: ____

Reflection:

Supervisor's Signature

SDL 3.3

Name of Facilitator: ____________________ Date: ____________

Time Allotted: ____________________ Competency: ____________

Topic: ____

Exercise given: ____

Details of activity: ____

Reflection:

Supervisor's Signature

SDL 3.4

Name of Facilitator: ______________________ Date: ______________

Time Allotted: ______________________ Competency: ______________

Topic: ____

Exercise given: ____

Details of activity: ____

Reflection:

Supervisor's Signature

SDL 3.5

Name of Facilitator: ______________________ Date: ______________

Time Allotted: ______________________ Competency: ______________

Topic: ____

Exercise given: ____

Details of activity: ____

Reflection:

Supervisor's Signature

SDL 3.6

Name of Facilitator: ______________________ Date: ______________

Time Allotted: ______________________ Competency: ______________

Topic: ____

Exercise given: ____

Details of activity: ____

Reflection:

Supervisor's Signature

SDL 3.7

Name of Facilitator: ____________________ Date: ____________

Time Allotted: ____________________ Competency:____________

Topic: ____

Exercise given: ____________________________________

Details of activity: ________________________________

Reflection:

Supervisor's Signature

SDL 3.8

Name of Facilitator: ______________________ Date: ______________

Time Allotted: ______________________ Competency: ______________

Topic: ____

Exercise given: ____

Details of activity: _____________________________________

Reflection:

Supervisor's Signature

SDL 3.9

Name of Facilitator: ____________________ Date: __________

Time Allotted: ____________________ Competency: __________

Topic: ____

Exercise given: ____

Details of activity: ____

Reflection:

Supervisor's Signature

SDL 3.10

Name of Facilitator: ____________________ Date: __________

Time Allotted: ____________________ Competency: __________

Topic: ______________________________

Exercise given: ______________________________

Details of activity: ______________________________

Reflection:

Supervisor's Signature

SDL 3.11

Name of Facilitator: ____________________ Date: __________

Time Allotted: ____________________ Competency: __________

Topic: ______________________________

Exercise given: ______________________________

Details of activity: ______________________________

Reflection:

Supervisor's Signature

SDL 3.12

Name of Facilitator: ______________________ Date: ______________

Time Allotted: ______________________ Competency: ______________

Topic: ____

Exercise given: ______________________________________

Details of activity: ___________________________________

Reflection:

Supervisor's Signature

SDL 3.13

Name of Facilitator: ______________________ Date: ______________

Time Allotted: ______________________ Competency: ______________

Topic: ____

Exercise given: ____

Details of activity: ____

Reflection:

Supervisor's Signature

SDL 3.14

Name of Facilitator: ____________________ Date: ____________

Time Allotted: ____________________ Competency: ____________

Topic: ____

Exercise given: ____

Details of activity: ____

Reflection:

Supervisor's Signature

SDL 3.15

Name of Facilitator: ______________________ Date: ______________

Time Allotted: ______________________ Competency: ______________

Topic: ____

Exercise given: ____

Details of activity: ____

Reflection:

Supervisor's Signature

SDL 3.16

Name of Facilitator: ______________________ Date: ______________

Time Allotted: ______________________ Competency: ______________

Topic: ____

Exercise given: ____

Details of activity: ____

Reflection:

Supervisor's Signature

SDL 3.17

Name of Facilitator: ______________________ Date: ______________

Time Allotted: ______________________ Competency: ______________

Topic: ____

Exercise given: ______________________________________

Details of activity: ___________________________________

Reflection:

Supervisor's Signature

SDL 3.18

Name of Facilitator: ______________________________ Date: __________________

Time Allotted: ______________________________ Competency: __________________

Topic: ____

Exercise given: ____

Details of activity: ____

Reflection:

Supervisor's Signature

SDL 3.19

Name of Facilitator: ______________________ Date: ______________

Time Allotted: ______________________ Competency: ______________

Topic: ____

Exercise given: ______________________________________

Details of activity: ____________________________________

Reflection:

Supervisor's Signature

SDL 3.20

Name of Facilitator: ______________________ Date: ______________

Time Allotted: ______________________ Competency: ______________

Topic: ______________________

Exercise given: ______________________

Details of activity: ______________________

Reflection:

Supervisor's Signature

Section VIII

Logbook

General Instructions

1. The logbook is a record of the academic / co-curricular activities of the designated student, who would be responsible for maintaining his/her logbook.
2. The student is responsible for getting the entries in the logbook verified by the Faculty in charge regularly.
3. Entries in the logbook will reflect the activities undertaken in the department and have to be scrutinized by the Head of the concerned department.
4. The logbook is a record of various activities by the student like:
   (a) Overall participation and performance
   (b) Attendance
   (c) Participation in sessions
   (d) Record of completion of pre-determined activities
   (e) Acquisition of selected competencies

Section VIII: Logbook

Contents

Chapter 1

Certificate

This is to certify that the candidate Mr/ Ms ______________________________,

Univ Reg No. ____________, admitted in the year 20 ____- ____ in the ______________________

______________________ Medical College, ______________________ has satisfactorily completed / has not completed all assignments /requirements mentioned in this logbook for MBBBS course in the subject of Community Medicine /AETCOM/Foundation Course during the period from ______________________ to______________________ .

She / He is /is not eligible to appear for the summative (University) assessment as on the date given below.

Signature of Faculty
Name and Designation

Countersigned by Head of the Department

Principal/Dean of the College

Date: ____________

Place: ____________

Chapter 2

Eligibility for Appearing in University Exams

ATTENDANCE

(a) Attendance requirements are 75% in theory and 80% in practical /clinical for eligibility to appear for the examinations in the subject. In subjects that are taught in more than one phase – the learner must have 75% attendance in theory and 80% in practical in each phase of instruction in that subject.

(b) 75% attendance in Professional Development Programme (AETCOM Module) is required for eligibility to appear for final examination in each professional year.

(c) 75% attendance in the electives and submission of log book maintained during elective is required for eligibility to appear in the final MBBS examination.

Internal Assessment:

1. Regular periodic examinations shall be conducted throughout the course. There shall be no less than three internal assessment examinations in each Preclinical / Para-clinical subject and no less than two examinations in each clinical subject in a professional year. An end of posting clinical assessment shall be conducted for each clinical posting in each professional year.
2. Learners must secure at least 50% marks of the total marks (combined in theory and practical/ clinical; not less than 40 % marks in theory and practical separately) assigned for internal assessment in a particular subject in order to be eligible for appearing at the final University examination of that subject.

Students Signature **Parent's Signature**

Name: **Name:**

Roll Number: **Phone Number:**

Phone Number:

Chapter 3

Record of Self Directed Learning

The SSDL model

Stage	Student	Teacher	Examples
Stage 1	Dependent	Authority Coach	Coaching with immediate feedback. Drill, Informational lecture. Overcoming deficiencies and resistance
Stage 2	Interested	Motivator, Guide	Inspiring lecture plus guided discussion. Goal-setting and learning strategies
Stage 3	Involved	Facilitator	Discussion facilitated teacher who participates as equal, Seminar, Group projects
Stage 4	Self Directed	Consultant Delegator	Internship, dissertation, individual work or self directed study-group

The Staged Self Directed Learning Model, G. Grow

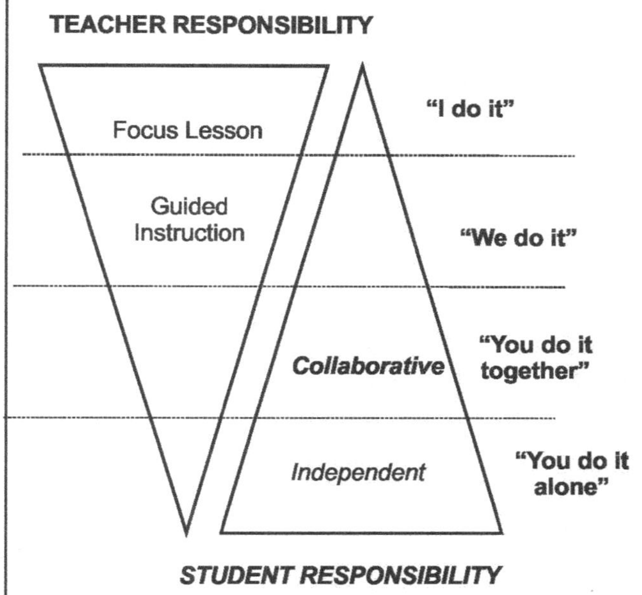

A Model for Success for All Students

Fisher D. and Frey N. (2008). *Better learning through structured teaching: A framework for the gradual release of responsibility.* Alexandria, VA: Association for Supervision and Curriculum Development.

Source: Academic Cell, Medical Council of India, 2019

A. SDL Grading Second Professional Year (10 Hours)

1	2	3	4	5	6	7	8	9	10
S. No.	Comptency addressed	Name of activity	Date completed dd-mm-yyyy	Attempt at activity First or Only(F)/ Repeat (R)/ Remedial (Re)	Rating Below expectations (B)/Meets expectations (M)/Exceed expectations (E)	Decision of faculty Completed (C)/Repeat (R)/ Remedial (Re)	Initial of faculty and date	Feedback received Initial of learner	Page no.

B. SDL Grading Third Professional Year Part I (20 Hours)

1	2	3	4	5	6	7	8	9	10
S. No.	Comptency addressed	Name of activity	Date completed dd-mm-yyyy	Attempt at activity First or Only(F)/ Repeat (R)/ Remedial (Re)	Rating Below expectations (B)/Meets expectations (M)/Exceed expectations (E)	Decision of faculty Completed (C)/Repeat (R)/ Remedial (Re)	Initial of faculty and date	Feedback received Initial of learner	Page no.

1	2	3	4	5	6	7	8	9	10
S. No.	Comptency addressed	Name of activity	Date completed dd-mm-yyyy	Attempt at activity First or Only(F)/ Repeat (R)/ Remedial (Re)	Rating Below expectations (B)/Meets expectations (M)/Exceed expectations (E)	Decision of faculty Completed (C)/Repeat (R)/ Remedial (Re)	Initial of faculty and date	Feedback received Initial of learner	Page no.

Chapter 4

Instructions for Attitude, Ethics and Communication Module (AETCOM)

According to Gazette notification, "Regulations on Graduate Medical Education (Amendment), 2019":

1. This will be a longitudinal programme spread across the continuum of the MBBS programme including internship,
2. Learning experiences may include – small group discussions, patient care scenarios, workshop, seminars, role plays, lectures etc.
3. Attitude, Ethics andCommunication Module (AETCOM module) developed by Medical Council of India should be used longitudinally for purposes of instruction.
4. 75% attendance in Professional Development Programme (AETCOM Module) is required for eligibility to appear for final examination in each professional year.
5. Internal Assessment will include:
   (a) Written tests comprising of short notes and creative writing experiences,
   (b) OSCE based clinical scenarios / viva voce.
6. At least one question in each paper of the clinical specialties in the University examination should test knowledge competencies acquired during the professional development programme.
7. Skill competencies acquired during the Professional Development Programme must be tested during the clinical, practical and viva voce.

CHAPTER 5

Instructions for Pandemic Management Module

Longitudinal Module on Management of Pandemics for MBBS Course

Period	Module	Broad areas	No. of hours	Major department(s) to coordinate
Phase II	2.2	Emerging and Re-emerging infections, early identification and control of new infections	6	Community Medicine
	2.4	Vaccination strategies including vaccine development and Implementation	6	Community Medicine, Biochemistry
Phase III Part 1	3.1	Outbreak Management including Quarantine, Isolation, Contact Tracing	5	Community Medicine
	3.2	Interdisciplinary Collaboration, Principles of Public Health Administration, Health Economics, International Health	5	Community Medicine
	3.3	Operational Research, Field work, Surveillance	8	Community Medicine
Electives		Epidemiology and research Components		Community Medicine

(Ref: Medical Council of India, Module on Pandemic Management, August 2020)

CHAPTER 6

Record of DOAP/Shows–How Competencies Including AETCOM Module and Pandemic Management Module

Millers Pyramid Clinical Competence

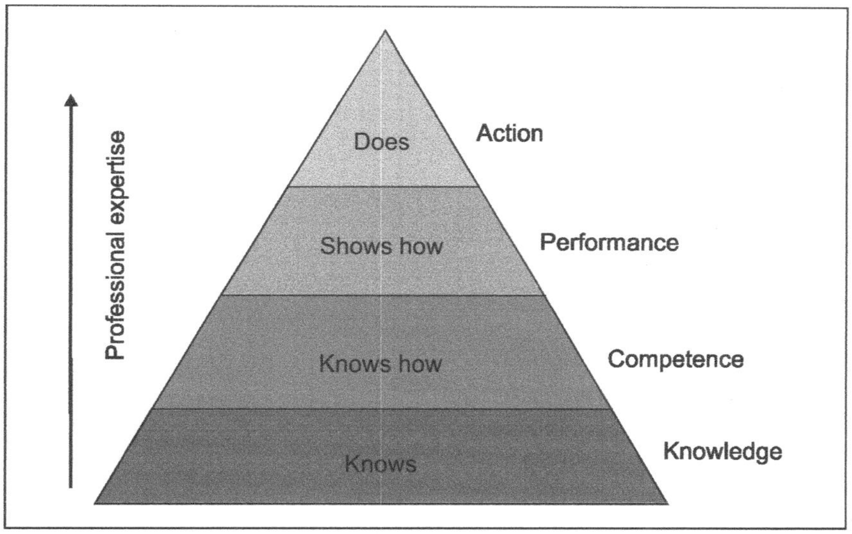

Note: As per "Competency Based Undergraduate Curriculum for the Indian Medical Graduate", 2018:

In the table of competency - the highest level of competency acquired is specified and implies that the lower levels have been acquired already. Therefore, when a student is able to SH - Show how, it is presumed that the preceding steps - the knowledge, the analytical skills, the skill of communicating have all been obtained.

It may also be noted that attainment of the highest level of competency may be obtained through steps spread over several subjects or phases and not necessarily in the subject or the phase in which the competency has been identified. Therefore, the 'Logbook' includes only higher level of competencies.

Certifiable Competencies

1	2	3	4	5	6	7	8	9
S. No.	Competency addressed	Name of activity	Date completed dd-mm-yyyy	Attempt at activity First or Only (F)/ Repeat (R)/ Remedial (Re)	Rating Below expectations (B)/Meets expectations (M)/Exceed expectations (E)	Decision of faculty Completed (C)/Repeat (R)/ Remedial (Re)	Initial of faculty and date	Feedback received Initial of learner

Certifiable Competencies

1	2	3	4	5	6	7	8	9
S. No.	Competency addressed	Name of activity	Date completed dd-mm-yyyy	Attempt at activity First or Only (F)/ Repeat (R)/ Remedial (Re)	Rating Below expectations (B)/Meets expectations (M)/Exceed expectations (E)	Decision of faculty Completed (C)/Repeat (R)/ Remedial (Re)	Initial of faculty and date	Feedback received Initial of learner

Certifiable Competencies

1	2	3	4	5	6	7	8	9
S. No.	Competency addressed	Name of activity	Date completed dd-mm-yyyy	Attempt at activity First or Only (F)/ Repeat (R)/ Remedial (Re)	Rating Below expectations (B)/Meets expectations (M)/Exceed expectations (E)	Decision of faculty Completed (C)/Repeat (R)/ Remedial (Re)	Initial of faculty and date	Feedback received Initial of learner

Certifiable Competencies

1	2	3	4	5	6	7	8	9
S. No.	Competency addressed	Name of activity	Date completed dd-mm-yyyy	Attempt at activity First or Only (F)/ Repeat (R)/ Remedial (Re)	Rating Below expectations (B)/Meets expectations (M)/Exceed expectations (E)	Decision of faculty Completed (C)/Repeat (R)/ Remedial (Re)	Initial of faculty and date	Feedback received Initial of learner

Certifiable Competencies

1	2	3	4	5	6	7	8	9
S. No.	Competency addressed	Name of activity	Date completed dd-mm-yyyy	Attempt at activity First or Only (F)/ Repeat (R)/ Remedial (Re)	Rating Below expectations (B)/Meets expectations (M)/Exceed expectations (E)	Decision of faculty Completed (C)/Repeat (R)/ Remedial (Re)	Initial of faculty and date	Feedback received Initial of learner

Certifiable Competencies

1	2	3	4	5	6	7	8	9
S. No.	Competency addressed	Name of activity	Date completed dd-mm-yyyy	Attempt at activity First or Only (F)/ Repeat (R)/ Remedial (Re)	Rating Below expectations (B)/Meets expectations (M)/Exceed expectations (E)	Decision of faculty Completed (C)/Repeat (R)/ Remedial (Re)	Initial of faculty and date	Feedback received Initial of learner

Chapter 7

Attendance Record

S. No.	From and to Date	Theory (%)	Practical (%)	Sign of student	Sign of teacher
1	First MBBS				
2	Second MBBS				
3	Third MBBS Part I				
	Total				

Signature of Head of the Department

A. Record of Assessment (Theory)

S. No.	Phase	Activity	Date of Assessment	Marks Obtained	Maximum Marks

B. Record of Assessment (Practical)

S. No.	Phase	Activity	Date of Assessment	Marks Obtained	Maximum Marks

Signature of Head of the Department

CHAPTER 8

Records of Internal Assessment

Final Internal Calculation	
Theory (Out of 100)	
Practical (Out of 100)	

Signature of Head of the Department

Chapter 9

Electives (If Applicable)

1. Elective is the brief course made available to learner during undergraduate study period. Students can choose from available options depending upon:
   - Their interest
   - Career preferences
2. The learner shall rotate through two elective blocks of 04 weeks each. In 1st four of the eight weeks of electives, regular clinical postings shall be accommodated.

   Block-1

   Preclinical/ para-clinical/ other basic sciences laboratory

   OR

   Under a faculty researcher in an ongoing research project

   Block-2

   Clinical department (including specialties, super-specialties, ICUs, blood bank and casualty) from a list of electives developed and available in the institution

   OR

   Supervised learning experience at a rural/ urban community clinic
3. 75% attendance mandatory in Electives
4. Students to be assessed in between and at end of elective posting
5. Feedback, comments and /or grades by faculty mentor
6. Performance of students in electives to contribute towards internal marks

   Examples of Electives Settings in Community Medicine

Block 1

1. Community outreach experience

Assisted living

Hospice care

School Health programs

Community outreach for National Health Programs

Maternal and child health outreach

2. **Research**

Community and epidemiologic surveys

Block 2

Urban or Rural Community Experience

- Rural Community Health Centtre
- Primary Health Centre
- Corporation Health Centre
- Selected Private Primary Care Clinic

Source: Medical Council of India. Electives for the Undergraduate Medical Education Training Program, 2020: p 1- 30.

Other Suggested Areas for Electives:

- Research Methods (Quantitative, Qualitative, Mixed-Methods)
- Data Handling and Management
- Inventory Techniques

Chapter 10

Details of Elective

1. **Name of Block:**
2. **Title of Elective:**
3. **Duration:**
4. **Location of Elective:**
5. **Name of Internal Preceptor(s):**
6. **Name of External Preceptors (if any):**
7. **Learning Objectives:**
8. **Prerequisite:**
9. **Learning Resources:**
10. **List of activities in which student participated:**
11. **Portfolio Entry (Portfolio to be submitted separately):**
12. **Log-book entries (Completed /Not completed):**
13. **Assessment:**
14. **Comments:**

*Assessment Details to be entered in the logbook by the Preceptor

Signature of Head of the Department

STUDENT'S NOTES

STUDENT'S NOTES

Supervisor's Signature

CHAPTER 11

Family Adoption Logbook

Professional year	Visit number	Date	Objective	Rating by supervisor Below expectation (B), meets expectation (M), exceed expectation (E)	Faculty signature

Professional year	Visit number	Date	Objective	Rating by supervisor Below expectation (B), meets expectation (M), exceed expectation (E)	Faculty signature

Professional year	Visit number	Date	Objective	Rating by supervisor Below expectation (B), meets expectation (M), exceed expectation (E)	Faculty signature

[redacted]

Professional year	Visit number	Date	Objective	Rating by supervisor Below expectation (B), meets expectation (M), exceed expectation (E)	Faculty signature

References

1. Census report 2011, census schedule 2021, NFHS-5 report, MCH indicators
2. SRS Bulletin, Volume 53 No. 1. Delhi: Office of the Registrar General and Census Commissioner, India; May 2020. 9 p.
3. Vital Statistics of India based on the Civil Registration System 2019. Delhi: Office of Registrar General, India. June 2021. 145 p.
4. Special bulletin on maternal mortality in India 2016-18. Delhi: Office of Registrar General, India. July 2020. 4 p.
5. Office of the Registrar General and Census Commissioner, India, Census 2011 [Internet]. India: Ministry of Home Affairs; [reviewed 2021 Oct 20; cited 2021 Oct 20]. Available from: https://censusindia.gov.in/2011-Common/Archive.html
6. Manual on integrated vector management India. Delhi: Directorate of National Vector Borne Disease Control Programme, DGHS, MoHFW, India. 2015. 248 p.
7. National Centre for Disease Control. Delhi. A Brief note on the NICD desert cooler: NICD, Delhi; [reviewed 2021 Oct 20; cited 2021 Oct 20]. Available from: http://www.nvbdcp.gov.in/Doc/brief-NICD-cooler.pdf.
8. Guidelines for Management of healthcare waste as per biomedical waste management rules, 2016. Central Pollution Control Board, Ministry of Environment, Forest and Climate Change, India. 2018.
9. ICMR-National Institute of Nutrition. Nutrition, Lifestyle and Immunity: NIN, Hyderabad; [reviewed 2021 Oct 20; cited 2021 Oct 20]. Available from: https://www.nin.res.in/downloads/Nutrition_Lifestyle_and_Immunity.pdf
10. ICMR-National Institute of Nutrition. Nutrition, Nutrition requirements for Indians, A report of Expert Group, 2020: NIN, Hyderabad; [reviewed 2021 Oct 20; cited 2021 Oct 20]. Available from: https://www.nin.res.in/RDA_Full_Report_2020.html
11. Central Pollution Control Board, National air quality index. [Internet]. India: Ministry of Environment, Forest and Climate Change; [reviewed 2021 Oct 20; cited 2021 Oct 20]. Available from: https://cpcb.nic.in/National-Air-Quality-Index/
12. Bhalwar R, Dudeja P, Jindal AK, Bhatnagar A. Textbook of Community Medicine. 4th edition. New Delhi: Walter Kluwer; 2021.
13. Park K. Textbook of Preventive and Social Medicine. 26th ed. Jabalpur: Banarsidas Bhanot,2021.
14. Suryakantha AH. Community Medicine with Recent Advances. 6th ed. New Delhi: Jaypee Brothers Medical Publishers Ltd; 2021.
15. Nutritive Value of Food Stuffs- Gopalan C, Ramashashtri BV, Balasubramanium SC- Nutritive Value of Indian Foods. Revised 1st ed. Hyderabad: National Institute of Nutrition, Indian Council of Medical Research; 2010
16. Dietary Guidelines for Indians- a Manual. 2nded.Hyderabad: National Institute of Nutrition, Indian Council of Medical Research; 2011.
17. A Dictionary of Epidemiology, Fourth Edition- Edited by John M Last, Robert A Spasoff and Susan S Harris
18. Gordis L Epidemiology 2014 Epidemiology 5th Edition Elsevier Saunders
19. K R Sundaram S N Dwivedi V Sreenivas 2010 Medical Statistics : Principles and Methods Tunbridge Wells : Anshan New Delhi B I Publications Pvt Ltd
20. Jatinder Bali Anil Kant 2017 Basics of Biostatistics A Manual for Medical Practitioners Jaypee Brothers Medical Publishers
21. Adapted from Health research methodology: a guide for training in research methods. 2nd ed., WHO http://www.anusandhan.net/fin_for_tech/main_template.jsp?file=icmr_11.htm)
22. http://www.cdc.gov/csels/dsepd/ss1978/lesson6/section2.html
23. *Number of doses received in pulse polio programme on National and Sub-national immunization days.
    Zero Dose –YES/NO.